Smokeless Tobacco and its Effects on Periodontal Health

Fawad Javed • Saman Warnakulasuriya
Editors

Smokeless Tobacco and its Effects on Periodontal Health

Springer

Editors
Fawad Javed
Department of Orthodontics and Dentofacial Orthopedics, Eastman Institute for Oral Health
University of Rochester
Rochester, NY, USA

Saman Warnakulasuriya
Faculty of Dentistry, Oral & Craniofacial Sciences
King's College London
London, UK

ISBN 978-3-032-16408-7   ISBN 978-3-032-16409-4 (eBook)
https://doi.org/10.1007/978-3-032-16409-4

This Springer imprint is published by the registered company Springer Nature Switzerland AG
The registered company address is: Gewerbestrasse 11, 6330 Cham, Switzerland

Foreword

Smokeless tobacco (ST) encompasses a wide array of products used across various cultures and regions. Several forms of ST products are widely consumed, including gutka/gutkha/ghutka, mainpuri, toombak, naswar/niswaar, khaini, and snuff (or *snus*). ST is also used as an additive to betel-quid. These products are not only prevalent in their regions of origin but have also gained significant accessibility in countries such as the United Kingdom, the United States, and Australia, largely due to global trade and their popularity among immigrant communities.

The health implications of ST use have been extensively studied in relation to oral premalignant and malignant conditions. However, a considerable gap remains in the scientific literature regarding its specific effects on periodontal and peri-implant health. Given the increasing diversity of patient populations and the growing use of these products, it is imperative for healthcare professionals, particularly oral healthcare providers, to develop a comprehensive understanding of the types of ST products, prevalence of use in different regions, their chemical characteristics, and their potential to compromise periodontal health.

This textbook, *Smokeless Tobacco and Its Effects on Periodontal Health*, aims to fill this crucial knowledge gap. It provides evidence-based insights and clinical perspectives to help oral health professionals, researchers, and students recognize the periodontal implications of these widely used yet often overlooked products. The significance of this book lies not only in its contribution to oral science but also in its potential to enhance patient education, diagnosis, cessation methods, and long-term care in diverse clinical settings. This textbook on the periodontal health effects of existing ST products would help caution practitioners to look for potential periodontal health effects of novel emerging ST products that the industry is releasing periodically.

Prakash C. Gupta
Director
Healis Sekhsaria Institute for Public Health,
Navi Mumbai, Maharashtra, India
April 2025

Contents

Global Epidemiology of Smokeless Tobacco Use

1

Ravi Mehrotra, Rewa Malhotra, Kamran Siddiqi, and Deepika Mishra

Abbreviations

AN	Areca nut
ANVISA	Agência Nacional de Vigilância Sanitária (Brazilian National Health Surveillance Agency)
ASTRAMOD	Asia-specific Tobacco Risk Assessment Model
BQ	Betel quid
BRFSS	Behavioural Risk Factor Surveillance System
CDC	Centres for Disease Control and Prevention
CI	Confidence Interval
COTPA	Cigarettes and Other Tobacco Products Act
FCTC	Framework Convention on Tobacco Control
FDA	Food and Drug Administration
FM	Frequency Modulation (in context of FM radio)
GATS	Global Adult Tobacco Survey
GST	Goods and Services Tax
GTSS	Global Tobacco Surveillance System
GYTS	Global Youth Tobacco Survey

R. Mehrotra (✉)
Centre for Health, Innovation and Policy Foundation, Noida, India

Hull York Medical School, University of York, York, UK
e-mail: ravi.mehrotra@ohsl.us

R. Malhotra · D. Mishra
Division of Oral Pathology and Microbiology, Centre for Dental Education and Research, All India Institute of Medical Sciences, New Delhi, India
e-mail: rewamalhotra@aiims.edu; deepikamishra@aiims.edu

K. Siddiqi
Hull York Medical School, University of York, York, UK
e-mail: kamran.siddiqi@york.ac.uk

F. Javed, S. Warnakulasuriya (eds.), *Smokeless Tobacco and its Effects on Periodontal Health*, https://doi.org/10.1007/978-3-032-16409-4_1

HNC	Head and neck cancer
HSE	Health Survey for England
NHANES	National Health and Nutrition Examination Survey
NHIS	National Health Interview Survey
OPMD	Oral potentially malignant disorders
PAHO	Pan-American Health Organization
SEAR	South-East Asia Region
ST	Smokeless Tobacco
USA	United States
WHO	World Health Organization

Learning Goals

- Understand the global distribution and regional disparities in smokeless tobacco (ST) use.
- Identify age-specific and gender-specific trends in ST consumption.
- Recognize the sociocultural factors contributing to the initiation and continuation of ST use.
- Analyse the role of socioeconomic status, education level, and psychosocial stressors in influencing patterns of ST use across various populations.
- Evaluate the public health impact of ST use, particularly its strong association with periodontal disease, oral cancer, and other oral health conditions.
- Evaluate the effectiveness of national and international regulatory frameworks, such as taxation, advertising bans, and packaging regulations, in controlling ST use.
- Compare the epidemiological patterns of ST use between high-income and low- to middle-income countries.
- Explore data collection methodologies and major surveillance tools for tracking ST use globally.
- Discuss the influence of marketing practices, product affordability, and accessibility on the promotion and prevalence of ST use.
- Develop critical insights into policy and intervention gaps, and propose targeted public health strategies for reducing the burden of ST-related diseases.

1.1 Global Epidemiology of Smokeless Tobacco Use

1.1.1 Global Statistics and Trends

The prevalence of smokeless tobacco (ST) use varies considerably across geographic regions, age cohorts, and gender demographics. These disparities are intricately influenced by cultural practices, socioeconomic factors, public health policies, and the availability of tobacco products. A detailed analysis of these multifaceted differences, including age- and gender-specific patterns, is presented below.

Key Points
- Prevalence of ST use varies across the globe
- Cultural practices, socioeconomic factors, and public health policies affect ST use.

1.1.2 Global and Regional Prevalence Variation in ST Use

The geographical distribution of ST use is notably diverse. These intricate patterns are deeply shaped by historical traditions, pervasive cultural norms, and specific national regulatory frameworks. Understanding these influences is crucial for comprehending the global landscape of ST use.

The World Health Organization (WHO) South-East Asia Region (SEAR), which includes countries with the highest prevalence, such as India and Bangladesh, accounts for strikingly more than 80% of all global ST users (WHO 2019). Within this vibrant and populous South Asian region, the consumption of chewable tobacco forms, including but not limited to gutkha, betel quid (BQ) with tobacco, naswar, and khaini, is not merely common but deeply ingrained in daily life. For instance, in India, current estimates are staggering, indicating that about 200 million individuals actively consume ST, characterized by high prevalence among men and a discernible, albeit comparatively smaller, increase in usage observed among women, signalling evolving consumption patterns (GATS 2016). Both India and Bangladesh consistently rank among the nations with the highest global prevalence of ST use, underscoring the severity of the public health challenges they face. In India alone, 21.4% of the entire adult population reports current ST use. In India, prevalence among men can be as high as 30–40% in rural areas, especially in the northern and central parts of India, where BQ with tobacco is often consumed (Bharati et al. 2023). In certain specific Indian states, notably Bihar and Uttar Pradesh, this prevalence escalates even further, reaching alarming levels where ST is often considered an intrinsic and common part of daily life, particularly within rural settings.

The ST products in South Asia, encompassing the BQ with tobacco (a distinct combination of betel leaf, areca nut (AN), and slaked lime, frequently augmented with added tobacco) (Javed et al. 2013); and the commercially manufactured gutkha/gutka and pan masala are typically either chewed or sucked. These products are extensively marketed, often aggressively targeting and penetrating low-income communities, a strategy that directly contributes to and exacerbates the already elevated usage rates observed across the region (Niaz et al. 2017).

In countries of the region such as Sri Lanka, Nepal, and Pakistan, ST use is also widely prevalent, contributing to national health challenges. Notably, Sri Lanka was ranked among the top ten countries globally for a high prevalence of chewing ST in 2019, with distinct gender disparities evident: rates were higher in males (13.6%)

compared to females (5.15%) (Dhanapriyanka et al. 2022). These traditional products, incorporating betel leaves and AN, are commonly consumed alongside tobacco in various forms across these regions, amplifying their addictive potential and health consequences. ST use is highly prevalent in Indonesia, especially among rural communities, with both men and women commonly consuming BQ and chewing tobacco.

Southeast Asian nations, including Thailand, Myanmar, and Indonesia, also report substantial and concerning rates of ST use. Within this diverse region, products such as BQ are customary, often, but not exclusively, combined with tobacco and AN. It is critically important to acknowledge that while BQ may or may not contain tobacco, the consumption of BQ itself, even in its tobacco-free form, carries inherent and documented health risks. The consumption of ST in these areas is profoundly and historically culturally ingrained, extending beyond mere habit to become a part of the social fabric, with younger demographics increasingly adopting and perpetuating the practice. Similarly, Vietnam and Thailand report high rates of ST use in rural areas, where it is often paired with betel nut in Vietnam. In Myanmar, ST use is widespread, with betel chewing deeply rooted in cultural traditions (Lee et al. 2012). Figure 1.1 presents a heat map showcasing the diverse prevalence of smokeless tobacco (ST) use across different regions of the globe.

Key Points

- South-East Asia is the global epicenter of ST use, with India and Bangladesh alone accounting for over 80% of the world's users.
- ST consumption is deeply embedded in the cultural and daily practices of rural and low-income communities.
- In India, the prevalence of ST use is alarmingly high, with approximately 200 million users and male usage reaching up to 40% in some rural regions.
- Gender disparities in ST use are evident but evolving, with men typically showing higher prevalence.
- ST use is emerging among women in countries including India and Sri Lanka.

In stark contrast, ST use is significantly less widespread in Western countries, although it unequivocally remains a persistent public health concern, particularly within the United States (USA). In the Americas, ST use is primarily dominant in North America (USA and Canada) and parts of South America, notably in Brazil (Chang et al. 2016). In the Latin American region, ST represents an emerging, yet frequently overlooked, public health concern that warrants greater attention. In Latin America, while overall ST use is comparatively low, certain indigenous and rural communities persistently employ traditional forms, often deeply intertwined with ancient cultural practices. In a systematic review and meta-analysis, Pedroso et al. (2023) assessed the prevalence of ST use and its association with oral

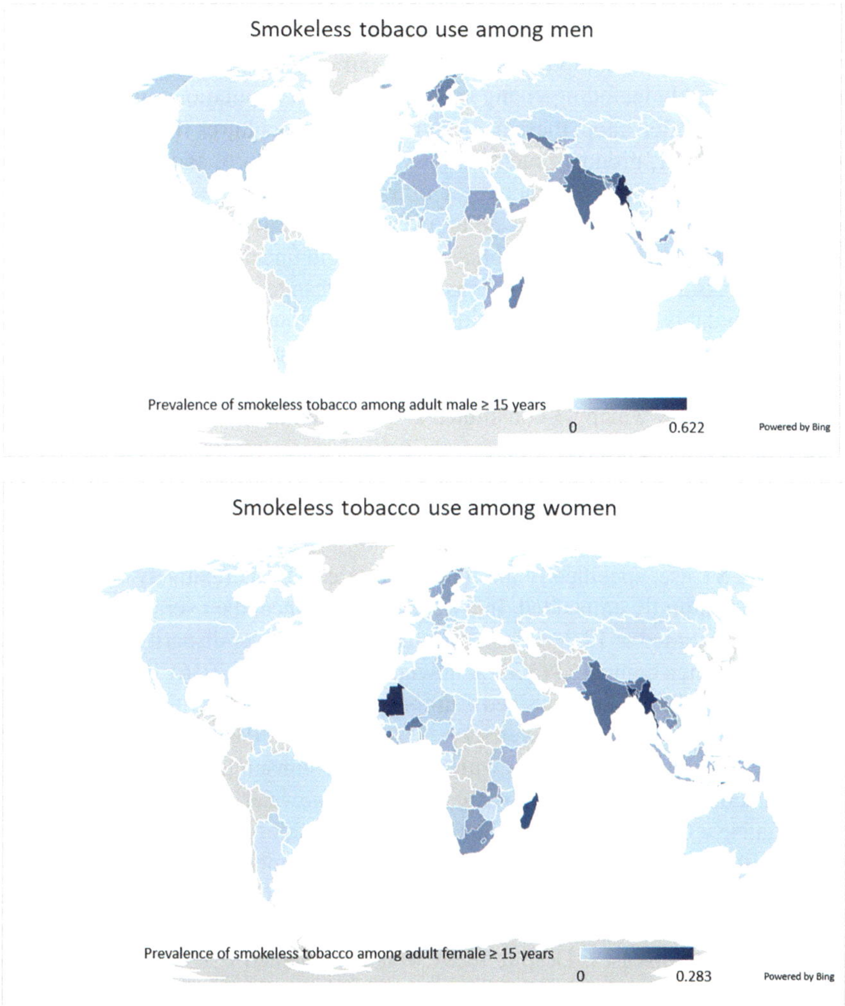

Fig. 1.1 A heat map showcasing the diverse prevalence of smokeless tobacco use across different regions of the world. (Adapted from Siddiqi et al. (2020). Figure caption (from [x.y], licensed under CC-BY 4.0). Powered by Bing. ©GeoNames, HERE, MSFT, Microsoft, NavInfo, Thinkware Extract, Wikipedia)

potentially malignant disorders (OPMD) and head and neck cancer (HNC) across countries in the Pan-American Health Organization (PAHO) region. Data from 59 studies across six countries revealed an overall ST use prevalence of 15%, higher in adults (17%) than in paediatric populations (11%), with Venezuela showing the highest national prevalence. The analysis found a significant association between ST use and increased risk of HNC (Pedroso et al. 2023). Among OPMD, only leukoplakia showed a significant association with ST use. In summary, the findings highlight substantial ST use in the PAHO region and its potential role in oral carcinogenesis, especially HNC (Pedroso et al. 2023).

In the USA, ST consumption is most concentrated among specific demographic subgroups, notably including young males and distinct populations such as military personnel, who often adopt these habits within their subcultures (Dai and Leventhal 2023). In the USA, products such as snus, chewing tobacco, and dipping tobacco enjoy popularity among a minority of users. Nevertheless, contemporary trends across the nation generally indicate an overall decline in ST use, a positive shift largely attributed to increasing public awareness and understanding of the substantial health risks associated with its consumption. Despite this decline, the USA still harbours a notably high user population. Data meticulously collected from the 2020 National Health Interview Survey (NHIS) indicated that an estimated 47.1 million US adults (19.0% of the adult population) reported currently using any commercial tobacco product, of which ST constituted 2.3% of all tobacco users. (Cornelius et al. 2022). ST remains particularly common in rural areas, where cultural norms and accessibility often differ from urban centres, with chewing tobacco and snuff being the most frequently consumed products in these communities.

Scandinavia stands as a compelling exception within the broader European context, where ST use, specifically the form known as snus, is relatively common and profoundly culturally embedded. In Sweden, for instance, the overall prevalence of ST use was recorded at 12.3%, demonstrating a clear gender disparity with a 20.7% prevalence in men compared to 3.5% in women (Leon et al. 2016). This figure contrasts sharply with other combined European countries, where the corresponding overall estimate was a much lower 1.1% (1.2% in men, 1.1% in women), underscoring Sweden's unique relationship with snus and ST consumption

The Pacific Islands report substantially higher prevalence, notably exemplified by Papua New Guinea, where over half the population of adults reportedly use BQ mixed with or without tobacco—a habit that is not merely common but deeply ingrained in daily social interactions and rituals (WHO 2013). This widespread habit is strongly associated with alarmingly high rates of oral cancers and other debilitating oral diseases. Despite these well-documented risks, public awareness campaigns, regulatory oversight, and systematic surveillance of ST use remain regrettably limited in both regions, necessitating more robust public health interventions.

In Sub-Saharan Africa, in countries such as Kenya, Tanzania, and Uganda, ST use is less prevalent than in South Asia, yet it is experiencing a concerning growth trajectory, particularly among younger demographics. Products like khat (a psychoactive plant that is chewed) and nasal snuff are utilized in some East African nations, forming part of local traditions.[28] In these countries, khat use is common, particularly in rural areas, where it is often used in conjunction with alcohol (in regions like Ethiopia) (Hirpa et al. 2023; Ngaruiya et al. 2018). The increasing availability of various ST products, often unregulated and easily accessible, coupled with insufficient regulatory controls, has directly contributed to this concerning rise in consumption. In Sudan, ST is widely used in the form of *toombak*, a homemade product with extremely high nicotine and carcinogen levels, contributing to alarming rates of oral cancer. In Nigeria, ST use is less prevalent but still present, especially in rural areas and among older populations, where products like *snuff* are commonly used nasally or orally. Among men in the region, smoking prevalence rates were notably high in Sierra Leone (37.7%), Lesotho (34.1%), and Madagascar (28.5%). The prevalence of ST use, however, was below 10% in the majority of these countries, except Madagascar, which recorded a significantly higher prevalence of 24.7%, and Mozambique at 10.9%, highlighting specific regional hotbeds of ST use within the continent (Sreeramareddy et al. 2014).

Key Points

- ST use is less widespread in Western countries but remains a significant public health concern in the USA, especially among young males and military personnel.
- In the PAHO region, ST prevalence is around 15%, with a strong association found between ST use and head and neck cancers.
- ST consumption in the USA is declining overall, yet remains prominent in rural areas; the 2020 NHIS reported that 2.3% of tobacco users consumed ST products.
- Sweden stands out in Europe with high ST use, particularly snus, showing a marked gender disparity (20.7% in men vs. 3.5% in women), unlike the low prevalence in other European nations.
- ST use in Latin America and the Pacific Islands, though generally low, is substantial among indigenous and rural populations, with Papua New Guinea reporting over 50% adult prevalence.
- In Sub-Saharan Africa, ST use is increasing, especially among youth in rural areas, with products like toombak in Sudan contributing to high oral cancer rates.

1.2 Age Differences in ST Use

The prevalence of ST use exhibits considerable variation across distinct age groups, with younger populations frequently acting as the primary initiators of use. However, it is also important to acknowledge that older adults contribute significantly to the overall burden of ST consumption, often due to long-standing habits and addiction.

1.2.1 Adolescents and Young Adults

According to the comprehensive Global Youth Tobacco Survey, meticulously conducted across 138 countries between 2010 and 2019, the overall prevalence of current ST use among adolescents was recorded at 4.4% (with a 95% confidence interval [CI] ranging from 4.0% to 4.9%). Specifically, it was 5.7% (5.1–6.3) for boys, 3.1% (2.6–3.5) for girls, 3.9% (3.5–4.4) for adolescents aged 12–14 years, and 5.4% (4.8–5.9)1 for those aged 15–16 years. The highest prevalence in this age group was consistently observed in the Southeast Asian region, reaching 6.1% (4.4–7.7), while the lowest was in the Western Pacific region at 2.0% (1.7–2.4%) (Yang et al. 2022).

Adolescents and young adults are especially vulnerable to starting ST use, a vulnerability worsened in areas where these products are aggressively promoted through highly appealing flavours, attractive packaging, and widespread social media campaigns. Peer pressure, innate curiosity, and the dangerous misconception that ST is a safer alternative to smoking also push its widespread use in this impressionable group, potentially leading to lifelong addiction and significantly higher health risks. In India, adolescent ST use is a major public health issue. A recent study among school children in Delhi found that 11% of all students surveyed used ST, and 27.9% of these students did so between 6 and 9 days per month. Concerningly, most student-initiated use occurs at the young age of 10–11 years. Among the many ST products available, pan masala combined with zarda was identified as the most commonly consumed product, utilized by a significant 70.8% of ST users in that study (Sharma et al. 2023).

Key Points

- Adolescents and young adults are the primary initiators of ST use, often beginning consumption at an early age due to peer influence, curiosity, and misperceptions about its safety.
- The Global Youth Tobacco Survey (2010–2019) reported a global ST use prevalence of 4.4% among adolescents, with higher usage among boys (5.7%) than girls (3.1%) and greater prevalence in older adolescents aged 15–16 years.
- Marketing tactics such as flavoured products, attractive packaging, and social media campaigns exacerbate ST initiation among youth by increasing product appeal.
- In India, ST use among adolescents is a growing concern, with 11% of surveyed schoolchildren in Delhi reporting use, and initiation commonly occurring as early as 10–11 years of age.
- Pan masala with zarda is the most prevalent form of ST used by Indian adolescents, consumed by approximately 70.8% of school going children.

1.2.2 Adults

Among adults, ST use consistently shows a tendency to be more common among men, especially in countries with high overall tobacco consumption rates. The prevalence of ST use among middle-aged adults is notably high in South Asian countries, where the practice is widely accepted and normalized both culturally and socially. Based on all available data from Bhutan, India, Myanmar, Nepal, and Sri Lanka, ST use was consistently higher among males than females. However, a different pattern appears in Bangladesh, Indonesia, and Thailand, where ST use was unexpectedly higher among females. Among males, the prevalence of ST use ranges from a striking 51.4% in Myanmar to a much lower 1.1% in Thailand. For females, the figures vary from 27.9% in Bangladesh to 1.9% in Timor-Leste (Sinha et al. 2012). Of all ST products, BQ with tobacco is the most prevalent in many countries, including Bangladesh and Thailand, reflecting deeply rooted cultural habits. Conversely, khaini chewing is the most common form of ST in India, highlighting national preferences. In the USA, the highest rates of ST use are found among men aged 18–34, with 6.5% reporting regular use in the past month, as documented by the 2020 National Health Interview Survey (Cornelius et al. 2022).

Key Points

- ST use among adults is predominantly higher in men, particularly in South Asian countries like India, Bhutan, Myanmar, Nepal, and Sri Lanka, where it is culturally and socially normalized.
- An exception to this trend is observed in Bangladesh, Indonesia, and Thailand, where female ST use exceeds or closely rivals that of males, indicating region-specific gender dynamics.
- Product preferences vary by region, with BQ + tobacco being most common in countries such as Bangladesh and Thailand, while gutka/gutkha and khaini chewing is the preferred form in India.
- In the U.S., ST use is most prevalent among men aged 18–34.

1.2.3 Older Adults

Older adults, generally defined as individuals aged 50 and above, represent a significant and often overlooked portion of ST users, particularly in Scandinavian countries such as Sweden. Here, snus is frequently utilized as a widely accepted alternative to smoking, contributing to its sustained prevalence. In Sweden, the prevalence of snus use remarkably remains relatively stable even in older age groups, with some estimates indicating that approximately 15–20% of older men continue to use snus, reflecting a persistent habit throughout the life course (Foulds et al. 2003). In stark contrast, in countries like India and Bangladesh, older adults who have consumed ST for many years are considerably more likely to continue its use due to established addiction patterns, notwithstanding the well-documented and severe health risks they face from prolonged exposure. Figure 1.2 depicts age-specific patterns of smokeless tobacco use and outlines potential factors contributing to its prevalence across different age groups.

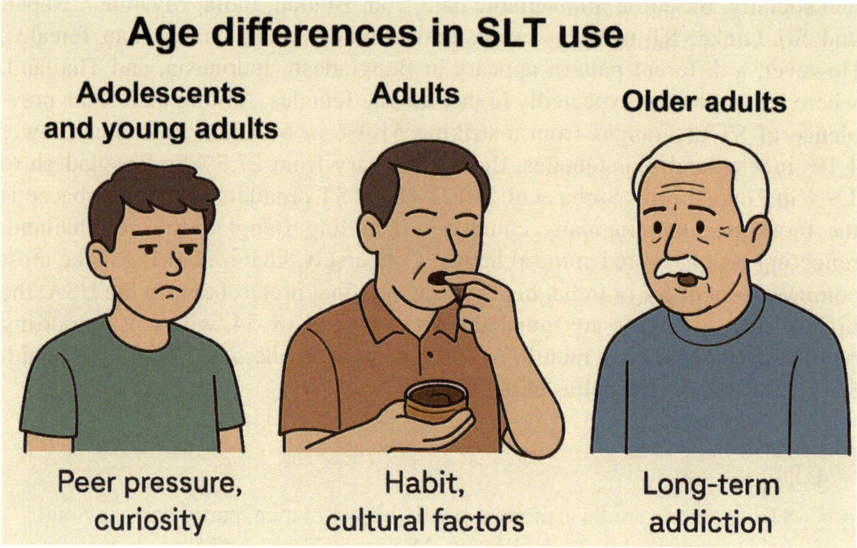

Fig. 1.2 Age-specific patterns of smokeless tobacco use and outline of potential factors contributing to its prevalence across different age groups

Key Points

- In Sweden, snus use among older adults remains relatively stable, with 15–20% of older men continuing its use, reflecting its cultural acceptance and role as a smoking alternative.
- In contrast, in India and Bangladesh, long-term smokeless tobacco use among older adults persists due to entrenched addiction, despite known severe health risks.

1.3 Gender Differences in Smokeless Tobacco Use

The gender gap in ST use constitutes a significant epidemiological feature, with men generally exhibiting substantially higher usage rates than women across most regions. While both genders engage in ST consumption, men typically do so more frequently, except for notable exceptions observed in Bangladesh, Indonesia, and Thailand, where female usage patterns deviate from the norm. Data from the Global Adult Tobacco Survey (GATS) for India meticulously showed that 29.6% of men and 12.1% of women were current ST users, revealing a clear disparity. The broader GATS for the years 2016–2017 for India further indicated that 42.4% of men and 14.2% of women were current all-tobacco users, encompassing both smoked and smokeless forms. Despite these general trends, it is crucial to recognize that exceptions exist, and in certain countries, ST use among women is notably high and warrants specific public health attention.

Key Points

- GATS data from India has shown that 29.6% of men and 12.1% of women are current ST users.
- Despite the overall gender disparity, countries like Bangladesh, Indonesia, and Thailand report higher or comparable rates of ST use among women, highlighting the need for gender-specific public health strategies.

1.3.1 Men

Men undeniably constitute the vast majority of ST users across virtually all global regions, with the aforementioned exceptions. In South Asia, especially in India and Pakistan, ST is predominantly and culturally used by men, with prevalence rates soaring as high as 30–40% in certain rural areas, reflecting deeply entrenched social norms. In the USA, ST is most prevalent among young adult men, with reported rates of 7–8% among 18–29-year-old men, as documented by the 2020 National Health Interview Survey. Scandinavian countries also demonstrate a consistently high prevalence of ST use among men, particularly snus in Sweden, where approximately 20% of men engage in regular snus use as part of their daily routine (Foulds et al. 2003).

Key Points

- In India and Pakistan, ST is predominantly and culturally used by men, with prevalence rates soaring as high as 30–40%.
- In the USA, ST is most prevalent among young adult men, with reported rates of 7–8% among 18–29-year-old men.

1.3.2 Women

In most of South Asia, while overall rates are lower than men, ST use is becoming increasingly common among women. This trend is particularly pronounced in countries such as Bangladesh, Indonesia, and Thailand, where female prevalence often exceeds that of males. Overall, across the 16 GATS countries surveyed, 6.7% of women reported using ST, indicating a significant global burden (Giovino et al. 2012). Historically, the use of ST by women was largely confined to Southeast Asian countries, but it is now rapidly increasing across diverse global regions, necessitating broader public health responses. In the USA during 2004–2005, 3% of adults used ST, breaking down to 6% of men and 0.4% of women (SAMSHA 2004–2005). However, more recent NHIS 2020 data, while reporting an overall decrease in incidence to 2.3%, regrettably, does not specify gender-disaggregated data for this latest figure. According to a comprehensive 2019 European Commission report on the health effects of ST products, 20.7% of Swedish men and 3.5% of Swedish women used snus daily, showcasing a unique pattern of female ST use in a high-income setting.

Key Point

- ST use among females is emerging globally, including in high-income settings like Sweden, where 3.5% of women use snus daily, and in the USA, where earlier data showed 0.4% female prevalence.

1.4 Data Sources and Methods

The accurate assessment and monitoring of ST use prevalence constitute a critical public health concern. To this end, the World Health Organization (WHO) and various national and international bodies diligently and regularly monitor and report on this pervasive issue. The core of this surveillance relies on key data sources and rigorous methodologies employed to measure ST use, with a particular emphasis on comprehensive WHO reports, nationally representative health surveys, and pertinent academic literature.

1.4.1 World Health Organization Reports

The WHO consistently generates authoritative global reports on tobacco use, comprehensively encompassing ST, through meticulously conducted surveys and the collation of country-specific data. Pivotal sources in this endeavour include the Global Tobacco Surveillance System (GTSS), an overarching framework that integrates two foundational components: the Global Youth Tobacco Survey (GYTS) and the GATS. These surveys are systematically conducted periodically in numerous countries worldwide to gather robust data on tobacco use patterns among both youth and adult populations. The GATS, launched in February 2007 as a new, integral component of the ongoing GTSS, stands as a nationally representative household survey. Since its inception, GATS has been meticulously implemented in over 30 countries, providing highly detailed and invaluable information on the prevalence of ST use and its precise demographic distribution, serving as a cornerstone for policy development.

The GYTS is a self-administered, school-based survey specifically targeting students in grades typically associated with 13–15 years of age. Its primary objective is to enhance the capacity of countries to accurately monitor tobacco use among youth and to provide actionable guidance for the effective implementation and rigorous evaluation of tobacco prevention and control programmes. The GYTS adheres to a strict standard methodology encompassing the construction of sampling frames, the selection of schools and classes, the preparation of questionnaires, the adherence to consistent field procedures, and the application of uniform data management processes for both data processing and analysis. While the GYTS maintains a stronger focus on smoking, it consistently includes pertinent questions on ST use, providing a broader understanding of youth tobacco habits.

Key Points

- The WHO monitors tobacco use globally through the GTSS, which includes the GATS and the GYTS.
- GATS is a nationally representative household survey that collects data on the prevalence and demographic patterns of ST use.
- GYTS is a school-based survey targeting 13–15-year-old students, aiming to track youth tobacco use and support the development of prevention and control programmes.
- GATS and GYTS use standardized methodologies to ensure consistency and accuracy.

1.4.2 National Health Surveys

Beyond global initiatives, numerous countries independently conduct national health surveys that meticulously track tobacco use patterns, including specific data on ST. Some key examples illustrate the breadth of this data collection. The National Health Interview Survey (NHIS) in the USA comprehensively collects data on a wide spectrum of health behaviours and conditions, encompassing tobacco use. Within this survey, detailed data on ST is gathered as part of broader questions on overall tobacco use, and specific information on distinct types of ST (e.g. chewing tobacco, snuff) is rigorously included. The Behavioural Risk Factor Surveillance System (BRFSS), adeptly managed by the Centres for Disease Control and Prevention (CDC), also incorporates questions about ST use, providing invaluable state-specific data on tobacco use patterns, including whether individuals consume ST products like chewing tobacco or snuff.

The Health Survey for England (HSE) is an annual survey that diligently collects extensive data on the health and lifestyle behaviours of the population in England, consistently including ST use as part of its broader tobacco consumption assessment. Furthermore, the National Health and Nutrition Examination Survey (NHANES) in the USA tracks the health and nutritional status of Americans, with ST inclusion in the survey primarily focused on examining its association with diet, overall health status, and other critical lifestyle factors. India's GATS yields particularly comprehensive data on the prevalence of ST use, which is notably high in certain regions and specific demographic groups, rendering this data crucial given India's immense population and the widespread use of ST products within its borders.

Key Points

- The National health surveys in several countries independently track ST use, providing detailed and region-specific data that complement global surveillance efforts.
- In the USA, the NHIS and the BRFSS collect extensive data on various forms of ST (e.g., chewing tobacco and snuff).
- The HSE includes ST use as part of its annual assessment of population health and lifestyle behaviours, contributing to national tobacco control strategies.

1.4.3 Relevant Literature and Academic Research

The prevalence of ST use has been the subject of numerous rigorous studies published in highly respected academic journals, significantly contributing to the collective understanding of this public health issue. Key research themes consistently emerge within this body of work. Many academic studies are singularly focused on dissecting the prevalence of ST use across diverse demographic groups, including age, gender, and geographic region. These studies frequently employ robust population-based surveys, analyse longitudinal data, and utilize other sophisticated statistical methods to accurately track trends in ST use over time.

Cross-national studies represent another vital area, meticulously comparing ST use patterns across different countries, thereby providing profound insights into the complex cultural, social, and regulatory factors that exert influence on usage patterns. For instance, ST use is demonstrably more common in South Asia and specific parts of Europe, leading to numerous comparative studies on usage patterns in countries like India, Sweden, and the USA.

Furthermore, several studies delve into the behavioural and health risks intimately associated with ST use, exploring its association with other forms of tobacco consumption, alcohol consumption, and its unequivocal impact on oral health and cancer risk. These studies are intrinsically important for comprehending the broader public health implications of ST use. Finally, systematic reviews and meta-analyses serve a crucial role, providing a comprehensive summary of findings meticulously extracted from multiple studies, thereby offering invaluable insights into overarching trends in ST use across varying populations and historical periods. These comprehensive reviews frequently highlight the inherent challenges in accurately measuring ST prevalence, largely owing to the vast variety of products used and the methodological differences in survey administration across distinct regions.

In summation, the prevalence of ST use is meticulously tracked through a sophisticated combination of global surveys, exemplified by the WHO's GTSS components

(GATS and GYTS), nationally conducted health surveys (such as NHIS and BRFSS), and rigorous academic research. The methodologies employed typically involve self-reported questionnaires, with some surveys strategically focusing on specific age groups or particular geographic regions to capture granular data. This wealth of collected data serves as a vital and indispensable guide for informing public health strategies and formulating effective regulatory measures, all aimed at significantly reducing tobacco use and mitigating its devastating associated health risks.

Key Points

- Studies have focused on the demographic patterns of ST use, analysing differences by age, gender, and geographic region
- Cross-national studies have highlighted the cultural, social, and regulatory factors influencing ST use, particularly in high-prevalence regions like South Asia and specific parts of Europe.
- Several studies have established the behavioural and health risks of ST use, including its association with alcohol use, oral diseases, and increased cancer risk.
- Systematic reviews, meta-analyses, and global/national health surveys such as WHO's GATS/GYTS and NHIS/BRFSS provide critical data that guide public health strategies and tobacco control policies.

1.5 Factors Affecting the Prevalence of ST

1.5.1 Sociocultural Factors in ST Use

ST consumption is profoundly and intrinsically influenced by a complex tapestry of cultural and societal norms, which exhibit remarkable variation across different regions of the world. From the deeply ingrained traditions of South Asia to the diverse practices found in Africa, the Middle East, America, and Europe, ST use is meticulously shaped by historical practices, entrenched social structures, deeply held religious beliefs, and society-defined gender roles. These multifaceted factors collectively determine the acceptability, overall prevalence, and specific patterns of ST consumption within each distinct region. This section will thoroughly explore how ST is culturally accepted and intricately integrated into the social practices across these remarkably diverse regions.

1.5.2 Cultural Acceptance and Practices

In South Asia, ST has for centuries been an integral part of cultural, social, and even religious practices, leading to a significant portion of the population consuming products such as BQ, gutkha, pan masala, and khaini. In countries including India,

Sri Lanka, and Bangladesh, the act of chewing BQ, which very often contains AN (commonly known as betel nut) and frequently includes tobacco, is not merely a habit but a deeply rooted tradition interwoven into religious ceremonies, various social rituals, and the fabric of daily life itself. While betel leaves and AN have been traditionally consumed for centuries across South and Southeast Asia, the widespread incorporation of tobacco into this mixture is largely attributed to a complex colonial legacy. This addition was primarily introduced during European colonization, particularly by the Portuguese and British empires, who actively promoted tobacco cultivation and trade, thereby embedding it into local customs and practices. This crucial colonial influence, though rarely explicitly acknowledged in public discourse, plays a critical role in understanding the historical roots of pervasive ST use and its enduring, severe public health consequences in the region. The consumption of BQ is often seamlessly integrated into marriage ceremonies, various religious festivals, and casual social gatherings, where the act of offering betel to guests is a traditional and revered form of hospitality, symbolizing warmth, respect, and community bonding. Passed down through generations, its use is deeply ingrained and often begins in adolescence, heavily influenced by prevailing family norms and peer practices within the community.

Key Points

- In countries including India, Sri Lanka, and Bangladesh, the act of chewing BQ, which very often contains AN and frequently powdered tobacco, is not merely a habit but a tradition interwoven into religious ceremonies, rituals, and daily life.
- The incorporation of tobacco into traditional BQ is largely a colonial legacy, introduced and promoted by European powers, particularly the Portuguese and British, which has contributed significantly to the widespread and enduring public health burden in the region.

Unlike smoking, which often carries social stigmas, ST often enjoys greater social acceptability among women, particularly those engaged in agricultural or labour-intensive roles, where it is often mistakenly believed to relieve fatigue and suppress hunger, offering a perceived functional benefit. Additionally, many users hold erroneous beliefs that ST possesses medicinal or spiritual benefits, such as alleviating headaches, toothaches, or even morning sickness during pregnancy, or that it can be used in offerings to ancestors or deities. These deeply held misconceptions contribute to its sustained use, often with very little awareness of its scientifically documented health risks. Furthermore, in India, products like gutkha and pan masala (which combine chewing tobacco with a mixture of spices and other flavourings) are profoundly prevalent, especially in rural areas. These products are culturally accepted as commonplace, everyday consumables, frequently enjoyed during casual social interactions, such as family gatherings, during travel, or throughout long communal activities, further embedding them into the daily routine (Croucher and Islam 2002; Warnakulasuriya and Peters 2002). Even though their severe health risks are now well documented and widely publicized, they continue to retain significant cultural importance, particularly among men.

Key Points

- ST is socially accepted among women in labour-intensive roles due to misconceptions about its functional and medicinal benefits, such as relieving fatigue, hunger, and minor ailments, despite the lack of scientific support for these beliefs.
- In rural India, products such as gutkha/gutka and pan masala are ingrained in social and cultural practices, making them widely accepted and commonly used during daily interactions, despite their well-documented health risks.

In the Middle East and Africa, ST products such as snuff, various forms of chewing tobacco, Shamah, and naswar are commonly encountered. These regions possess their distinct sociocultural factors that profoundly shape the acceptance and patterns of ST use. In many countries across the Middle East, particularly within Arab nations, ST is often used more discreetly than in the highly public settings of South Asia, yet it remains culturally accepted. Naswar, a specific form of ST widely consumed in Pakistan and Afghanistan, is notably gaining popularity in Iran and Turkey, particularly among younger men, and is used in both private settings and during social gatherings (Khan et al. 2019). In many Middle-Eastern societies, tobacco use (including ST) is often interpreted through unique religious and cultural lenses. In some communities, it is associated with masculinity and adulthood, signalling a transition or affirmation of social status. However, the severe health risks associated with ST may be regrettably overlooked within these cultures due to a prevailing perception of lesser harm compared to smoking cigarettes, a misconception that public health campaigns strive to correct.

Key Points

- In many Middle-Eastern societies, tobacco use (including ST) is often associated with masculinity and social status, and its serious health risks are frequently underestimated.
- Naswar, a specific form of ST widely consumed in Pakistan and Afghanistan, is gaining popularity in Iran and Turkey, particularly among younger men.

In East Africa, specifically in Tanzania and Kenya, the chewing of tobacco products, whether loose leaf or prepared snuff, represents a longstanding traditional practice. In these areas, chewing tobacco is often sold in small, affordable packets in informal markets, making it widely accessible to the general population. It is particularly common among men, though its use among women has been steadily rising in recent years, indicating changing consumption patterns (Quadri et al. 2019). In Sub-Saharan Africa, ST use is frequently influenced by powerful peer pressure and broad community acceptance. The traditional use of ST is often intrinsically tied to community rituals, such as significant gatherings or ceremonies, where it is customarily shared among peers, reinforcing social bonds. In some regions, snuff is consumed as a communal social activity, passed from person to person during group meetings or broader community events, highlighting its role in social cohesion. While gendered patterns often show snuff predominantly used by men in certain African countries, in some parts of West Africa, notably Nigeria and Ghana, women also actively participate in ST consumption. In these specific cultures, women may use ST products as part of traditional beauty rituals or to communicate elevated social status and authority, reflecting diverse and complex cultural motivations (Quadri et al. 2019).

Key Points

- In East and Sub-Saharan Africa, ST use is deeply rooted in tradition, with its communal consumption during gatherings reinforcing social cohesion and peer acceptance.
- In parts of West Africa, ST use among women is increasing; where the habit is tied to cultural practices such as beauty rituals and expressions of social status.

In the West, ST use has undergone significant cultural shifts over time. In North America, ST use, particularly chewing tobacco and snuff, has historically been deeply associated with sports culture (especially baseball) and has subsequently disseminated into less urbanized areas, forming part of regional identities. However, over the past few decades, its use has become considerably more stigmatized, a transformation largely driven by increasingly effective public health campaigns that vividly highlight the dangers of oral cancers, debilitating gum disease, and profound nicotine addiction. In the USA, ST products are frequently and strategically marketed to young men and boys, particularly those residing in rural or semiurban areas. This targeted marketing has inadvertently contributed to a concerning normalization of use within specific subcultures, including those centred around traditional outdoor activities such as hunting, fishing, and various sports (Mejia and Ling 2010). Both Canada and the USA have proactively implemented stringent restrictions on advertising and sales to minors, and both mandate conspicuous warning labels on product packaging. Canada has further advanced tobacco control by implementing plain packaging requirements for certain tobacco products, including specific ST forms, to diminish their appeal. While ST use in the USA has traditionally been more common among men, recent trends indicate an increasing pattern of use among young women, particularly within adolescent and college-age populations, signalling a demographic shift (CDC 2023). Studies have rigorously explored ethnic differences in ST use in the USA, with findings suggesting a higher prevalence among non-Hispanic White males (Roberts et al. 2016).

Key Points

- ST use in North America, once culturally associated with sports and rural identity, has become stigmatized due to public health campaigns emphasizing its health risks.
- Despite regulatory efforts like advertising bans and warning labels, ST use persists among young rural males; and is now showing a rising trend among adolescent and college-aged females.

Scandinavian countries such as Sweden and Norway represent distinctive cases where snus, a unique form of moist ST, is widely accepted and has become an entrenched component of the national culture. Unlike most other forms of ST, snus use in Scandinavia is often actively promoted and perceived as a harm-reduction strategy when compared to smoking, a notion supported by some public health arguments, leading to it being considerably less stigmatized. Snus is notably popular among men but is also utilized by some women, reflecting its broader social integration. The Swedish government, recognizing its unique context, has taken specific steps to promote snus as a less harmful alternative to smoking, consequently leading to relatively high rates of use in comparison to other European countries, which largely prohibit its sale (Foulds et al. 2003). In other European countries like Spain, Italy, and France, ST use is less common but persists, particularly within immigrant communities. Snuff is occasionally used in countries such as Poland and Portugal, although the overall rates of consumption are relatively low when compared to prevalent smoking habits (Leon et al. 2016).

Key Points

- In Scandinavian countries such as Sweden and Norway, moist snus is widely accepted and has become an entrenched component of the national culture
- The Swedish government, recognizing its unique context, has taken specific steps to promote snus as a less harmful alternative to smoking.
- ST use is relatively low in some European countries, including France, Italy, Poland, Portugal, and Spain.

1.6 Economic and Education Levels

ST use shows a clear association with income status. It is often more affordable than cigarettes, making it a common choice among lower-income groups. In many settings, ST serves as a cheaper alternative to smoking, particularly in areas where cigarettes are more expensive or less accessible. Individuals with lower incomes may also face greater stress and economic instability, which can lead some to use tobacco products as a coping mechanism. Additionally, limited access to healthcare and tobacco cessation programmes can contribute to continued use in these populations (Azam et al. 2016). In contrast, people in higher income brackets generally have more access to education, health resources, and support for quitting tobacco, resulting in a lower prevalence of ST use (Shaikh and Saikia 2022). However, this pattern is not universal. Certain high-income individuals, particularly in specific regions or cultural groups, such as some affluent subcultures in the USA or parts of India may continue using/chewing ST due to social or cultural influences (Shaikh and Saikia 2022; Hiscock et al. 2012).

Key Points

- In many settings, ST serves as a cheaper alternative to smoking.
- ST use is more common among economically or financially deprived individuals than among those in higher income brackets.

1.7 Education Levels

Similarly, education level also plays a crucial role in ST use (Javed et al. 2013, 2015). Lower educational attainment is associated with higher rates of ST use (Javed et al. 2013, 2015). Individuals with a deprived education status may lack awareness about the health risks of ST and have less engagement with public health campaigns aimed at reducing its use. Moreover, people with deprived education levels may not have adequate access to information or support systems to help them quit, which can perpetuate the cycle of use. Conversely, higher levels of education are generally linked to a better understanding of the risks associated with ST, including its links to cancer, gum disease, and other serious health conditions. Educated individuals are also more likely to have access to resources like health campaigns, tobacco cessation programmes, and medical support that can help them quit or avoid starting ST use (Lund et al. 2022).

Key Points

- An underprivileged education status is associated with increased ST use.
- Individuals with a deprived education status may lack awareness about the health risks of ST.
- People with deprived education levels may not have adequate access to information or support systems to help them quit.

1.8 Psychosocial Factors

Many individuals use ST as a means of coping with stress, anxiety, or other mental health challenges (Javed et al. 2008, 2015). In such cases, the use of ST can act as a form of self-medication, providing temporary relief from negative emotions or difficult life circumstances. This pattern is often observed in populations facing high levels of stress, whether due to economic hardship, personal trauma, or occupational pressures (Solhi et al. 2021; Rollins et al. 2017). Unfortunately, while ST might offer momentary solace, it ultimately exacerbates health risks and can contribute to a cycle of dependence. Additionally, the perceived social acceptance of ST use within certain communities or peer groups can significantly impact its prevalence. In settings where tobacco chewing or BQ use is culturally normalized or even seen as a rite of passage, individuals may be more likely to initiate and continue use. Conversely, in communities where tobacco use is stigmatized or actively discouraged by social norms and public health messaging, rates of ST use tend to be lower.

Key Points
- Many individuals use ST to cope with psychological stress, anxiety, or other mental health challenges.
- This pattern is often observed in populations facing high levels of stress, whether due to economic hardship, personal trauma, or occupational pressures.

1.9 Genetic and Behavioural Factors

The presence of nicotine in ST makes it highly addictive, and individuals with a genetic predisposition to nicotine dependence may be at greater risk of developing a strong addiction once they begin using these products (Fowler et al. 2008). The risk is especially pronounced for those who start at an early age, as early initiation often leads to long-term use and greater difficulty quitting. Behavioural influences also play a critical role. People with a personal history of smoking, or those who have family members or close contacts who use ST products, are more likely to start using ST products. Such behaviours can reinforce social learning and make quitting even harder, particularly given the addictive properties of nicotine in these products. The interplay of genetic vulnerability and behavioural exposure underscores the need for targeted prevention and cessation strategies.

Key Points
- Individuals with a genetic predisposition to nicotine dependence are at greater risk of developing a strong addiction once they begin using these products than their counterparts.
- The interplay of genetic vulnerability and behavioural exposure underscores the need for targeted prevention and cessation strategies.

1.10 Regulatory Factors

Regulatory factors play a critical role in shaping the epidemiology of ST use. Government policies, taxation, advertising restrictions, and public health regulations collectively influence the accessibility, affordability, and social acceptability of these products. Taxation is among the most powerful tools for reducing tobacco consumption. By raising taxes on ST products, governments increase their price, making them less affordable, especially for price-sensitive groups such as youth and low-income individuals. This can deter initiation and encourage cessation. For instance, higher taxes on products like chewing tobacco or snuff have been shown to reduce use, particularly in low- and middle-income countries where demand is more elastic.

A meta-analysis of 36 studies across 15 countries found that a 10% price increase in ST led to an average 2.1% reduction in consumption (95% CI: −0.6% to 4.8%) (Nazar et al. 2021). In countries such as India and Bangladesh, where ST is prevalent, studies report own-price elasticity estimates ranging from −0.39 to −0.64 for products such as Zarda, suggesting that a 10% price hike could reduce consumption by 3.9–6.4% (Nazar et al. 2021; Kostova and Dave 2015). Moreover, tobacco taxes generate revenue that can be reinvested in public health programmes, supporting cessation services and anti-tobacco campaigns. In India, for example, ST products like gutka and pan masala fall under the highest Goods and Services Tax (GST) slab of 28%, with additional cess on certain items. While this has curbed open promotion under COTPA 2003, challenges in enforcement—especially in rural areas—highlight the need for complementary strategies (Rout and Parhi 2020).

Advertising and marketing restrictions further impact ST use. Bans on tobacco advertising in media, print, and digital platforms limit marketing exposure, particularly among vulnerable groups like youth (Singh et al. 2022). Mandatory packaging regulations, including graphic health warnings and plain packaging, reduce product appeal and inform consumers of the risks associated with ST. Restrictions on tobacco company sponsorship of public and cultural events also diminish the glamorization of these products. Public smoking and tobacco use restrictions, though primarily focused on smoking, increasingly extend to ST. Several countries and regions prohibit ST use in public spaces, workplaces, and youth-centric venues, helping to shift social norms and reduce exposure. For example, Norway enforces public smoking bans that also cover certain forms of ST, reducing visibility and acceptability, particularly among young people (Linnansaari et al. 2023).

Regulations on the composition of ST products are another critical area. Governments can require disclosure of ingredients, limit harmful additives, and regulate nicotine levels to reduce addictiveness. Some countries have banned flavoured ST products, which are particularly appealing to youth, as a measure to prevent initiation.

Health education and awareness campaigns also form a core regulatory strategy. Public health initiatives highlighting the dangers of ST—such as its links to oral cancer and gum disease—help reduce prevalence by shifting attitudes and increasing awareness. These campaigns often target high-risk populations and may be complemented by community outreach programmes that provide cessation resources and support. Thailand's national campaigns exemplify how such efforts can contribute to declining ST use among youth.

Finally, access restrictions—including minimum age laws and limits on points of sale—further reduce the availability of ST. Laws prohibiting sales to individuals under 21, regulating vending machine distribution (primarily to adult-only venues), and restricting illicit bulk sales are common measures in countries like the USA, where compliance is closely monitored.

Key Points

- Taxation is a powerful deterrent to ST use, particularly in low- and middle-income countries, where a 10% price increase can reduce consumption by 3.9–6.4%.
- Advertising bans and packaging regulations, such as graphic warnings and plain packaging, limit the appeal and visibility of ST products.
- Public use restrictions and enforcement in public spaces, including schools and workplaces, help reduce social acceptability and overall exposure to ST products.
- Health education campaigns and sales access restrictions can play a critical role in raising awareness and reducing ST product availability.

1.11 Public Health Impact

The public health impact of ST use is profoundly significant and multifaceted, contributing substantially to a wide array of debilitating diseases across the globe. ST use is unequivocally and strongly associated with alarmingly high rates of oral cancers, severe gum disease, and a spectrum of other debilitating dental issues, posing a direct threat to oral health. The overarching burden of tobacco-related diseases is particularly onerous in India, where ST stands as a major causative factor in the alarming incidence of oral cancers, tragically establishing India as home to one of the highest numbers of oral cancer cases worldwide (Gupta et al. 2022; Bharati et al. 2023; Mehrotra and Lauby-Secretan 2025). This underscores the critical need for targeted interventions.

In Southeast Asia, the pervasive use of ST is a primary driver of persistently high oral cancer rates. For instance, in Thailand, oral cancer ranks among the leading causes of cancer death, with ST unequivocally identified as a major risk factor. The widespread practice of betel chewing in this region is also significantly linked to the development of oral precancerous lesions and widespread periodontal disease, contributing to a substantial burden of oral morbidity.

In Africa, the health ramifications of ST use tragically include oral cancers, gum disease, and entrenched nicotine addiction. Oral malignancies are increasingly recognized as a major public health concern in countries where ST is widely used, though the full extent of the disease burden often remains severely underreported due to limitations in surveillance systems. For example, in Sudan, the widespread consumption of toombak, a homemade ST product characterized by extremely high nicotine and carcinogen levels, directly contributes to alarming rates of oral cancer, presenting a severe public health crisis in the region.

Key Points

- India bears a particularly high burden, with ST use being a leading cause of its alarmingly high incidence of oral cancers, making it one of the countries most affected worldwide.
- In Southeast Asia, especially Thailand, ST use is a major driver of oral cancer and oral precancerous lesions.
- In Africa, ST use contributes to rising rates of oral cancers and nicotine addiction, with products such as toombak in Sudan playing a significant role due to their high carcinogenic content.
- The full impact of ST-related diseases in some regions is underreported, primarily due to weak surveillance systems, hindering effective public health responses.

1.12 Government Policies

Government policies are a critical and indispensable pillar in efforts to control ST use, though their effectiveness is profoundly influenced by regional contexts and the consistency of enforcement. In South Asia, while some countries, most notably India and Pakistan, have commendably implemented bans on gutkha/gutka and various other ST products. In specific regions, the consistent and effective enforcement of such regulations remains a significant and ongoing challenge. This is often hampered by entrenched cultural practices and logistical difficulties. Public health campaigns in India have strategically targeted youth with compelling messages about the severe harms of ST, yet formidable challenges persist in significantly reducing consumption due to deep-seated cultural acceptance and often insufficient resources for widespread implementation.

In Southeast Asia, several countries have proactively commenced rigorous enforcement of bans on advertising and the public consumption of these harmful products. Thailand, for instance, has implemented notably strong tobacco control laws, including mandatory and prominent health warnings displayed conspicuously on product packaging, demonstrating a commitment to public health messaging (Bhatia and Sarkar 2023). However, the deeply ingrained traditional use of BQ with tobacco remains a powerful cultural force, posing substantial difficulties for effective enforcement as public health efforts contend with centuries-old customs.

In Africa, ST use is regrettably and generally under-regulated across many countries, reflecting a broader challenge in comprehensive tobacco control across the continent. Public health initiatives specifically targeting ST use are frequently constrained by severe resource limitations and a pervasive lack of public awareness regarding its profound health risks (Hirpa et al. 2023; Ngaruiya et al. 2018). This necessitates increased investment and targeted educational campaigns.

In the Americas, the US Food and Drug Administration (FDA) regulates ST products under the Family Smoking Prevention and Tobacco Control Act (Deyton 2011). Similarly, in Brazil, tobacco use is regulated through the National Health Surveillance Agency (ANVISA), which requires warning labels on ST products (da Silva et al. 2020). In the USA and Canada, strict minimum age laws prohibiting the sale of ST to minors are crucial preventive measures against initiation. These laws are rigorously enforced through stringent age verification requirements at all points of sale, whether online or in physical retail stores. Additionally, comprehensive sales restrictions, such as prohibiting ST sales in specific sensitive locations (e.g. near schools or youth centres) or limiting bulk sales, further contribute to reducing accessibility and, consequently, usage rates (Chang et al. 2016). The USA meticulously regulates the sale of ST to individuals under 21 and robustly enforces restrictions on the distribution of these products in vending machines and other public places where they could be easily accessed by minors. Canada has demonstrated progressive leadership by further implementing plain packaging requirements for certain tobacco products, including specific ST forms, an initiative designed to diminish their allure and health appeal, thereby protecting vulnerable populations.

Key Points

- While bans on products like gutka/gutkha exist in countries such as India and Pakistan, effective enforcement is hampered by cultural acceptance and logistical difficulties.
- India has implemented targeted campaigns to raise awareness among youth about ST-related harms, though cultural normalization and limited resources hinder broader impact.
- Thailand has enforced stringent ST policies, including advertising bans and graphic health warnings, but face challenges from deeply entrenched cultural practices like betel quid use.
- ST use remains largely unregulated in many African nations due to limited public health infrastructure, insufficient awareness, and scarce resources.
- The US FDA and Brazil's ANVISA impose strict laws, including health warnings and age restrictions, to control ST use; enforcement includes sales limits near schools and rigorous age verification.
- The USA bans ST sales to individuals under 21 and restricts access in vending machines; Canada mandates plain packaging to reduce product appeal.
- High taxation (e.g., India's GST on ST products) is widely employed to reduce affordability and discourage consumption, especially among vulnerable groups.
- Many countries implement cross-platform advertising bans and mandatory graphic warnings on ST packaging as core strategies to reduce appeal and promote health awareness.

Table 1.1 Comparative overview of taxation, advertising restrictions, and key observations on smokeless tobacco control in selected countries

Country	Taxation on ST	Advertising restrictions	Key observations
India	28% GST + additional cess	The total ban (COTPA 2003), includes surrogate ads	Strong legal framework; enforcement weaker in rural areas
Bangladesh	55% of retail price	Total ad ban; mandatory pictorial warnings	High rural use; informal sector undermines taxation
Pakistan	Excise tax on gutkha, naswar	Ad ban exists but are weakly enforced	Widespread informal production
Nepal	High excise duty	90% graphic warnings; full ad ban	Strong packaging laws reduce the appeal
Myanmar	Low excise tax	Partial ad restrictions; informal promotion common	ST is culturally ingrained; rural use remains high
Thailand	Uniform excise tax (by price/volume)	Total ad ban including point-of-sale	ST use is low; strong tobacco control policies
Indonesia	Minimal tax on ST	Weak ST-specific rules; local ads common	ST less regulated than cigarettes
USA	Federal and state taxes (vary widely)	Partial ad bans; FDA regulation	Stronger controls in some states, especially youth protections
UK	ST taxed as tobacco	Total ad ban; plain packaging required	ST use is minimal; Snus banned
Sweden	Moderate tax on snus (EU exemption)	Marketing restricted; health warnings required	Snus regulated under food laws
Norway	High tax on snus	Full ad ban; age restrictions; labelling required	Snus widely used as a cigarette alternative
Australia	ST import ban; taxed if imported	Total ad ban; ST not legally sold	One of the strictest tobacco control environments globally
Saudi Arabia	High tobacco tax (includes ST)	Total ad ban; plain packaging	Strong recent regulatory push
Sudan	ST taxed under general law	Some ad restrictions; weak enforcement	Toombak is widely used; informal production is common
South Africa	ST tax; regulated under tobacco laws	Ad and sponsorship ban	Use concentrated in rural, low-income groups

Source: WHO Report on the Global Tobacco Epidemic 2023 including WHO MPOWER report and WHO FCTC implementation report. Adapted from https://www.who.int/publications/i/item/9789240077164 & https://fctc.who.int/resources/publications/m/item/2023-global-progress-report

Various countries implement a diverse range of taxation and regulatory policies to control ST use, reflecting distinct national contexts and approaches to public health (Chugh et al. 2023). These policies in selected countries are summarized in Table 1.1. Taxation stands out as a powerful tool, with governments like India imposing high Goods and Services Tax (GST) on ST products to increase prices and deter consumption, particularly among vulnerable groups (Coyle et al. 2025) Beyond taxation, stringent advertising and marketing restrictions, including bans across media platforms and mandatory graphic health warnings on packaging, are common strategies to reduce product appeal and inform consumers (Abdullah et al. 2024).

Some nations, such as Canada, have gone further by implementing plain packaging requirements for certain ST forms. Public use restrictions, though primarily for smoking, are increasingly extended to ST in countries such as Norway, aiming to shift social norms. Furthermore, regulatory measures often include controlling product composition, requiring ingredient disclosure, limiting harmful additives, and banning appealing flavours to prevent initiation. Despite these efforts, consistent and effective enforcement often remains a challenge, particularly in regions like South Asia and Africa, where deep-seated cultural practices and resource limitations can hinder policy impact (Mehrotra et al. 2019, 2020).

1.13 Conclusions

Habitual use of ST products represents a significant and persistent global public health challenge, with its prevalence varying considerably across different regions, demographics, and age groups. Despite a common misconception that ST is less harmful than smoking, these products—including chewing tobacco, snuff, and other forms—pose serious, scientifically documented health risks such as oral cancer, severe gum disease, and profound nicotine addiction.

Our analysis indicates that ST use remains particularly prevalent among specific populations, notably young adults, men, and individuals in rural areas. Its deep cultural integration in regions like South Asia, alongside its growing adoption as a perceived "safer" alternative to smoking in other areas, fuels its continued use. This persistence is often exacerbated by less stringent tobacco control policies and insufficient public awareness campaigns regarding its dangers. The concerning trend of flavoured ST products, designed to appeal to younger users, further contributes to rising usage rates.

In essence, while smokeless tobacco use is widespread, its severe health consequences must not be underestimated. Mitigating its global public health impact necessitates a concerted effort involving comprehensive public health campaigns, robust regulatory frameworks, and significantly increased awareness of the inherent harms associated with these products.

Key Points

- Habitual ST use is a global health concern.
- ST use is particularly prevalent among young adults, men, and rural populations, driven by cultural acceptance, perceived safety compared to smoking, weak regulations, and aggressive marketing
- Effective mitigation requires coordinated public health efforts, including strong regulatory policies, targeted awareness campaigns, and global education to dispel misconceptions about ST.

References

Abdullah SM, Huque R, Siddiqi K, Kanaan M, Huque S, Ullah S, Garg S, Singh MM, Deshmukh C, Borle AL, Iqbal R, Mazhar L, Parascandola M, Mehrotra R, Croucher R, Khan Z (2024) Non-compliant packaging and illicit smokeless tobacco in Bangladesh, India and Pakistan: findings of a pack analysis. BMJ Tob Control 33(3):333–340

Azam MN, Shahjahan M, Yeasmin M, Ahmed NU (2016) Prevalence of smokeless tobacco among low socioeconomic populations: a cross-sectional analysis. PLoS One 11(6):e0156887

Bharati B, Sahu KS, Pati S (2023) Prevalence of smokeless tobacco use in India and its association with various occupations: a LASI study. Front Public Health 11:1005103

Bhatia G, Sarkar S (2023) Tobacco industry and surrogate advertising in South East Asia region: moves and countermoves. Indian J Psychol Med 45(2):185–188

Centers for Disease Control and Prevention (CDC) (2023) Tobacco product use among middle and high school students — United States, 2022. Morb Mortal Wkly Rep 72(6):133–140. https://www.cdc.gov/mmwr/volumes/72/wr/pdfs/mm7206a3-H.pdf

Chang JT, Levy DT, Meza R (2016) Trends and factors related to smokeless tobacco use in the United States. Nicotine Tob Res 18(8):1740–1748

Chugh A, Arora M, Jain N, Vidyasagaran A, Readshaw A, Sheikh A, Eckhardt J, Siddiqi K, Chopra M, Mishu M, Kanaan M, Rahman MA, Mehrotra R, Huque R, Forberger S, Dahanayake S, Khan Z, Boeckmann M, Dogar O (2023) The global impact of tobacco control policies on smokeless tobacco use: a systematic review. Lancet Glob Health 11(6):e953–e968

Cornelius ME, Loretan CG, Wang TW, Jamal A, Homa DM (2022) Tobacco product use among adults – United States, 2020. MMWR Morb Mortal Wkly Rep 71(11):397–405

Coyle K, Singh PK, Kaushik R, Huque R, Khan Z, Mehrotra R, Siddiqi K, Pokhrel S (2025) The lifetime health and economic burden of smokeless tobacco use in Bangladesh, India and Pakistan: results from ASTRAMOD. Nicotine Tob Res 27(4):684–692

Croucher R, Islam S (2002) Socio-economic aspects of areca nut use. Addict Biol 7(1):139–146

da Silva ALO, Grilo G, Branco PAC, Fernandes AMMS, Albertassi PGD, Moreira JC (2020) Tobacco industry strategies to prevent a ban on the display of tobacco products and changes to health warning labels on the packaging in Brazil. Tob Prev Cessat 6:66

Dai HD, Leventhal AM (2023) Use of traditional smokeless, snus, and dissolvable tobacco among U.S. Youth. Am J Prev Med 64(2):204–212

Deyton LR (2011) FDA tobacco product regulations: a powerful tool for tobacco control. Public Health Rep 126(2):167–169

Dhanapriyanka M, Kanthi RDFC, Jayasekara P, Ha DH (2022) Tobacco chewing and associated factors among a vulnerable youth population in Sri Lanka. BMC Public Health 22(1):2209

Foulds J, Ramstrom L, Burke M, Fagerström K (2003) Effect of smokeless tobacco (snus) on smoking and public health in Sweden. Tob Control 12(4):349–359

Fowler CD, Arends MA, Kenny PJ (2008) Subtypes of nicotinic acetylcholine receptors in nicotine reward, dependence, and withdrawal: evidence from genetically modified mice. Behav Pharmacol 19(5–6):461–484

GATS (2016) (Global Adult Tobacco Survey) Fact Sheet India 2016–17. Tata Institute of Social Sciences (TISS), Mumbai and Ministry of Health and Family Welfare, Government of India (2016). Available online at: https://www.tobaccofreekids.org/assets/global/pdfs/en/GATS_India_2016-17_FactSheet.pdf

Giovino GA, Mirza SA, Samet JM, Gupta PC, Jarvis MJ, Bhala N et al (2012) Tobacco use in 3 billion individuals from 16 countries: an analysis of nationally representative cross-sectional household surveys. Lancet 380:668–679

Gupta AK, Siddiqi K, Kanaan M, Sinha DN, Mehrotra R (2022) Oral cancer risk assessment for different types of smokeless tobacco products sold worldwide: a review of reviews and meta-analyses. Cancer Prev Res (Phila) 15(11):733–746

Hirpa S, Fogarty AW, Addissie A, Bauld L, Frese T, Unverzagt S, Kantelhardt EJ, Getachew S, Deressa W (2023) Prevalence and risk factors for tobacco, khat, and alcohol consumption among high school students in Ethiopia. BMC Public Health 23(1):226

Hiscock R, Bauld L, Amos A, Fidler JA, Munafò M (2012) Socioeconomic status and smoking: a review. Ann N Y Acad Sci 1248:107–123

Javed F, Altamash M, Klinge B, Engström PE (2008) Periodontal conditions and oral symptoms in gutka-chewers with and without type 2 diabetes. Acta Odontol Scand 66(5):268–273

Javed F, Tenenbaum HC, Nogueira-Filho G, Qayyum F, Correa FO, Al-Hezaimi K, Samaranayake LP (2013) Severity of periodontal disease in individuals chewing betel quid with and without tobacco. Am J Med Sci 46(4):273–278

Javed F, Al-Kheraif AA, Al Amri MD, Mikami T, Vohra F, Warnakulasuriya S, Romanos GE (2015) Periodontal parameters and whole salivary cytokine profiles among habitual gutka chewers and non-chewers. J Periodontol 86(5):689–695

Khan Z, Suliankatchi RA, Heise TL, Dreger S (2019) Naswar (smokeless tobacco) use and the risk of oral cancer in Pakistan: a systematic review with meta-analysis. Nicotine Tob Res 21(1):32–40

Kostova D, Dave D (2015) Smokeless tobacco use in India: role of prices and advertising. Soc Sci Med 138:82–90

Lee CH, Ko AM, Warnakulasuriya S, Ling TY, Sunarjo, Rajapakse PS, Zain RB, Ibrahim SO, Zhang SS, Wu HJ, Liu L, Kuntoro, Utomo B, Warusavithana SA, Razak IA, Abdullah N, Shrestha P, Shieh TY, Yen CF, Ko YC (2012) Population burden of betel quid abuse and its relation to oral premalignant disorders in South, Southeast, and East Asia: an Asian Betel-quid Consortium Study. Am J Public Health 102(3):e17–e24

Leon ME, Lugo A, Boffetta P, Gilmore A, Ross H, Schüz J, La Vecchia C, Gallus S (2016) Smokeless tobacco use in Sweden and other 17 European countries. Eur J Public Health 26(5):817–821

Linnansaari A, Ollila H, Pisinger C, Scheffels J, Kinnunen JM, Rimpelä A (2023) Towards tobacco-free generation: implementation of preventive tobacco policies in the Nordic countries. Scand J Public Health 51(8):1108–1121

Lund L, Bast LS, Rubæk M, Andersen S (2022) Exploring factors associated with smokeless tobacco use among young people: a systematic scoping review. Drug Alcohol Depend 240:109627

Mehrotra R, Lauby-Secretan B (2025) Smokeless tobacco is a major risk factor for oral cancer in South and Southeast Asia. Oral Dis 31(5):1473–1478

Mehrotra R, Yadav A, Sinha DN, Parascandola M, John RM, Ayo-Yusuf O, Nargis N, Hatsukami DK, Warnakulasuriya S, Straif K, Siddiqi K, Gupta PC (2019) Global scenario of smokeless tobacco control: call to action for full implementation of WHO FCTC measures. Lancet Oncol 20(4):e208–e217

Mehrotra R, Kaushik N, Kaushik R (2020) Why smokeless tobacco control needs to be strengthened. Cancer Control 27(1):1073274820914659

Mejia AB, Ling PM (2010) Tobacco industry consumer research on smokeless tobacco users and product development. Am J Public Health 100(1):78–87

Nazar GP, Sharma N, Chugh A, Abdullah SM, Lina S, Mdege ND, John RM, Huque R, Bauld L, Arora M (2021) Impact of tobacco price and taxation on affordability and consumption of tobacco products in the South-East Asia Region: a systematic review. Tob Induc Dis 19:97

Ngaruiya C, Abubakar H, Kiptui D, Kendagor A, Ntakuka MW, Nyakundi P, Gathecha G (2018) Tobacco use and its determinants in the 2015 Kenya WHO STEPS survey. BMC Public Health 18(Suppl 3):1223

Niaz K, Maqbool F, Khan F, Bahadar H, Ismail Hassan F, Abdollahi M (2017) Smokeless tobacco (*paan* and *gutkha*) consumption, prevalence, and contribution to oral cancer. Epidemiol Health 39:e2017009

Pedroso CM, Normando AGC, Siracusa CS, Lauby-Secretan B, Nethan ST, Tomasi RA, Lopes MA et al (2023) Pan-American prevalence of smokeless tobacco use and association with oral potentially malignant disorders and head and neck cancer: a systematic review and meta-analysis. Oral Surg Oral Med Oral Pathol Oral Radiol 136:322–332

Quadri MFA, Tadakamadla SK, John T (2019) Smokeless tobacco and oral cancer in the Middle East and North Africa: a systematic review and meta-analysis. Tob Induc Dis 17:56

Roberts ME, Colby SM, Lu B, Ferketich AK (2016) Understanding tobacco use onset among African Americans. Nicotine Tob Res 18 Suppl 1(Suppl 1):S49–S56

Rollins K, Lewis C, Goeckner R et al (2017) American Indian knowledge, attitudes, and beliefs about smokeless tobacco: a comparison of two focus group studies. J Community Health 42(6):1133–1140

Rout SK, Parhi A (2020) Has tax reforms in India been effective in tobacco control: evidences on affordability of cigarette after introduction of Goods and Service Tax. J Family Med Prim Care 9(12):5927–5932

SAMHSA, Office of Applied Studies, National Survey on Drug Use and Health (2004–2005)

Shaikh R, Saikia N (2022) Socioeconomic inequalities in tobacco cessation among Indians above 15 years of age from 2009 to 2017: evidence from the Global Adult Tobacco Survey (GATS). BMC Public Health 22:1419

Sharma AD, Garg S, Singh MM, Deshmukh C, Mishra A, Singh V, Sharma R (2023) Pattern of smokeless tobacco initiation and use among school going adolescents in Delhi, India: a mixed method study. Asian Pac J Cancer Prev 24(9):3187–3193

Siddiqi K, Husain S, Vidyasagaran A et al (2020) Global burden of disease due to smokeless tobacco consumption in adults: an updated analysis of data from 127 countries. BMC Med 18:222

Singh PK, Jain R, Tyagi A, Yadav A, Singh S (2022) Smokeless tobacco industry's brand stretching through FM radio: a study from Delhi National Capital Region, India. Front Public Health 10:999552

Sinha DN, Gupta PC, Ray C, Singh PK (2012) Prevalence of smokeless tobacco use among adults in WHO South-East Asia. Indian J Cancer 49(4):342–346

Solhi M, Fattahi E, Manzari ZS, Gupta PC, Kargar M, Kasmaei P, Barati H (2021) The reasons for using smokeless tobacco: a review. Iran J Public Health 50(3):492–501

Sreeramareddy CT, Pradhan PM, Sin S (2014) Prevalence, distribution, and social determinants of tobacco use in 30 sub-Saharan African countries. BMC Med 12:243

Warnakulasuriya S, Peters T (2002) Introduction: biology, medical and socio-economic aspects of areca nut use. Addict Biol 7(1):75–76

World Health Organization (2013) Review of areca (betel) nut and tobacco use in the Pacific: a technical report

World Health Organization (2019) WHO global report on trends in prevalence of tobacco use 2000–2025

Yang H, Ma C, Zhao M, Magnussen CG, Xi B (2022) Prevalence and trend of smokeless tobacco use and its associated factors among adolescents aged 12–16 years in 138 countries/territories, 1999–2019. BMC Med 20(1):460

Description of Smokeless Tobacco Products, Their Chemical Composition, and Practices

2

Karishma M. Desai and Vinay K. Hazarey

Abbreviations

BQ	Betel quid
MNBA	4-(methylnitrosamino) butyric acid
MNPA	3-(methylnitrosamino) propionic acid
N. glauca	*Nicotiana glauca*
N. rustica	*Nicotiana rustica*
N. tabacum	*Nicotiana tabacum*
NAB	N′-nitrosoanabasine
NAT	N′-nitrosoanatabine
NDMA	N-nitrosodimethylamine
NKK	4-(methylnitrosamino)-1-(3-pyridyl)-1-butanone
NMOR	N-nitrosomorpholine
NNN	N′-nitrosonornicotine
NPIP	N-nitrosopiperidine
NPYR	N-nitrosopyrrolidine
NSAR	N-nitrososarcosine
PAH	Polycyclic Aromatic Hydrocarbons
ST	Smokeless Tobacco
TSNA	Tobacco-Specific Nitrosamines

K. M. Desai
Tokyo Dental College, Misakicho, Chiyoda-ku, Tokyo, Japan
e-mail: desaikarishma@tdc.ac.jp

V. K. Hazarey (✉)
Dr. D. Y. Patil Dental College and Hospital, Dr. D. Y. Patil Vidyapeeth, Pune, India

Datta Meghe Institute of Medical Sciences, Wardha, India

Manav Rachana Dental College, Faridabad, New Delhi, India
e-mail: vinay.hazarey@dpu.edu.in

F. Javed, S. Warnakulasuriya (eds.), *Smokeless Tobacco and its Effects on Periodontal Health*, https://doi.org/10.1007/978-3-032-16409-4_2

Learning Goals

- Understand the historical evolution of smokeless tobacco (ST), including its origin, global trade routes, and cultural integration over centuries.
- Identify and classify different types of smokeless tobacco products (e.g., paan/betel quid, gutkha/gutka, mishri, shammah, snuff, khaini, snus, toombak) based on their composition, method of use, and regional prevalence.
- Comprehend the chemical composition of ST, including nicotine content, pH, alkaloids, additives, and the role of processing methods like curing and fermentation in altering tobacco's pharmacological profile.
- Recognize the carcinogenic and toxic constituents of ST, especially tobacco-specific nitrosamines, polycyclic aromatic hydrocarbons, aldehydes, heavy metals, and radioelements.
- Assess the role of pH and moisture in determining nicotine bioavailability in ST products and how additives like slaked lime influence nicotine absorption through the oral mucosa.
- Distinguish between the pharmacological and sensory properties of various ST forms and how they are tailored using sweeteners, spices, flavourings, and texture-modifying agents.
- Evaluate the impact of manufacturing, storage, and packaging practices on the chemical stability and toxicity of smokeless tobacco products.
- Understand the oral and systemic health effects associated with ST use, including its role in the aetiology of oral cancers, periodontal disease, and mucosal damage.
- Analyse the sociocultural and gender-related patterns of ST use and their implications for public health policies.
- Differentiate between oral and nasal forms of ST, including methods of preparation, routes of administration, and regional variations in use.
- Assess the role of ST as a dentifrice in various cultures and evaluate the associated health risks of such practices.
- Develop foundational knowledge to contribute to regulatory frameworks and tobacco control programmes targeting ST through evidence-based strategies and culturally sensitive interventions.

2.1 Sweep Across the Time: Classification and Evolution of Smokeless Tobacco (ST) Products

ST is described as "a large variety of commercially or noncommercially available products and mixtures that contain tobacco as the principal constituent and are used either orally or nasally without combustion (IARC monographs, 2007)". ST products are commonly derived from plants species, namely, *Nicotiana tabacum* (*N. tabacum*) and *Nicotiana rustica* (*N.rustica*), belonging to genus *Nicotiana*

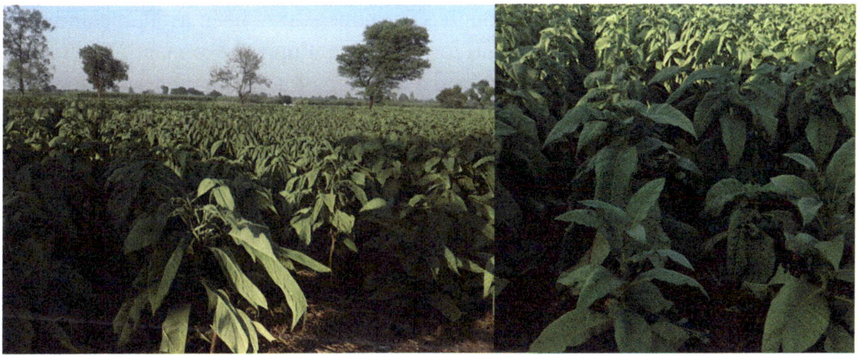

Fig. 2.1 Tobacco cultivations in Karnataka, India. (Courtesy: Dr. Pushpak Shah and Dr. Abhilasha Jha)

Smokeless tobacco products

Based on route of intake

Oral route

(a) Tobacco alone (with aromatics and flavouring agents)
- Creamy snuff
- Gudhaku
- Gul
- Mishri
- Red tooth powder
- Tuibur
- Khiwam
- Loose-leaf
- Dry/Moist snuff
- Twist/roll

(b) Tobacco with other components (pH modifiers)
- Chimo'
- Iq'mik
- Khaini
- Maras
- Nass/Naswar
- Zarda

(c) Betel quid with tobacco–Paan, Gutkha, Mawa

Nasal route

Snuff
- Dry Snuff
- Liquid snuff

Based on use

Applied to teeth & gums
- Creamy snuff
- Gudhaku
- Gul
- Mishri
- Red tooth powder
- Tuibur

For sucking
- Chimo'
- Dry Snuff
- -Moist snuff
- Gutkha
- Khaini
- Looseleaf
- Maras
- Mishri
- Naswar
- Plug
- Shammah
- Snus
- Tobacco tablets
- Toombak

For chewing

- Betel quid with tobacco
- Gutkha
- Iq'mik
- Khaini
- Khiwam
- Looseleaf
- Mawa
- Plug
- Tobacco chewing gum
- Twist/roll
- Zarda

Based on processing

Natural
Fermented
Cured
(using air, flue, fire)

Fig. 2.2 Smokeless tobacco products

(Solanaceae) (Fig. 2.1). Archaeological excavations in parts of Mexico and Peru have found tobacco seeds dating back to 3500 BC (Voges 1984). Worldwide, several variations in ST forms (Fig. 2.2), curing, and consumption methods have evolved. STs have been classified based on their usage and method of preparation. Oral STs can be either dipped/sucked or chewed and are commonly placed in the vestibular areas of lip and cheek. STs are also available as pastes or fine powders that are rubbed onto the teeth or gingiva. Another common form includes snuff or fine mixture of tobacco that is inhaled and absorbed through the nasal passage. The frequency, duration of habit, method of consumption, and close contact of STs with the oral and/or nasal mucosa determine its effects on oral and system health. Several forms of STs have been adopted across the world and even incorporated in various cultural and religious practices. Though ST products have been available and used for over hundreds of years, its use and forms have multiplied exponentially over the recent years necessitating a thorough understanding of its history, chemical composition, effects, and global practices.

Key Points

- ST use dates back to at least 3500 BC and has evolved globally through different preparation and usage methods
- ST use is deeply rooted in many cultural and religious practices.
- ST products include both commercial and traditional forms and are primarily derived from the *N. tabacum* and *N. rustica* species.
- ST products exist in multiple forms—chewed, sucked, dipped, rubbed on oral tissues, or inhaled as snuff—each with distinct methods of consumption that influence their health effects.

2.1.1 History of Tobacco Chewing: Influence of Trade

The word "tobacco" originated from "*tobago*" or "*tobaca*", which was a Y-shaped hollow pipe or cone-like instrument used by the American Indians for inhaling powered leaves of a plant. The Spaniards later named the device as "tobacco" (Christen et al. 1982) and commercialized the tobacco in West Indies and the European markets between 1531 and 1575. Prior to this, tobacco chewing was prevalent amongst the Indians who lived off the coast of Venezuela, on the Margita Island. Amerigo Vespucci in 1499 described that the American Indians used the herb to reduce thirst and hunger, increase salivation, and clean their teeth (IARC 2007a, b; Heimann 1960; Stewart 1967; Voges 1984). In the 1500s, the practice of tobacco consumption expanded to Latin America, particularly in south and central America (Voges 1984). American Indians travelled long distances and used the dry herb as a means to alleviate hunger, thirst, and fatigue. Native and other American tribes further adapted finely powdered tobacco by mixing it with lime and burnt, fresh- or saltwater molluscs (Curtis 1935). They perceived tobacco as a remedy for toothache, insect/spider/snake bite, and wound disinfection by mixing tobacco juice and saliva (Axton 1975).

Alongside the Spaniards, the Portuguese propagated tobacco on a large scale. The generic name *Nicotiana* is derived from Jean Nicot, who was the French Ambassador to Portugal in 1559. The French Ambassador propagated this plant in England for its "Cure-all" medicinal properties. It had applications ranging from prophylactic in plague to a cleanser for brushing teeth (Brooks 1952).

As a major export commodity, tobacco products spread all over in countries such as Europe, Turkey, Russia, Arabia, China, and others (Axton 1975). ST gained remarkable popularity and swiftly spread across the Central and South East Asian countries. During the Ching Dynasty, the Chinese also believed in the medicinal properties of tobacco and stored it in precious materials such as ivory, amethyst, amber, amongst several others. The Portuguese traders further carried tobacco to the Indian subcontinent between the late sixteenth and early seventeenth century. During this period, the South Indian Kingdom of Adil Shah, North India Kingdom of Asad Beg, and others popularized the tobacco practice. Moghul King Akbar was advised by his physicians to filter tobacco through water and thus the "Hookah culture" came into existence. From the early smoked tobacco forms, eventually snuff and chewing tobacco practices came into use. Tobacco was also broadcasted through art, poetry and literary work, and music (Smokeless Tobacco and Public Health in India 2016). The earliest ST practice was chewing tobacco in betel leaf (*Piper betle*) as *paan/pan*/betel quid (BQ). Paan chewing (without tobacco) is an ancient custom which advanced for more than 2000 years. It was referred to as *tambula* and deeply embraced as a cultural and social custom in India. It was considered amongst the eight *bhogas* or enjoyments of life. One of the regular additives in paan was areca nut (*Areca Catechu*). During the European trade and colonization period, "*Chuna*" or slaked lime, i.e. calcium hydroxide, was included as a component of BQ. Gradually, a myriad of other methods for the use of ST were developed. Post-independence of India, the use of pan masala came into being in the seventeenth century. It was believed to be an easier and less time-consuming alternative to paan. Due to its nature of being user-friendly, less cumbersome, and portable, it spread rapidly amongst the youth and elderly. When trade was affected in 1776 due to American Revolution, the British (East India Co.) expanded tobacco cultivation in India (Smokeless Tobacco and Public Health in India 2016). The seventeenth century observed marked rise in tobacco cultivations across regions such as Bengal, Bihar, Orissa, and other northern and central parts of India.

Thereafter, in 1860s, the Americans introduced a variation in the chewable form of tobacco by developing the plug or twist (Heimann 1960). Herein the leaf was bundled and laced with a sweetener such as brandy or cane sugar, which on fermentation produced a tasty chew (Axton 1975). Chewing tobacco remained a common practice in America before the rise of cigarette practice in 1918 and resurged between 1960 and 1970 (Gottsegen 1940; Christen and Glover 1981). Similarly, the use of ST in India is considerably higher compared to smoked tobacco.

Key Points

- Indigenous communities used tobacco for various purposes, including hunger suppression, oral hygiene, and traditional medicine, such as pain relief and wound treatment.
- The Spanish and Portuguese played a major role in spreading tobacco globally, with Jean Nicot introducing the plant to France, leading to the name *Nicotiana*.
- In India, the traditional practice of BQ (*paan*) chewing dates back over 2000 years.
- In the 1860s, Americans introduced new chewable forms like plug and twist tobacco sweetened with brandy or sugar.

2.1.2 History of Snuff

Snuff or the ground powdered form of tobacco was first used by Brazilians. They used a rosewood cup and pestle to grind the tobacco leaves to acquire a delicate whiff from rosewood. This powder was held in an ornate bone tube that is plugged at one end for retention of the fragrance (Curtis 1935). The American Indians used Tobago, wherein, the forked ends of the Y-shaped device were placed in both nostrils and the other end close to the snuff (Christen et al. 1982). Similarly, the use of snuff by Caribbean Indians in lesser Antilles was reported by Columbus's co-traveller and monk, Friar Ramón Pané in 1493. He propagated the practice in Spain and the rest of the Europe. As with chewing tobacco, snuff was used for medicinal purposes such as clearing of the nasal passages, analgesia, burns wound-healing, and as a sleep inducer in various regions such as Haiti and Mexico in the early 1500s (Stewart 1967). Jean Nicot recommended snuff to the Queen of France, Catherine de Medici as a cure for headaches. It was in 1560 that the Dutch used powdered tobacco and gave it the commonly recognized name "Snuff" (Christen et al. 1982).

During the early 1600s, tobacco snuff was an expensive, widely commoditized product that spread through South America, Africa, and Asian countries of Japan and China. Various terms such as "carotte" and "rappee" associated with its preparation process originated. By 1650s, snuff reached England, Scotland, and Ireland. In Ireland, the appellation for snuff was "powder" or "smutchin", while in Scotland it was "sneeshin" (Harrison 1964). Usage of ready-made snuff peaked in England from 1702 to 1714 during Queen Anne's reign; wherein it was called "the final reason for human nose". Many members of the royal family continued using snuff, and snuff boxes came to be recognized as a symbol of wealth and rank of its possessor (Christen et al. 1982). While homemade snuff was common, shops provided special blends such as King's morning mix, plain, and carotte (Ryan 1980). The carotte, i.e. tightly rolled tobacco in a carrot-like form, was often soaked in agents such as cinnamon, lavender, or almond oil. It is often dried and pulverized using an iron hand-grater. The technique used for inhaling snuff comprised of placing small quantity of snuff on the backside of hand for sniffing via nostrils such that it induced a sneeze (Christen et al. 1982). By the 1800s, three varieties of snuff were largely popular in Europe, namely Scotch snuff which was a stronger, unscented powder; Maccaboy which was moist and scented, frequently consumed by sucking or inhalation; and Rapee or the Swedish Snuff which was coarsely grated form of snuff, commonly used by inhalation. In Sweden, snuff usage grew from the mid-1700 to early-1800s, especially amongst the aristocrats at the court of King Gustav III. The city of Gothenburg was considered as the chief snuff producer in Sweden (Loewe 1981).

From the twentieth century, snuff usually drifted from nasal to oral route. Similarly in North America, the colonists took to oral manner of snuff consumption in contrast to nasal sniffing. In Virginia, snuff mills were established in 1730s and in New York in 1760s. However, major boom in snuff production in the USA occurred between 1880 and 1930 (Garner 1951). Snuff was processed from dried, dark tobacco made by curing with air or fire. The stem and tobacco leaves were preconditioned and aged in large wooden barrels or hogsheads, cut and fermented for

2 months to bring out an aromatic odour. This processed form was then dried, ground, and filtered using a silk cloth to obtain fine powder for retail packaging. These dried and moist forms of snuff were frequently used for dipping and placing in mouth.

Though tobacco use promulgated largely due to its perceived medicinal benefits, various communities studied the adverse effects and formulated punishments, prohibitions, and laws against the use of tobacco. To understand the effects, a thorough knowledge of its chemical composition is of paramount importance.

Key Points

- Snuff, a powdered form of ST, originated in Brazil and was initially used through specialized tools like rosewood pestles and ornate bone tubes for nasal inhalation.
- American and Caribbean Indians used snuff not only for recreational purposes but also for medicinal applications, including relieving headaches, clearing nasal passages, and promoting sleep.
- The term "snuff" was popularized in 1560 by the Dutch, and its use spread rapidly throughout Europe, partly due to Jean Nicot's endorsement to the French royal court.
- In the seventeenth to eighteenth century Europe, especially during Queen Anne's reign, snuff became a luxury item symbolizing status and wealth.
- By the 1800s, multiple regional snuff variants emerged, with Sweden's city Gothenburg becoming a major production hub favoured by aristocrats.
- From the twentieth century onward, snuff use transitioned from nasal to oral routes, especially in North America, where it became commercially mass-produced and consumed through dipping.

2.2 Chemical Composition

Overview

Composition of tobacco varies based on source or type of tobacco leaf, environment, processing (Tso 1990), curing (air/flue/fire-cured), and storage conditions (Burton et al. 1983, 1989a, b; Peele et al. 1995; Walton et al. 1995; Wiernik et al. 1995; Peele et al. 2001; Bush et al. 2001). The earliest known chemical information on tobacco components and its smoke was given in 1968. Thereafter, additional information was given by Roberts in 1988 and Hoffman et al. in 2001 (23 N-nitrosamines and 28 pesticides) which brought the numbers to 3095. Diverse ST preparations have ingredients blended together to achieve definite concentration of nicotine, pH, and taste. These enhance user acceptance, bioavailability of nicotine (Djordjevic et al. 1995; Henningfield et al. 1995; Richter and Spierto 2003), and influence of nitrosamines (Fischer et al. 1989; Burton et al. 1994; Hoffmann et al. 1995). Majority of commercial ST are produced from the *N. Tabacum* in North America and globally. The alkaloid content of *N. Tabacum* varies between 0.17% and 4.93% depending on the type, parts of plant used, maturity, and fertilizer treatments. Cured *N. Tabacum* varieties consist of 0.2–4.75% of nicotine by weight (Tso 1990; Stratton et al. 2001). Whereas, in Europe, Asia, and Africa, the cured leaves of *N. rustica* species contain high levels of tobacco-specific *N*-nitrosamines (TSNA) and nicotine ranging up to 12%. Curing causes physical and chemical changes in the composition of tobacco. Curing via thermal effects or desiccation of leaves causes arrest of the biochemical processes in the metabolically active tobacco leaves. Curing largely reduces the starch content and increases sugar content by 100%. Protein and nicotine contents reduce marginally. Furthermore, fermentation reduces the carbohydrates and polyphenol content of the leaves. This necessitates processing with molasses, liquorice, and other flavourings or extracts to improve taste, flavour, enhance shelf-life, and meet the consumers' need (Mookherjee and Wilson 1988; Roberts 1988; Sharma et al. 1991). Other components of tobacco comprise 0.5–5% alkaloids (nicotine (85–95%), nornicotine, cotinine, anabasine, and anatabine), 0.5–4.5% polyphenols, 0.1–3% terpenes, 0.1–2.5% phytosterols, <1% of carboxylic acids and alkanes, aromatic and heterocyclic hydrocarbons, aldehydes, ketones, amines, nitriles and alkali nitrates, pesticides, and other metallic compounds (Brunnemann and Hoffmann 1992; IARC 2004a, b). Additives commonly used include β-citronellol, menthol, eugenol, salicylates, benzoate, 1,8-cineole, and many others. Antimicrobial agents such as ascorbic acid and fungicides such as sodium propionate are also added in commercial preparations of tobacco.

Key Points

- *N. tabacum* and *N. rustica* differ in alkaloid and TSNA content.
- N. tabacum (common in North America) has 0.2–4.75% nicotine, while *N. rustica* (more common in Asia, Africa, and Europe) can contain nicotine levels up to 12% and higher concentrations of carcinogenic TSNAs.
- Over 3000 chemical constituents have been identified in tobacco products, including 23 tobacco-specific nitrosamines and 28 pesticides.
- The chemical makeup of ST includes adjustments in pH to increase the availability of free nicotine.
- Tobacco contains a wide range of harmful compounds, such as alkaloids (nicotine, nornicotine, cotinine), polyphenols, terpenes, phytosterols, aldehydes, hydrocarbons, pesticides, heavy metals, and added antimicrobial and flavouring agents.

Carcinogens and Toxins in ST

As of 2013, ST products contain about 28 carcinogens that include non-volatile TSNA and nitrosamino acids (most abundant), volatile compounds like *N*-nitrosamines and aldehydes, ethyl carbamate, polycyclic aromatic hydrocarbons (PAH), metals (Group I carcinogens—arsenic and cadmium, Group 2B carcinogen—lead and nickel, and Group 3—chromium), radioelements such as uranium and polonium 210 (Sharma et al. 1985), and mycotoxins (Table 2.1).

Table 2.1 Major carcinogens in smokeless tobacco (ST) products and their carcinogenic potential as per WHO International Agency for Research on Cancer (IARC) (IARC 2007a, b; Sharma et al. 1985; Hoffmann and Djordjevic 1997)

	Type of compound	IARC Group	ST products
1	Tobacco-specific nitrosamine		
	N-Nitrosonornicotine	Group 1	Most ST products (Chewing tobacco and snuff)
	4-(Methylnitrosamino)-1-(3-pyridyl)-1-butanone	Group 1	Khaini, zarda, snuff, gutkha
	N-Nitrosoanabasine	Group 3	Moist snuff, Indian products
	N-Nitrosoanatabine	Group 3	Canadian moist snuff, others
2	Volatile N-nitrosamine		
	N-nitrosodimethylamine	Group 2A/B	Snuff, chewing tobacco
	N-nitrosodiethylamine	Group 2A	Snuff, chewing tobacco
	N-nitrosopyrrolidine	Group 2B	Snuff, chewing tobacco
	N-nitrosomorpholine	Group 2B	Snuff, chewing tobacco
3	Nitrosamino Acids		
	Nitrosarcosine	Group 1	Snuff
4	Polycyclic aromatic hydrocarbons		
	Benzo[a]pyrene	Group 1	Natural tobacco, Iq' mik, moist snuff, dry snuff
	Dibenz[a,h]anthracene	Group 2A	US/Swedish products
5	Volatile aldehyde		
	Acetaldehyde	Group 2B	Majority of ST products
	Formaldehyde	Group 1	Additive in ST
	Crotonaldehyde	Group 3	
6	Heavy and trace metals		
	Arsenic	Group 1	Absorbed via soil (Natural tobacco)
	Cadmium	Group 1	Moist snuff
	Lead	Group 2B	All ST
	Cobalt, chromium, nickel	Group 2B/3	Moist snuff and dry snuff
	Beryllium	Group 1	Various ST
7	Chemical contaminant		
	Hydrazine	Group 2A	Rare
8	Radioactive elements		
	Uranium-235/238, Polonium-210	Sufficient carcinogenicity in animals and humans	Natural tobacco, snuff, common Indian/US ST products

ST smokeless tobacco, *US* United States

Amongst the nitroso compounds in ST the three most common ones include (a) TSNA such as 4-(methylnitrosamino)-1-(3-pyridyl)-1-butanone (NNK) and N′-nitrosonornicotine (NNN) which are strong carcinogens (IARC group I carcinogen). TSNA are frequently linked carcinogens implicated in oral, oesophageal, and pancreatic cancers; (b) N-nitrosamino acids such as N-nitrososarcosine (NSAR), 3-(methylnitrosamino) propionic acids (MNPA) and 4-(methylnitrosamino) butyric acids (MNBA); (c) N-nitrosamines such as N-nitrosodimethylamine

Factors determining levels of TSNA in ST

A. Country, tobacco species and type of ST

N.tabacum	NNN	NNK
USA	0.39 ug/g	0.42 ug/g
India	0.035 ug/g	0.0115 ug/g

N. *rustica*	NNN	NNK
India	46.1 ug/g	2.34 ug/g

B. Precursor content and processing

Fermentation and curing

- Chemical changes in primary alkaloid precursors and nitrates leading to formation of TSNA
- ***Initial stage:*** Secondary amines → NAT & NAB
- ***Late stage:***Tertiary amines → NNK & NNN

Contaminants such as morpholine from additives & wax coated containers → NMOR

C. pH, moisture and temperature

At high temperature

Moist snuff → Progressively increases N-nitrosamines and nitrites

pH of oral cavity and stomach facilitate nitrosation of components and increase NNN (4 to 64 times)

Moist snuff products → Naswar and Toombak have high pH

D. Typeof ST

Moist snuff (High pH)

NNN	NNK
135 ug/g	17.8 ug/g
NDMA	NPYR
265 ng/g	860 ng/g

Moist snuff Sweden

NNN

0.15–0.61 μg/g wet wt

NNK

3.8 to 0.49 μg/g wet wt

Toombak

NNN	NNK
3085 ng/g dry wt	7870 ng/g dry wt

Fig. 2.3 Factors determining levels of TSNA (Bhide et al. 1987; Brunnemann et al. 1987; Brunnemann et al. 2004; Djordjevic et al. 1989)

(NDMA), N-nitrosopyrrolidine (NPYR), N-nitrosopiperidine (NPIP), and N-nitrosomorpholine (NMOR). Other carcinogens in ST include N′-nitrosoanabasine (NAB) which is a weak carcinogen and the inactive N′-nitrosoanatabine (NAT) (IARC 2012). Variations in the nitroso compounds are often determined by the leaves chosen (Bhide et al. 1987; Djordjevic et al. 1989), alkaloid precursor content and processing (Spiegelhalder and Fischer 1991; Henningfield et al. 1997; Hatsukami and Severson 1999), type of ST (Andersen et al. 1989; Connolly 2001; Djordjevic et al. 1993; Idris et al. 1998), region and method of manufacturing (Brunnemann et al. 1985; Brunnemann and Hoffmann 1992), and storage (Burton et al., 1989a, b, 1994; Fischer et al. 1989; Chamberlain and Chortyk 1992; Djordjevic et al. 1993; Peele et al. 2001; Li and Bush 2004) (Fig. 2.3).

Nicotine in tobacco is a known addictive agent and can occur in either acidic or basic form. The acidic form is bound, while the unprotonated basic form or "free nicotine" is the one that is easily absorbed by the mucosal lining of oral cavity. Agents like ammonia and carbonates are used to increase the pH and release unprotonated nicotine for quick absorption and circulation in blood (Djordjevic et al. 1995; Henningfield et al. 1995). The pH of ST products, moisture content, and its interaction with agents such as slaked lime or other alkalis also determines the absorption of nicotine (CDC 1999; Djordjevic et al. 1995; Richter and Spierto 2003). At high pH the absorption of nicotine increases, whereas at low pH, ionization of nicotine limits its absorption across the mucosal membranes. From amongst the 562 additives reported in smokeless tobacco (House of Representatives 1994), ammonium, sodium, and potassium salts, can alter the ST pH. Some ingredients are specifically designed to control how nicotine is delivered to the body (FDA 1996). Additionally, the way ST is used also affects the nicotine exposure. People who dip or chew 8–10 times/day can be exposed to as much nicotine as someone who smokes

30–40 cigarettes daily (DHHS 1986). A study (Lemmonds et al. 2005) showed that frequent and long-term use of smokeless tobacco is strongly linked to higher levels of cotinine (a nicotine breakdown product) in the body (Richter and Tricker 2002). Snuff dippers absorb about three times more nicotine per use than cigarette smokers (Hecht et al. 2005). This high nicotine exposure should be considered when recommending nicotine replacement therapies to people trying to quit snuff. Swallowing method causes significant ingestion of nitrate, nitrites, and secondary amines from ST. Additionally, studies show that alcohol can further increase nicotine absorption, especially for harmful compounds like NNN (Du et al. 2000). A recent report (Gupta and Sankar 2004) provided data on 14 types of smokeless tobacco in India which showed that certain STs had pH up to 10.1 and nicotine up to 10.2 mg/g. Similarly, a study in South Africa (Ayo-Yusuf et al. 2004) found that moist snuff had pH ranging from 7.1 to 10.1 and nicotine content from 0.8% to 1.6% (wet weight), with unprotonated nicotine making up 10.1–99.1% of the total nicotine.

PAHs such as benzo [a] pyrene (B[a]P) forms after fire-curing, pyrolyzation or burning of tobacco and is categorized as Group I carcinogen by the IARC. Aldehydes are suspected or known human carcinogens; tobacco contains aromatic alkyl aldehydes that are derived from heating of sugars and amino acids during tobacco processing (Coleman III and Perfetti 1997). The α- and β-angelica lactones have been reported in natural tobacco (Weeks et al. 1989). Natural tobacco also contains α- and β-angelica lactones, and scopoletin, a coumarin type polyphenol. Cured (air- and flue-cured) tobacco also contain hydrazines. Radioactive components such as polonium-210 are derived from soil that is treated with phosphates fertilizers containing radium-226 (Tso et al. 1966).

Key Points

- Approximately 28 carcinogens have been identified in ST products, including TSNAs, PAHs, volatile aldehydes, ethyl carbamate, toxic metals (e.g., arsenic, cadmium), radioactive elements (e.g., polonium-210), and mycotoxins.
- Compounds like NNN and NNK are strongly associated with cancers of the oral cavity, oesophagus, and pancreas, and are classified by the IARC as Group I carcinogens.
- Alkalizing agents in ST, such as ammonia and slaked lime, increase pH and facilitate nicotine absorption by oral mucosa.
- Daily use of ST (8–10 times) may result in nicotine exposure equivalent to smoking 30–40 cigarettes.
- Snuff users absorb up to 3x more nicotine per use compared to cigarette smokers.
- Swallowing ST can increase ingestion of harmful nitrosamines and nitrates, with alcohol use further enhancing absorption of toxic compounds like NNN.
- Carcinogenic compounds such as benzo[a]pyrene, aldehydes and hydrazines are generated during ST processing.
- The use of fertilizer during tobacco cultivation can introduce radioactive elements such as polonium-210 in the derived ST product.

2.3 Practices and Preparation of Various ST Products

Oral Use In the USA and Europe, chewable forms of tobacco are primarily available and consumed as a firm or moist plug, loose-leaf, and twist or roll (Rizio 1984). Each product is made through a distinct process and uses different forms of tobacco (dried, baked, or fermented) with additives that either increase absorption or make the product more palatable. Oral STs are placed in the mandibular groove or labial and buccal vestibules for chewing or sucking the tobacco. Frequently "chaw", which is a large, golf ball sized tobacco portion, is used for chewing tobacco; whereas, a smaller portion referred to as "quid" is held in mouth for sucking tobacco. In several south Asian countries, tobacco products were repurposed into formulations that were often used as dentifrice. Several products across countries were integrated as a part of their social or regional customs.

(a) *BQ/Paan with tobacco*: *Paan* is a chewable item that uses either raw or processed ST and is hand-made fresh at home or by the vendors at roadside small kiosks (Fig. 2.4).

Method of use: Chewable; placed in mouth as quid with or without ST

Components: Raw tobacco used is either finely chopped, powdered (roasted sun-dried) or paste-like (boiled) in consistency. Paan is not tobacco by itself but is often used as a carrier of tobacco, customized ingredients such slaked lime, catechu, volatile oils, sugar, starch, tannins and flavouring agents such as menthol, mint, rosewater, aniseed, cardamom, clove, amongst several others. The ingredients are often added as per regional customs or individual preferences.

Regional and commercial aspects: In northern parts of India, Zarda and Kiwam are popular choice for tobacco, whereas in Southern states such as Karnataka, powdered tobacco sticks, namely *Kaddipudi* and *hogesoppu* are crushed and used with *paan*. In Orissa and Bengal, "*Kadapan*" is prepared using a mixture called Gundi which comprises of tobacco, coriander seeds, and spices.

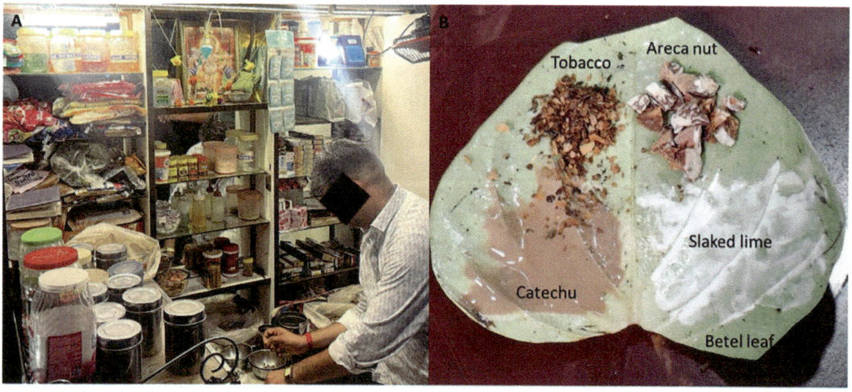

Fig. 2.4 (**a**) Roadside *paan* kiosks. (**b**) Betel leaf and components of BQ

Besides India, the practise of *Paan* chewing is also spread across central, eastern, and southern regions of the Asian subcontinent (Bhonsle et al. 1992; Mehta and Hamner 1993; Gupta and Ray 2003; Javed et al. 2015).

Key Point

- *Paan* is a culturally embedded chewable preparation in South Asia that often serves as a vehicle for ST, combining ingredients like slaked lime, spices, and flavourings.

(b) *Chimó*: Chimo is a peculiar form of concentrated ST that is found in Venezuela. *Method of use*: Chimó is typically placed in the vestibule (between lip, cheeks, and gingiva) and held for about 30 min then spat out.

Components: It is prepared as a mixture of tobacco leaves, sodium bicarbonate, sugar, Mamón tree, and flavouring agents. To obtain small quantities of highly concentrated Chimó, large quantities of leaves are boiled and seasoned. After reduction into a paste-like material (pasta), it is transferred into a carrier usually made from dried fruit ("*taparas*") or fruit (banana) leaves. The prepared paste is then made more suitable or palatable with seasoning ingredients.

Regional and commercial aspects: Chimó is often sold in portable, round metal tins or wrapped candy cylinders. Besides oil, Venezuela also exports chimó to other countries.

Key Point

- Chimó is a highly concentrated form of smokeless tobacco used in Venezuela, prepared by boiling large quantities of tobacco leaves with additives into a paste, and typically held in the oral vestibule for prolonged periods

(c) *Creamy snuff*: Creamy snuff is a ST product that is often packaged like a toothpaste (Fig. 2.5).

Method of use: Creamy snuff is rubbed onto the teeth by finger or toothbrush and is allowed to sit for about 3–4 min.

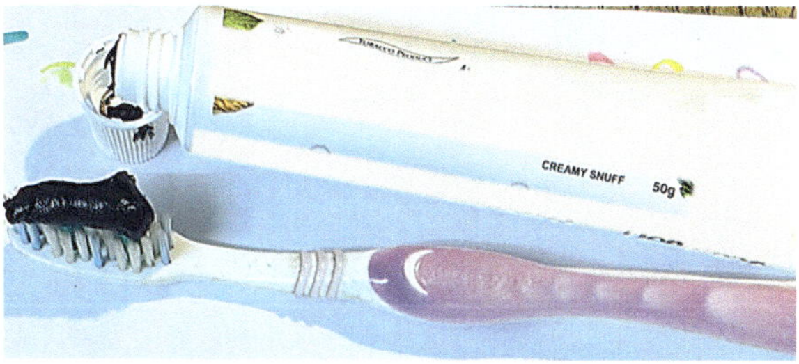

Fig. 2.5 Creamy snuff

Components: It is composed of fine, powdered and ground tobacco with aromatic components such as spearmint, menthol, and camphor. Other components include salt, clove oil, glycerine, and water.

Regional and commercial aspects: Though not all commercial products are marketed as a toothpaste, it is often used as a tooth cleanser and advertised for its antibacterial properties. Toothpaste containing creamy snuff are often marketed as herbal paste. Creamy snuff is often used as a "toothpaste" by South Asian women.

Key Point

- Creamy snuff is often used as a "toothpaste" by South Asian women.

(d) *Dry snuff*:

Method of use: Dry snuff is a powdered form of tobacco that is consumed by oral or nasal route. In the USA, a pinch or "dip" of dry snuff is held in the upper labial vestibule; whereas in Europe, it is used via the nasal route. In many regions of the world, dry snuff is used both orally and nasally. As with creamy snuff, it is commonly rubbed on the teeth and gums. Women tend to use it more frequently and several times during the day, due to its addictive properties.

Components and other details: In India, it is often prepared at home by roasting coarsely cut tobacco on a griddle and then powdering it (Fig. 2.6). This pyrolyzed snuff-like preparation known as "*Bajar*" or *Tapkeer/Tapkir* is used in cities like Goa, Maharastra, Gujarat, and eastern parts of India. In Europe and the USA, fire-cured tobacco (primarily Kentucky and Tennessee tobacco) is fermented and prepared into a powdered form. This dry, powdered tobacco has lower than 10% moisture content and is sold in small-sized, metal or glass containers. In northern Africa, dry snuff preparation is known as *naffa, tenfeha,* or *nufha* (Axéll et al. 1976). The Swedish moist snuff or snus is made of finely ground dried Kentucky and Virginia tobacco that is mixed with other components such as aromatics, humidifying agents, salts, and buffers.

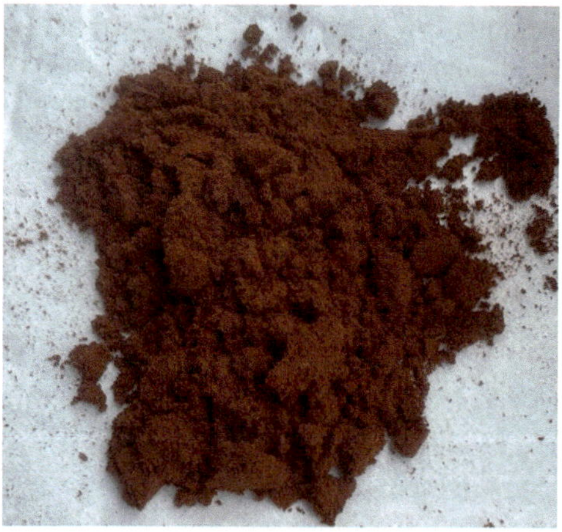

Fig. 2.6 Tapkir or dry snuff. Commonly used by women for brushing teeth

Key Point

- Dry snuff is a versatile, powdered tobacco product used both orally and nasally across different regions, with variations in preparation and cultural practices; it is particularly popular among women due to its addictive nature and frequent use.

(e) *Gudhaku*:

Method of use: Gudhaku is used by rubbing it on teeth and gums. Thereafter, it is either swallowed or spat out. Women are frequent users of Gudhaku.

Components: Gudhaku/Gurakhu is paste made of tobacco leaves, molasses, lime, and red soil (Smokeless Tobacco and Public Health in India 2016).

Regional and commercial aspects: It is commercially manufactured and packaged in metal containers (Fig. 2.7). The use of Gudhaku is popular in Indian states of Bihar (8.3% users), Orissa, Uttar Pradesh, and Uttaranchal (Mehta et al. 1971).

Key Points

- Gudhaku is used by rubbing it on teeth and gums. Thereafter, it is either swallowed or spat out.
- Women are frequent users of Gudhaku.

(f) *Gul*: Gul is a commercially manufactured fine form of tobacco (Fig. 2.8).

Method of use: This highly addictive form of tobacco is applied as a dentifrice and used several times in the day.

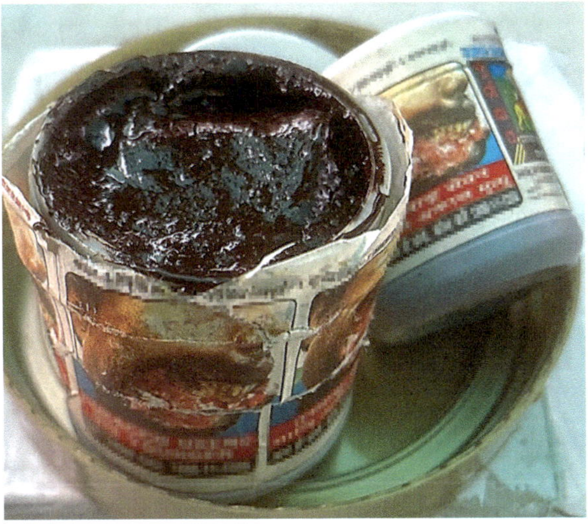

Fig. 2.7 Gudhaku paste. (Courtesy: Dr Amit Dalmia)

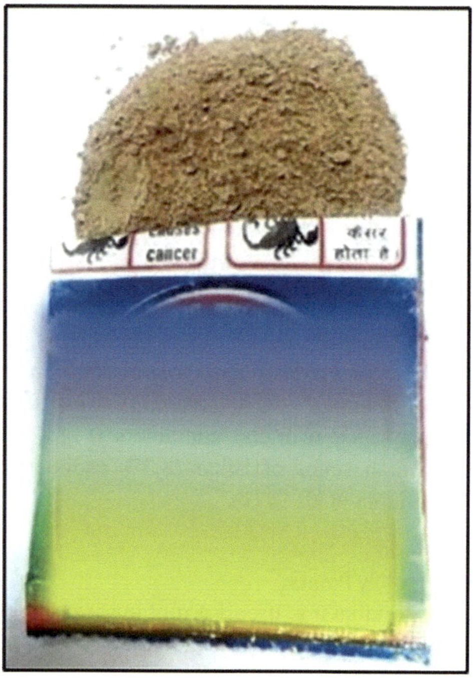

Fig. 2.8 Gul packet

Composition and other details: Motihari tobacco leaves with molasses, ash of tendu leaves, and other ingredients. Gul is used in South Asia, including the Indian subcontinent and Bangladesh.

Key Points

- Gul is a highly addictive form of ST product and is applied as a dentifrice and used several times in the day.
- Gul is used in South Asia, including the Indian subcontinent and Bangladesh.

(g) *Gutka/Ghutka*: Gutkha or gutka is a dehydrated substitute for *paan* that is mixed with tobacco. It is sold in easy-to-carry packets or small sachets. The average pH of gutkha is around 8.5 (Stanfill et al. 2011) and its consumption adversely affects oral health.

Method of use: It is held in the mouth, sucked, chewed, and either swallowed or spat out (Javed et al. 2015).

Composition: Gutkha/Gutka consists of sun-dried, roasted, finely chopped tobacco with areca nut, slaked lime, and catechu. Other ingredients such as sandalwood, saffron, clove and menthol may be used for flavouring. Sweeteners (saccharine, sorbitol) and humidifying agents such as glycerine and sodium propionate may be included in some commercial gutka/ghutka preparations.

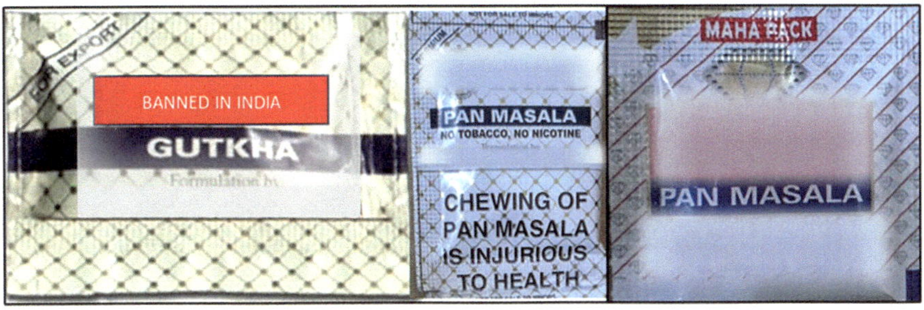

Fig. 2.9 Gutkha/gutka (banned in India) and pan masala (often used by people alone or by combining with chewable tobacco) packets. (Courtesy: Dr. Shruti Gundewar)

Regional and commercial aspects: Gutkha is used in India and by Asian expatriates in Canada, the UK, the USA, and several other countries (IARC 2004a). In India, several gutkha products were manufactured and packaged using the same brand names as pan masala (Fig. 2.9). Though gutkha is banned in India, people addicted to gutkha started to self-assemble it by mixing pan masala and chewable tobacco.

Key Points

- Gutkha/Gutka consists of sun-dried, roasted, finely chopped tobacco with areca nut, slaked lime and catechu. Other ingredients such as sandalwood, saffron, clove, and menthol may be used for flavouring.
- Gutka/gutkha is highly addictive, and its widespread use pose significant risks to oral and systemic health.
- The global export of Gutka/Gutkha has made this highly addictive ST product commercially available to users, primarily South Asian expatriates, in countries such as Canada, the UK and the USA.

(h) *Iq'mik*: Iq'mik is a ST product that is made by mixing fire-cured tobacco leaves (usually from *N. rustica*) with punk ash, which is derived from the charred fungus of birch trees or other wood sources. The ash increases the pH of the mixture, enhancing the absorption of nicotine through the oral mucosa.

Method of use: The users mix the ingredients and chew a small pinch of the Iq'mik. Sometimes, users store back the pre-chewed Iq'mik for reuse by others members of the household.

Composition: Iq'mik is made of fire-cured leaves of tobacco and punk ash from a woody birch tree fungus.

Regional and commercial aspects: Iq'mik is popular and often consumed by people from western Alaska and natives of north America. In some communities, pre-chewed Iq'mik may be shared among family members, including adolescents and children, raising serious public health concerns.

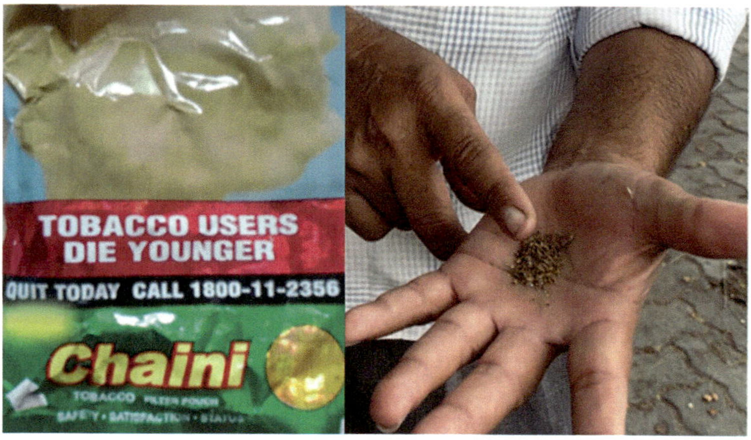

Fig. 2.10 (**a**) Commercial packet of khaini. (Courtesy: Dr. Shruti Gundewar); (**b**) Khaini mixed on palm of the hand (with or without lime)

Key Points

- Iq'mik is a ST product popular among Native communities in western Alaska.
- It combines fire-cured tobacco with punk ash to elevate pH and enhance nicotine absorption.
- Its communal use, poses significant public health risks, especially for users including children and adolescents.

(i) *Khaini*: Khaini (Fig. 2.10) is a ST typically consumed with lime.

Method of use: Small quantity of tobacco is mixed with slaked lime on the palm of the user's hand and rubbed with thumb. It is often held in the oral cavity and sucked for 10–15 min. It is rarely chewed; some users keep it on the tongue and others may even leave it overnight in the gingivo-buccal groove (Bhonsle et al. 1979). About 42% users hold khaini in the front of oral cavity, while others place it in either side of the buccal groove (Stich et al. 1982). Some users also add areca nut to khaini. Men use khaini more frequently than women.

Composition: It is made from *N. rustica* and/or *N. tabacum* leaves that are sun-dried or fermented and coarsely cut. It is packaged in a double-ended metal container containing tobacco on one side and slaked lime on the other.

Regional and commercial aspects: Khaini is frequently used in South Asian countries such as Nepal, India, and Bangladesh.

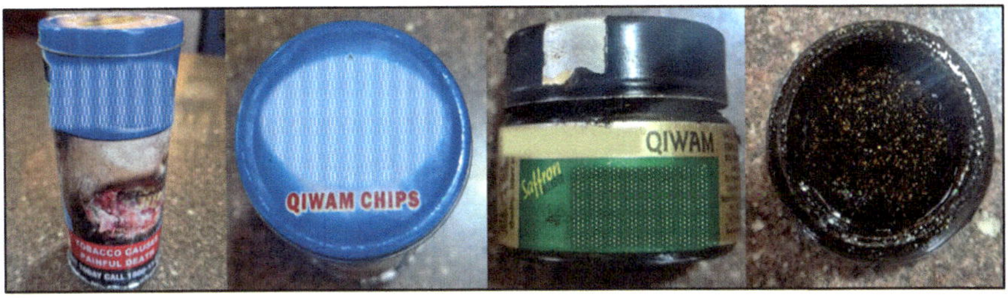

Fig. 2.11 Qiwam chips and paste. (Courtesy: Dr. Shruti Gundewar)

Key Points
- Khaini is a widely used smokeless tobacco product in South Asia.
- Khaini is typically prepared by mixing sun-dried or fermented tobacco leaves with slaked lime.
- It is commonly placed in the oral cavity for extended periods, significantly increasing mucosal exposure to nicotine and associated carcinogens

(j) *Khiwam*: Khiwam/qiwam is a thick paste preparation made from ST. Some manufacturers also market qiwam in the form of chips (Fig. 2.11).

Method of use: A thick qiwam paste is placed in the mouth and chewed.

Composition: It is prepared using extract from the leaves of *N. rustica* and/or *N. tabacum*, spices and additives. Boiled tobacco leaves are soaked in flavoured water containing spices such as saffron, cardamom, and aniseed. This mashed paste can be strained and dried.

Regional and commercial aspects: It is used in South Asia, including Bangladesh, India, and Pakistan.

Key Points
- Khiwam (or Qiwam) is a ST product commonly used in South Asia.
- It is prepared as a thick, chewable paste made from boiled tobacco leaf extracts (*N. rustica* and/or *N. tabacum*) mixed with aromatic spices such as saffron and cardamom.

(k) *Loose-leaf*:

Method of use: The loose leaves are used for smoking and chewing.

Composition: The leaves are air-cured, cut or granulated, and packed as strips of 0.75–1 inch diameter loose tobacco. Liquorice is often used as a sweetener.

Regional and commercial aspects: Most brands are sold as pouches weighing approximately 3 oz (Rizio 1984). Loose-leaf is used in Europe, India, and North America. In India, commercial loose-leaf bundles of 115 cm length and 5 cm thickness are available (Sinha 2004). It is also used as a component of BQ in Myanmar and Bangladesh. In the USA, loose-leaf or "scrap" is available commercially and consists of cigar tobacco leaves from Pennsylvania and Wisconsin.

Key Points
- Loose-leaf smokeless tobacco consists of air-cured, cut tobacco strips often sweetened with liquorice.
- It is widely used for chewing or smoking across Europe, India, North America, and parts of Southeast Asia.

(l) *Maras*:

Method of use: Small quantities of maras are used multiple times in a day. It is often placed between the lower gingiva and labial mucosa for about 5 min. Some users hold maras overnight in mouth.

Composition: It consists of dried powdered, sun-dried tobacco leaves derived from *N. rustica* L. and ash derived from oak tree, walnut, or grapevine tree wood (1:2 or 1:3 ratio). The product is often humidified prior to use.

Regional and commercial aspects: Maras is a popular ST used in south eastern cities of Turkey, namely Kahramanmaras and Gaziantep.

Key Points
- Maras is often placed between the lower gingiva and labial mucosa
- It consists of dried powdered, sun-dried tobacco leaves derived from *N. rustica* L. and ash derived from oak tree, walnut, or grapevine tree wood.
- Maras is a popular ST used in southeastern cities of Turkey.

(m) *Mawa*: Mawa is a self-assembled form of ST. In the state of Maharashtra, India, this preparation is also referred to as "Kharra".

Method of use: Mawa is chewed and held in the mouth for 10–20 min. Frequency of use varies from 5 to 25 times in a day.

Composition: Mawa consists of small flakes of sun-cured areca nut (95%), tobacco leaves, and slaked lime. It is sold in cellophane paper and tied using a thread into a small packet (Fig. 2.12) that is homogenized on the palm of user's hand.

Regional and commercial aspects: Mawa is extremely popular in India and is commonly used by young men, particularly in the state of Gujarat.

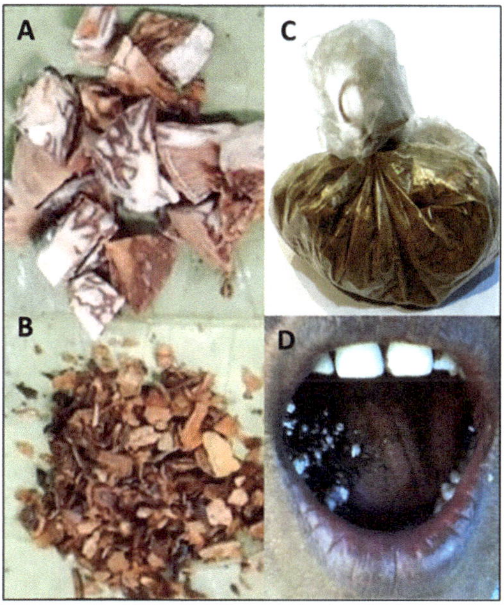

Fig. 2.12 (**a**) Areca nut. (**b**) tobacco. (**c**) Mixture homogenized in cellophane. (**d**) Mixture placement in buccal vestibule

Key Points

- Mawa is a widely used self-assembled smokeless tobacco product in India, particularly among young men.
- It is composed primarily of sun-cured areca nut, tobacco leaves, and slaked lime.

(n) *Mishri*:

Method of use: It is a substitute for chewing tobacco that is often used by women (Murdia et al. 1982). It is applied to the teeth and gums as a dentifrice (Fig. 2.13) (Mehta et al. 1972). Users apply it twice or multiple times and may even hold it for long durations in the mouth.

Composition: Mishri/Masheri/Misheri is powdered tobacco that is preprocessed by roasting leaves on a hot metal plate until brown or partially burnt.

Regional and commercial aspects: Mishri is used in South Asia, including the Indian Subcontinent. In Maharashtra, 38.9% women used mishri when compared to men (0.8%) (Mehta et al. 1972). In a survey conducted in Gujarat, 7.1% of population (mostly women) used mishri (Mehta et al. 1971). In Mainpuri, 0.24% of the population used tobacco to clean teeth (Wahi 1968).

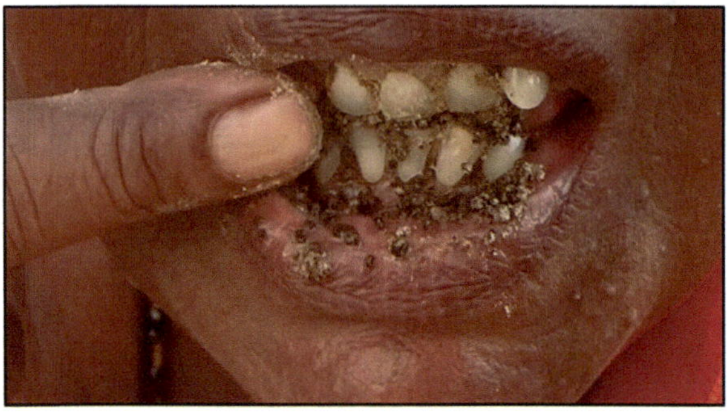

Fig. 2.13 Mishri applied to teeth

Key Points

- Mishri is a roasted, powdered form of ST commonly used by women in South Asia as a dentifrice.
- Mishri is applied multiple times daily to the teeth and gums, posing significant oral health risks due to prolonged mucosal exposure.

(o) *Naswar and Nass*:

Method of use: For oral sucking use, it is often mixed with water to form balls that are placed beneath the tongue (Mehta et al. 1969). Some users place it in the labial vestibule and rarely on the tongue dorsum.

Composition: These are partially cured form of powdered sun-dried tobacco frequently obtained from the *N. rustica* plant. It is processed by pouring water in a cavity that is lined by cement and further treated with lime and colouring like Indigo and flavouring agents like oils, cardamon, and menthol (Evstifeeva and Zaridze 1992). The mixture is then pound by a heavy wooden mallet and maybe packed as semi-dried pellets or powder (Fig. 2.14).

Regional and commercial aspects: Naswar is widely prepared and used in Afghanistan, Pakistan, Iran, Central Asian republics, and South Africa (Joint Iran-International Agency for Research on Cancer Study Group 1977). The composition varies and the primary difference is based on the content of lime used. Nass in Iran and central Asian republics is often made from local tobacco, ash, and oils such as cotton or sesame. Nass prepared in some areas of central Asian republics do not contain lime (Aleksandrova 1970), whereas those in other areas contain high amounts of lime. Users often consume nass for 10 min about 10–15 times per day (Aleksandrova 1970; Zaridze et al. 1985).

Fig. 2.14 Commercial preparation of Naswar. (Courtesy: Dr. Fawad Javed and Ms. Naureen Saqib)

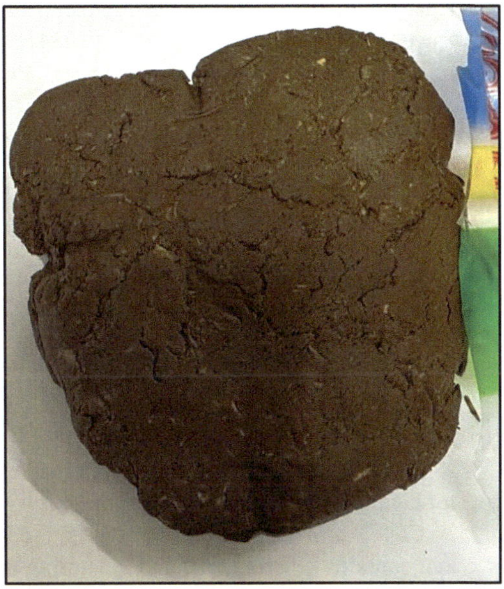

Key Points

- Naswar and nass are traditional ST products primarily used in Central and South Asia.
- Naswar and nass are characterized by their unique preparation involving sun-dried N. rustica tobacco, lime, and aromatic additives
- Users often consume nass for 10 min about 10–15 times daily.

(p) *Chewable plug and twist tobacco*:

Method of use: Plug is one of the oldest known forms of chewable tobacco.

Composition: Plug chewing tobacco typically refers to a firm or moist form of pressed-leaf or fragments of tobacco bars/rolls or plugs that are rolled in clear cellophane (Rizio 1984). The firm form of plug contains less moisture (<15%) and is more common compared to the moist plus that has over 15% moisture.

Plug is made from heavier grades of bright Burley or cigar tobacco leaves that are often located at the top part of the tobacco plant. After de-stemming, the leaves are soaked in liquorice or sugar and compressed into a plug that is covered by a wrapping leaf. Hence the sugar content of plugs is often 25%. The processed leaves are then re-shaped into flat bricks or blocks. Plugs are often chewed and placed in the gingiva-buccal or labial vestibule. The saliva may be spat or swallowed. As with plug, twist is made from air- or fire-cured burley leaves with sugar and flavouring agents. Twist is made by twisting the cured leaves into a rope-like form (Rizio 1984).

Regional and commercial aspects: Plugs are commonly used in North America.

Key Points

- Plug tobacco is one of the oldest forms of chewable tobacco.
- It is composed of firm or moist pressed tobacco leaves, commonly chewed and placed in the gingiva-buccal or labial vestibule.
- It is made from high-grade Burley or cigar tobacco leaves, which are de-stemmed, soaked in liquorice or sugar, and compressed into blocks or plugs

(q) *Red tooth powder*:

Method of use: In India it is often marketed as an herbal product and is used for cleansing teeth (*lal*—red, *dantmanjan*—dentifrice).

Composition: Red tooth powder is a red coloured, finely powdered tobacco that contains several herbs and flavouring agents.

Regional and commercial aspects: It is also used as a dentifrice in some parts of South Asia.

Key Points

- Red tooth powder is a red coloured, finely powdered tobacco that contains several herbs and flavouring agents.
- In India, red tooth powder is often marketed as an herbal product and used as a dentifrice.

(r) *Shammah*:

Method of use: The greenish-yellow powder is placed in the buccal or lower labial vestibule of the mouth and spat out.

Composition: Shammah is powdered tobacco mixed with ash, black pepper, sodium carbonate, oils, and flavouring agents.

Regional and commercial aspects: It is used in Saudi Arabia and Yemen (Salem et al. 1984).

Key Points

- Shammah is a form of ST product commonly used in Yemen and Saudi Arabia.
- The greenish-yellow powder is placed in the buccal or lower labial vestibule of the mouth
- Besides powdered tobacco, shammah contains ash, black pepper, sodium carbonate, oils, and flavouring agents

(s) *Tobacco tablets and chewing gum*:

Method of use: Tobacco tablets were designed to melt in the mouth. Chewing gum are designed similar to conventional gums but with tobacco.

Composition and other details: In 2002, compressed tobacco with mint and eucalyptus was launched in the form of tablets that were cased in a ten-piece blister card. Tobacco tablets formulations (Ariva® and Cigalett®) contain about 1.3 mg of nicotine per tablet and have a pH of 8.4. These tablets have enough buffering capacity to neutralize the acidic pH of saliva and increase bioavailability of nicotine (Nguyen et al. 2002). Another easy-to-use formulation created by the Swedish Match company in 2003 was the tobacco chewing gum. These were marketed under the brand name "Fire" and were test marketed in Tokyo, Japan. They were even propagated as an alternative tobacco product.

Key Points

- Tobacco tablets and gums are smokeless alternatives designed for oral use, with tablets dissolving in the mouth and gums mimicking conventional chewing gum.
- Tobacco tablets like Ariva® and Cigalett® contain 1.3 mg nicotine and a pH of 8.4.

(t) *Toombak*:

Method of use: Toombak is traditionally sold in plastic pouches (Fig. 2.15). It is manipulated by hand and usually shaped into a "ball" called *saffa,* which weighs approximately 10 g. It is often placed between the gingiva and buccal/labial mucosa, but some users also place toombak beneath the tongue. Toombak is usually held in the mouth for about 10–15 min and then either spat out or swallowed based on individual preference.

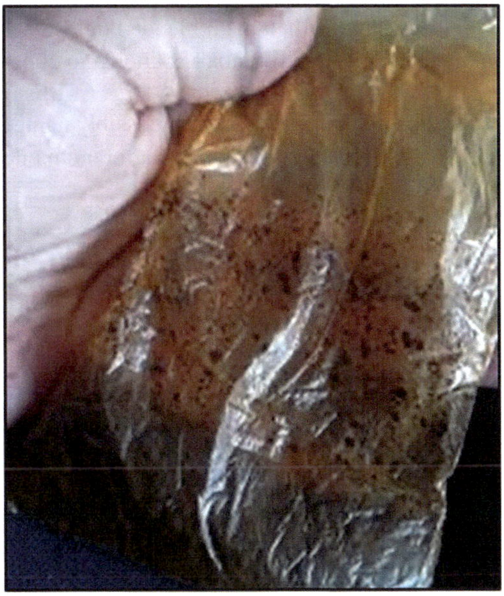

Fig. 2.15 Toombak being sold in plastic pouches. The complete content is shaped into a *saffa* ball which is then held in the oral cavity. (Courtesy: Dr. Salah Ibrahim)

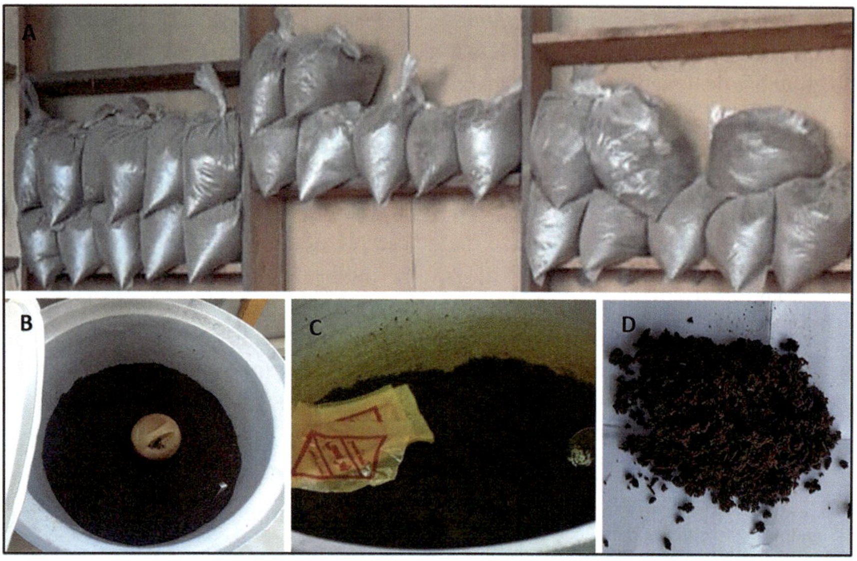

Fig. 2.16 Toombak storage and packaging prior to local distribution (**a**) Toombak powder packed after drying of ground tobacco leaves. (**b**) Toombak stored in containers in shop for distribution. (**c**) Yellow bags used for packaging. (**d**) Final product prepared by mixing 10 pounds of tobacco powder with 2 L of sodium bicarbonate solution. (Courtesy: Dr. Amir Afrogheh and Dr. Esraa Mosalleum)

Composition: The moist toombak preparation is commonly used in Sudan. It consists of tobacco (*N. rustica* and/or *N. glauca* [*N. glauca*]) and sodium bicarbonate. Tobacco leaves are dried uniformly in the field from where they are harvested. The leaves are then fermented at 30–45 °C under humid conditions for a couple of weeks. After prolonged maturation of about 1 year, the ground fermented product is packed (Fig. 2.16) with sodium bicarbonate (4:1) in bowls. The mixture is then hand blended until it achieves the right amount of moisture and consistency. Toombak is known to contain extremely high TSNA content.

Regional and commercial aspects: It is packaged in air-tight container prior to sale. El-Sanf, Wad Amari (possibly named after the person who introduced it) and Sultan El Khaif are popular brand names of Toombak (Idris et al. 1998).

Key Points

- Toombak is made from *N. rustica* and/or *N. glauca* mixed with sodium bicarbonate.
- Toombak is formed into 10 g balls called *saffa*, placed between the gingiva and buccal/labial mucosa or under the tongue for 10–15 min.
- Toombak is commonly used in Sudan and is commercially packaged in airtight containers.

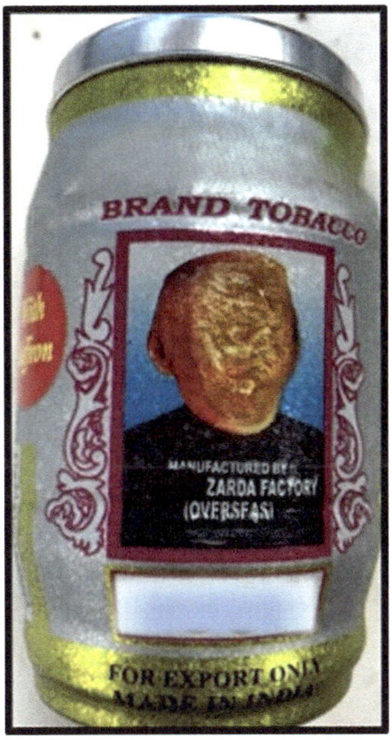

Fig. 2.17 Zarda smokeless tobacco being sold locally and internationally in glittery tins. (Courtesy: Dr. Fawad Javed)

(u) *Zarda*: Zarda is a form of ST product that is often used in BQ or chewed on its own.

Method of use: Chewable ST

Composition: Zarda consists of tobacco that is boiled with lime and spices until water is evaporated. Zarda is produced in both dry and wet forms. It may be used by mixing with finely chopped areca nut and spices. Two forms of Zarda are commonly available. The mild, yellow, granular version is referred to as *Pilapatti*; whereas, the stronger, black, loose version is called *Kalipatti*. Zarda flavoured with saffron is called Zafrani Zarda.

Regional and commercial aspects: Some manufacturers provide lime in the packaging. In West Bengal, India, Zarda is also known as "*Dokta*". It is commonly used in India, Bangladesh, Pakistan, Nepal, Myanmar, and the Middle East (Fig. 2.17).

Key Points
- Zarda is often used in BQ or chewed on its own.
- Zarda consists of tobacco that is boiled with lime and spices until water is evaporated.
- It is commonly used in India, Bangladesh, Pakistan, Nepal, Myanmar, and the Middle East.

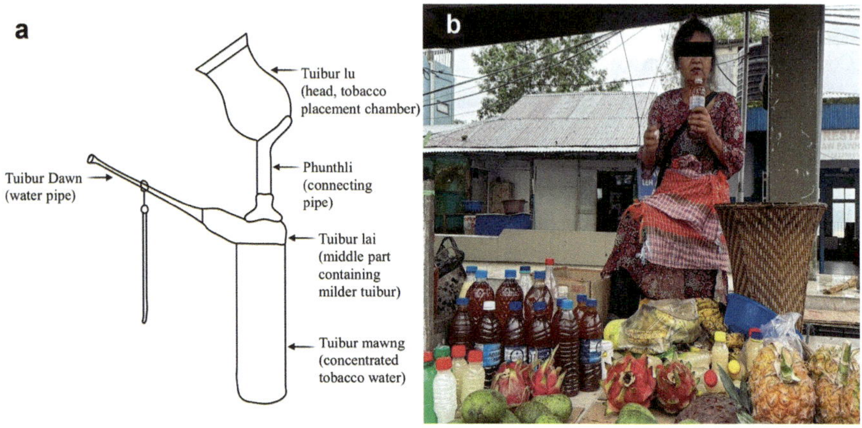

Fig. 2.18 (**a**) Tuibur waterpipe with detachable components (Created in BioRender. Desai, K. (2025) https://biorender.com/ct5d259) (legends in Mizo language). (**b**) Bottled cognac coloured tuibur sold by vendors in local markets of Mizoram. (Courtesy: Dr. C. Zirsangliana, Aizawl, Mizoram)

(v) *Tuibur: Liquid tobacco*

Method of use: Tuibur is used for gargling or sipping.

Composition: Tuibur or hidakphu is tobacco-smoke-infused water made for oral consumption. Using a traditional pipe, tobacco is burnt in the upper compartment and the smoke is passed through water in the lower chamber, which then turns into cognac coloured, pungent smelling, tobacco-infused water (Fig. 2.18a). While traditional preparations have become rare, commercial large-scale preparations of tuibur are common. The mass produce is often packaged in plastic bottles for local distribution and sale (Madathil et al. 2018) (Fig. 2.18b). Tuibur is often graded based on the concentration of tobacco smoke used to prepare the water; wherein high concentration is considered better.

Regional and commercial aspects: Tuibur is used in the north-eastern states of India including Tripura, Manipur, Sikkim, and Mizoram. Women are often seen distributing Tuibur in bottles in local market. In Manipur and Mizoram, the use of tobacco water has become an integral part of their social and cultural practices. The tribal community often served Tuibur as a welcome drink to their guests and visitors.

Nasal Use Finely powdered ST or snuff is frequently used by nasal inhalation. Snuff can be dry or liquid.

(a) *Dry snuff:* Tobacco for dry snuff is fire-cured, then fermented and processed into a powdered form and sold in metal or glass containers. The moisture content of the finished product is less than 10%. It is used both through oral and nasal routes. In Europe, dry snuff is commonly inhaled into the nostrils. In Europe, three methods are used for manufacturing snuff—the rapid method, the Paris method, and the Schmalzer method. In Thailand, the snuff preparation is different from that in Europe and the USA, and is referred to as "Oriental snuff". In north Africa, dry snuff is called "*tenfeha*" (Morocco) and "*nufha*" (Algeria). Some African snuff products may contain ash, region-specific plant products (aloe vera, *Amaranthus spinosus or Turbina oblongata*) and other agents such as oils and lemon juice.

(b) *Liquid snuff:* Liquid snuff is often used via nasal route. Consumption of liquid snuff is predominantly observed amongst the Nandi tribes in East Africa (Hou-Jensen 1964).

2.4 Summary

A detailed understanding and description of ST products, chemical composition, and practices is essential for risk assessment and the development of oral and general health interventions as well as regulatory policies.

References

Aleksandrova HM (1970) Role of nass in the development of pathological changes in the mouth. In: Epidemiology of malignant tumours. Nauka Publishing House, Alma-Ata, pp 243–246. (in Russian)

Andersen RA, Burton HR, Fleming PD, Hamilton-Kemp TR (1989) Effect of storage conditions on nitrosated, acetylated, and oxidized pyridine alkaloid derivatives in smokeless tobacco products. Cancer Res 49:5895–5900

Axéll T, Mörnstad H, Sundström B (1976) The relation of the clinical picture to histo pathology of snuff dipper's lesions in a Swedish population. J Oral Pathol 5:229–236

Axton WF (1975) Tobacco and Kentucky. University Press of Kentucky, Lexington, pp 8, 25, 58–59

Ayo-Yusuf OA, Swart TJP, Pickworth WB (2004) Nicotine delivery capabilities of smokeless tobacco products and implications for control of tobacco dependence in South Africa. Tob Control 13:186–189

Bhide SV, Nair J, Maru GB, Nair UJ, Kameshwar Rao BV, Chakraborty MK, Brunnemann KD (1987) Tobacco-specific N-nitrosamines [TNSA] in green mature and processed tobacco leaves from India. Beit Tabakforsch 14:29–32

Bhonsle RB, Murti PR, Daftary DK, Mehta FS (1979) An oral lesion in tobacco-lime users in Maharashtra, India. J Oral Pathol 8:47–52

Bhonsle RB, Murti PR, Gupta PC (1992) Tobacco habits in India. In: Gupta PC, Hamner JE III., Murti PR (eds) Control of tobacco-related cancers and other diseases (Proceedings of an international symposium January 15–19, 1990, TIFR, Bombay). Oxford University Press, Oxford, pp 25–46

Brooks JE (1952) The mighty leaf. Tobacco through the centuries. Little, Brown & Co., Boston, pp 109, 213, 277

Brunnemann KD, Hoffmann D (1992) Chemical composition of smokeless tobacco products. In: Smokeless tobacco or health. An international perspective (Smoking and tobacco control monograph no. 2; NIH Publ. No. 93-3461). National Cancer Institute, Bethesda

Brunnemann KD, Genoble L, Hoffmann D (1985) N-Nitrosamines in chewing tobacco: an international comparison. J Agric Food Chem 33:1178–1181

Brunnemann KD, Genoble L, Hoffmann D (1987) Identification and analysis of a new tobacco-specific N-nitrosamine, 4-(methylnitrosamino)-4-(3-pyridyl)-1-butanol. Carcinogenesis 8:465–469

Brunnemann KD, Qi J, Hoffmann D (2004) Levels of TSNA in oral moist snuff in the past 30 years and today (Abstract No. 38). In: 58th Tobacco Science Research conference proceedings. Tobacco Science Research, Winston-Salem

Burton HR, Bush LP, Hamilton JL (1983) Effect of curing on the chemical composition of burley tobacco. Recent Adv Tob Sci 9:91–153

Burton H, Bush L, Djordjevic M (1989a) Influence of temperature and humidity on the accumulation of tobacco-specific nitrosamines in stored burley tobacco. J Agric Food Chem 37:1372–1377

Burton HR, Childs GH Jr, Andersen RA, Fleming PD (1989b) Changes in chemical com position of burley tobacco during senescence and curing. 3. Tobacco-specific nitrosamines. J Agric Food Chem 37:426–430

Burton HR, Dye NK, Bush LP (1994) Relationship between tobacco-specific nitrosamines and nitrite from different air-cured tobacco varieties. J Agric Food Chem 42:2007–2011

Bush LP, Cui M, Shi H, Burton HR, Fannin FF, Lei L, Dye N (2001) Formation of tobacco-specific nitrosamines in air-cured tobacco. Recent Adv Tob Sci 27:23–46

CDC (Centers for Disease Control and Prevention) (1999) Determination of nicotine, pH, and moisture content of six U.S. commercial moist snuff products — Florida, January–February 1999. Mortal Morbid Wkly Rep 48:398–401

Chamberlain WJ, Chortyk OT (1992) Effects of curing and fertilization on nitrosamine formation in bright and burley tobacco. Beitr Tabakforsch 15:87–92

Christen AG, Glover ED (1981) Smokeless tobacco: seduction of youth. World Smoking Health 6:20–24

Christen AG, Swanson BZ, Glover ED, Henderson AH (1982) Smokeless tobacco: the folklore and social history of snuffing, sneezing, dipping, and chewing. J Am Dent Assoc 105:821–829

Coleman WM III, Perfetti TA (1997) The roles of amino acids and sugars in the production of volatile materials in microwave heated tobacco dust suspensions. Beit Tabakforsch 17:75–95

Connolly GN (2001) Establishing tolerance limits for tobacco specific nitrosamines (TSNAs) in oral snuff under the Massachusetts Hazardous Substance Act Mg L c 94 s-, Massachusetts Department of Public Health

Curtis MM (1935) The book of snuff and snuff boxes. Bramhall House, New York, pp 20–27, 67

DHHS (Department of Health and Human Services) (1986) The health consequences of using smokeless tobacco (NIH Publication No. 86-2874). Public Health Service, Washington, DC

Djordjevic MV, Gay SL, Bush LP, Chaplin JF (1989) Tobacco-specific nitrosamine accumulation and distribution in flue-cured tobacco alkaloid isolines. J Agric Food Chem 37:752–756

Djordjevic MV, Fan J, Bush LP, Brunnemann KD, Hoffmann D (1993) Effects of storage conditions on levels of tobacco-specific Nnitrosamines and N-nitrosamino acids in U.S. moist snuff. J Agric Food Chem 41:1790–4

Djordjevic MV, Hoffmann D, Glynn T, Connolly GN (1995) US commercial brands of moist snuff, 1994. I. Assessment of nicotine, moisture, and pH. Tob Control 4:62–66

Du X, Squier CA, Kremer MJ, Wertz PW (2000) Penetration of N-nitrosonornicotine (NNN) across oral mucosa in the presence of ethanol and nicotine. J Oral Pathol Med 29:80–85

Evstifeeva TV, Zaridze DG (1992) Nass use, cigarette smoking, alcohol consumption and risk of oral and oesophageal precancer. Eur J Cancer Part B Oral Oncol 28B(1):29–35

Fischer S, Spiegelhalder B, Preussmann R (1989) Preformed tobacco-specific nitrosamines in tobacco — role of nitrate and influence of tobacco type. Carcinogenesis 10:1511–1517

Food and Drug Administration (FDA) (1996) Regulations restricting sale and distribution of cigarettes and smokeless tobacco products to protect children and adolescents; final rule. Fed Reg 61:44395–44618

Garner WW (1951) The production of tobacco. The Blakiston Company, New York, pp 477–478

Gottsegen JJ (1940) A study of its consumption in the United States. Pitman, New York, p 3

Gupta PC, Ray CC (2003) Smokeless tobacco and health in India and South Asia. Respirology 8:419–431

Gupta I, Sankar D (2004) Tobacco consumption in India: a new look using data from the National Sample Survey. J Public Health Policy 24:233–245

Harrison DFN (1964) Snuff — its use and abuse. Br Med J ii:1649–1651

Hatsukami DK, Severson HH (1999) Oral spit tobacco: addiction, prevention and treatment. Nicotine Tob Res 1:21–44

Hecht SS, Murphy SE, Carmella SG, Jensen J, Le C, Joseph AM, Hatsukami DK (2005) Similar uptake of lung carcinogens by smokers of regular, light, and ultralight cigarettes. Cancer Epidemiol Biomarkers Prev 14:693–698

Heimann RK (1960) Tobacco and Americans. McGraw-Hill, New York, pp 8, 65, 118–119, 236

Henningfield JE, Radzius A, Cone EJ (1995) Estimation of available nicotine content of six smokeless tobacco products. Tob Control 4:57–61

Henningfield JE, Fant RV, Tomar SL (1997) Smokeless tobacco: an addicting drug. Adv Dent Res 11:330–335

Hoffmann DH, Djordjevic MV (1997) Chemical composition and carcinogenicity of smokeless tobacco. Adv Dent Res 11:322–329

Hoffmann DH, Djordjevic MV, Fan J, Zang E, Glynn T, Connolly GN (1995) Five leading U.S. commercial brands of moist snuff in 1994: assessment of carcinogenic N-nitrosamines. J Natl Cancer Inst 87:1862–1869

Hou-Jensen K (1964) On the occurrence of post nasal space tumours in Kenya. Br J Cancer 18:58–68

House of Representatives (1994) Smokeless tobacco ingredient list as of April 4, 1994. U.S. House of Representatives Report to Subcommittee on Health and Environment, Committee on Energy and Commerce. Patton, Boggs & Blow, Washington, DC

Idris AM, Ibrahim SO, Vasstrand EN, Johannessen AC, Lillehaug JR, Magnusson B, Wallstrom M, Hirsch JM, Nilsen R (1998) The Swedish snus and the Sudanese toombak: are they different? Oral Oncol 34:558–566

International Agency for Research on Cancer, IARC (2004a) IARC monographs on the evaluation of carcinogenic risks to humans, vol 85. Betel-quid and Areca-nut Chewing and Some Areca-nut Related Nitrosamines, Lyon

International Agency for Research on Cancer, IARC (2004b) IARC monographs on the evaluation of carcinogenic risks to humans, vol 83. Tobacco Smoke and Involuntary Smoking, Lyon

International Agency for Research on Cancer, IARC (2007a) Smokeless tobacco and some tobacco-specific N-nitrosamines. IARC monographs on the evaluation of carcinogenic risks to humans, vol 89. World Health Organization, International Agency for Research on Cancer, Lyon. http://monographs.iarc.fr/ENG/Monographs/vol89/index.php

International Agency for Research on Cancer, IARC (2007b) Tobacco habits other than smoking: betel-quid and areca nut chewing and some related nitrosamines. IARC monographs on the evaluation of carcinogenic risks to humans, vol 37. World Health Organization, International Agency for Research on Cancer, Lyon. http://monographs.iarc.fr/ENG/Monographs/Vol1-42/mono37.pdf

International Agency for Research on Cancer, IARC (2012) A review of human carcinogens. Part E: personal habits and indoor combustions. IARC monographs on the evaluation of the carcinogenic risk of chemicals to humans, vol 100E. International Agency for Research on Cancer, Lyon. Available from: http://momographs.iarc.fr/ENG/Monographs/vol100E

Javed F, Vohra F, Al-Kheraif A, Malmstrom H, Romanos GE (2015) Comparison of periodontal inflammatory conditions among habitual gutka chewers and betel quid chewers. Oral Dis 21(4):437–442

Joint Iran-International Agency for Research on Cancer Study Group (1977) Esophageal cancer studies in the Caspian littoral of Iran: results of population studies—a prodrome. J Natl Cancer Inst 59:1127–1138

Lemmonds CA, Hecht SS, Jensen JA, Murphy SE, Carmella SG, Zhang Y, Hatsukami DK (2005) Smokeless tobacco topography and toxin exposure. Nicotine Tob Res 7:469–474

Li X, Bush LP (2004) TSNA changes in cured powdered tobacco in short-time periods (Abstract No. 30). In: 58th Tobacco science research conference proceedings. Tobacco Science Research, Winston Salem

Loewe W (1981) Snuff in Gothenburg. Svenska Tobaks AB, Stockholm, pp 19–22

Madathil S, Senthil Kumar N, Zodinpuii D, Muthukumaran RB, Lalmuanpuii R, Nicolau B (2018) Tuibur: tobacco in bottle-commercial production of tonacco smoke-saturated aqueous concentrate. Addiction 113:577–580

Mehta FS, Hamner JE (1993) Tobacco-related oral mucosal lesions and conditions in India: a guide for dental students, dentists, and physicians. Basic Dental Research Unit, Tata Institute of Fundamental Research, Mumbai

Mehta FS, Pindborg JJ, Gupta PC, Daftary DK (1969) Epidemiologic and histologic study of oral cancer and leukoplakia among 50,915 villagers in India. Cancer 24:832–849

Mehta FS, Pindborg JJ, Hamnerje III et al (1971) Report on investigations of oral cancer and precancerous conditions in Indian rural populations, 1966–69. Munksgaard, Copenhagen

Mehta FS, Gupta PC, Daftary DK, Pindborg JJ, Choksi SK (1972) An epidemiologic study of oral cancer and precancerous conditions among 101,761 villagers in Maharashtra, India. Int J Cancer 10:134–141

Mookherjee JE, Wilson RA (1988) Tobacco constituents — their importance in flavor and fragrance chemistry. Recent Adv Tob Sci 14:114–168

Murdia US, Mehta FJ, Bhide SV (1982) Nitrate reductase activity and nitrite levels in the saliva of habitual users of various tobacco products. Food Chem Toxicol 20:269–271

Nguyen H, Lynch B, Dus J (2002) Review of Ariva — a compressed powdered tobacco product (Abstract). In: Proceedings of the 3rd International Conference on Smokeless Tobacco, 22–25 Sept 2002, Stockholm, Sweden

Peele DM, Danehower DA, Goins GD (1995) Chemical and biochemical changes during flue curing. Recent Adv Tob Sci 21:81–133

Peele DM, Riddick MG, Edwards ME (2001) Formation of tobacco-specific nitrosamines in flue-cured tobacco. Recent Adv Tob Sci 27:3–12

Richter P, Spierto FW (2003) Surveillance of smokeless tobacco nicotine, pH, moisture, and unprotonated nicotine content. Nicotine Tob Res 5:885–889

Richter E, Tricker AR (2002) Effect of nicotine, cotinine and phenethyl isothiocyanate on 4 (methylnitrosamino)-1-(3-pyridyl)-1-butanone (NNK) metabolism in the Syrian golden hamster. Toxicology 179:95–103

Rizio D (1984) Smokeless tobacco. Tabak-Jint 2:183–184

Roberts DL (1988) Natural tobacco flavor. Recent Adv Tob Sci 14:49–81

Ryan P (1980) Snuff? Snus? At least, an alternative to smoke. Smithsonian 10:176

Salem G, Juhl R, Schiødt T (1984) Oral malignant and premalignant changes in 'shammah' users from the Gizan region, Saudi Arabia. Acta Odontol Scand 42:41–45

Sharma PK, Lal N, Nagpaul KK (1985) Study of trace amounts of U in snuff. Health Phys 48:811–812

Sharma AK, Prokopczyk B, Hoffmann D (1991) Supercritical fluid extraction of moist snuff. J Agric Food Chem 39:508–510

Sinha DN (2004) Oral tobacco use and its implications in Southeast Asia region. WHO South East Asia Regional Office, New Delhi

Smokeless Tobacco and Public Health in India (2016). Available from: www.ntcp.mohfw.gov.in/assets/document/surveys-reports-publications/Smokeless-Tobacco-and-Public-Health-in-India.pdf

Spiegelhalder B, Fischer S (1991) Formation of tobacco-specific nitrosamines. Crit Rev Toxicol 21:241

Stanfill SB, Connolly GN, Zhang L, Jia LT, Henningfield JE, Richter P, Lawler TS, Ayo-Yusuf OA, Ashley DL, Watson CH (2011) Global surveillance of oral tobacco products: total nicotine, unionised nicotine and tobacco-specific Nnitrosamines. Tobacco control 20(3):e2. https://doi.org/10.1136/tc.2010.037465

Stewart GG (1967) A history of medicinal use of tobacco 1492–1860. Med Hist 11:228–268

Stich HF, Stich W, Parida BB (1982) Elevated frequency of micronucleated cells in the buccal mucosa of individuals at high risk of oral cancer: betel quid chewers. Cancer Lett 17:125–134

Stratton KS, Shetty P, Wallace R, Bondurant S (eds) (2001) Clearing the smoke: assessing the science base for tobacco harm reduction. National Academy Press, Washington, DC

Tso TC (1990) Production, physiology, and biochemistry of tobacco plant. Ideals, Beltsville, pp 55–64, 431, 595–614

Tso TC, Harley N, Alexander LT (1966) Source of lead-210 and polonium-210 in tobacco. Science 153:880–882

Voges E (1984) The pleasures of tobacco — how it all began and the whole story. Tob J Int 1:80–82

Wahi PN (1968) The epidemiology of oral and oropharyngeal cancer. A report of the study in Mainpuri District, Uttar Pradesh, India. Bull World Health Organ 38:495–521

Walton LR, Burton HR, Swetnam LD (1995) Effect of mechanization on the physical appearance and chemical composition of burley tobacco. Recent Adv Tob Sci 21:3–38

Weeks WW, Chaplin JF, Campbell CR (1989) Capillary chromatography: evaluation of volatiles from flue-cured tobacco varieties. J Agric Food Chem 37:1038–1045

Wiernik A, Christakopoulos A, Johansson L, Wahlberg I (1995) Effect of air-curing on the chemical composition of tobacco. Recent Adv Tob Sci 21:39–80

Zaridze DG, Kuvshinov JP, Matiakin E, Polakov BI, Boyle P, Blettner M (1985) Chemo prevention of oral and esophageal cancer in Uzbekistan, Union of Soviet Socialist Republics. Natl Cancer Inst Monogr 69:259–262

Effect of *Gutka* Chewing on Periodontal and Peri-implant Health

3

Fawad Javed and Georgios E. Romanos

Abbreviations

AN	Areca nut
BoP	Bleeding on probing
CAL	Clinical attachment loss
CBL	Crestal bone loss
GR	Gingival recession
IL	Interleukin
MBL	Marginal bone loss
MMPs	Matrix metalloproteinases
OPG	Osteoprotegerin
PD	Probing depth
PDL	Periodontal ligament
PI	Plaque index
RANKL	Receptor activator of nuclear factor kappa-B ligand
SRP	Scaling and root planing
ST	Smokeless tobacco
TNF-α	Tumour necrosis factor alpha

F. Javed (✉)
Department of Orthodontics and Dentofacial Orthopedics, Eastman Institute for Oral Health, University of Rochester, Rochester, NY, USA
e-mail: fawad_javed@urmc.rochester.edu

G. E. Romanos
Department of Periodontics and Endodontics, School of Dental Medicine, Stony Brook University, Stony Brook, NY, USA

F. Javed, S. Warnakulasuriya (eds.), *Smokeless Tobacco and its Effects on Periodontal Health*, https://doi.org/10.1007/978-3-032-16409-4_3

Learning Goals

- Definition of gutka and its composition, cultural prevalence, and patterns of use globally and within South Asian populations.
- Understand the chemical and biological mechanisms through which *gutka* components affect periodontal and peri-implant tissues.
- Identify the clinical and radiographic features of periodontal disease commonly observed among habitual *gutka* chewers.
- Describe the inflammatory pathways and cytokine profiles associated with *gutka*-induced periodontal destruction.
- Assess the current evidence on the impact of *gutka* chewing on the oral microbiome and the hypothesized increase in periodontopathogenic bacterial loads.
- Evaluate in vitro studies exploring the cytotoxic effects of smokeless tobacco products on gingival and periodontal cells.
- Discuss the potential implications of *gutka* use on peri-implant health.
- Patient and provider education including tobacco cessation strategies and patient counselling for users of smokeless tobacco products including *gutka*.

3.1 Background of *Gutka*

Gutka (also known as *ghutka*, and *gutkha*) is a smokeless tobacco (ST) product, which is widely consumed in many South Asian regions including Bangladesh, India, Nepal and Pakistan (Abdullah et al. 2024; Javed et al. 2015a, b; Khabir 2024; Muthukrishnan and Warnakulasuriya 2018; Sinha et al. 2015). However, the global export of *gutka* has made it commercially available to its consumers (predominantly migrant communities) in many foreign countries, including Thailand, the United Kingdom, and the United States (Changrani and Gany 2005; Chugh et al. 2023; Constance 2018) and Canada.

Gutka is addictive and typically contains powdered areca nut (AN) (also known as betel nut), tobacco, catechu (a tannin-rich extract from the *Acacia* tree, particularly the Acacia catechu), slaked lime (aqueous calcium hydroxide), and sweeteners, often flavoured with spices or menthol to enhance its appeal (Javed et al. 2013). It has also been claimed that some *gutka* manufacturers may even add crushed glass to the product (Baig et al. 2018). The crushed glass particles cause lacerations in the buccal mucosa, while slaked lime facilitates the extraction of alkaloids from the tobacco and AN, thereby enhancing the absorption of nicotine and arecoline through the oral mucosa into the bloodstream. *Gutka* is marketed in small, glittery and colourful sachets usually lacking a health warning (Fig. 3.1a); however, it seems that *gutka* manufacturers who export their product to other countries are obligated to print a health warning on *gutka* sachets (Fig. 3.1b).

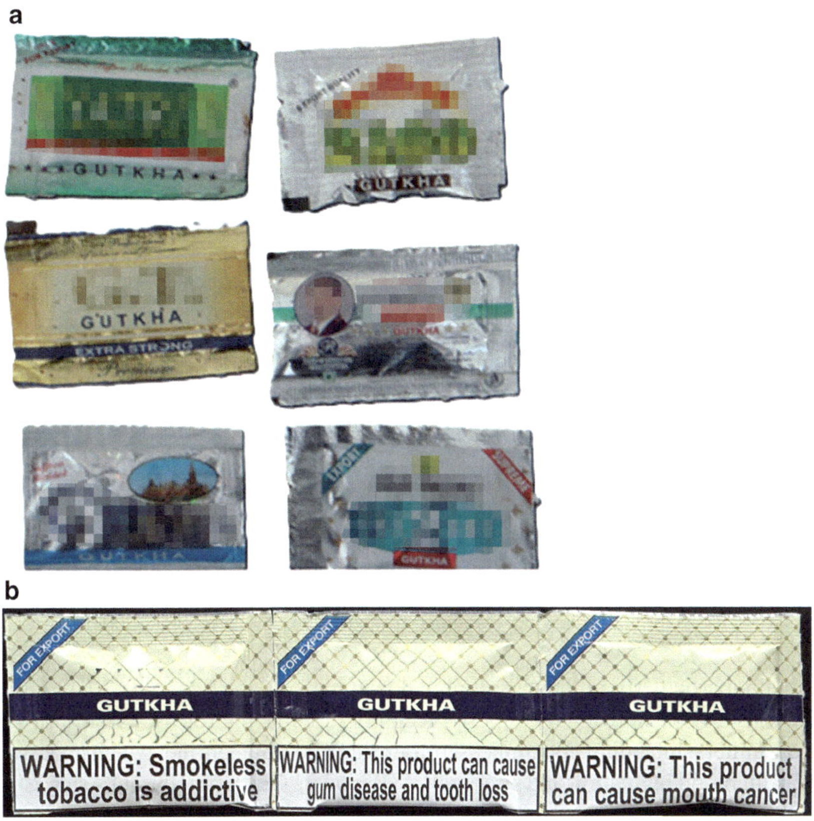

Fig. 3.1 (**a**) *Gutka* is sold in colourful and glittery sachets lacking a health warning. (**b**) *Gutka* being exported in colourful and glittery sachets with a health warning

Key Points

- *Gutka* is an addictive smokeless tobacco product composed of areca nut, tobacco, catechu, slaked lime, and sweeteners, often enhanced with flavourings to increase consumer appeal.
- Some *gutka* formulations may include harmful additives such as crushed glass, which can cause mucosal lacerations.
- *Gutka* is typically sold in attractive, unregulated sachets lacking health warnings.
- *Gutka* products that are exported may carry warning labels in compliance with international regulations.

3.2 Reasons for Gutka Chewing

In a cross-sectional study, GC reported that this form of ST helped them relieve "mental stress" (Javed et al. 2008). One explanation for this is that nicotine, the primary psychoactive component in ST, binds to nicotinic-acetylcholine receptors in

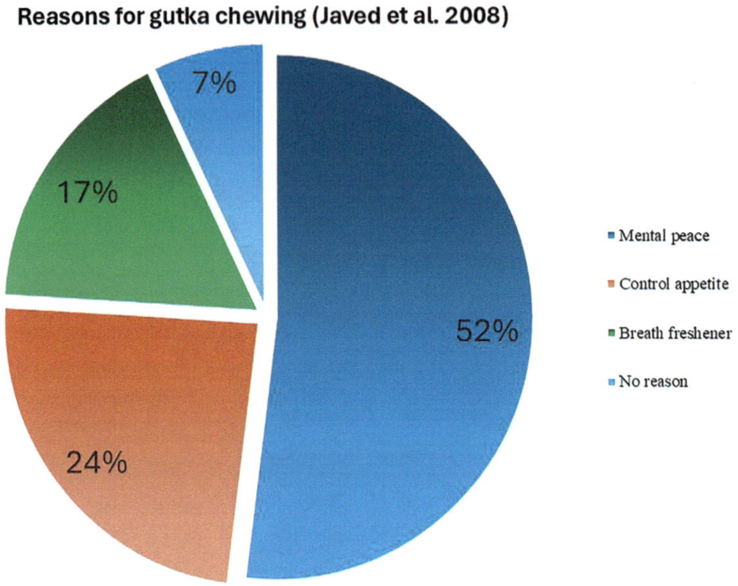

Fig. 3.2 Reasons for gutka chewing. (Modified from the study by Javed et al. (2008))

the brain, particularly in the mesolimbic dopamine system (Benowitz 2010; Ortells and Arias 2010). Activation of these receptors leads to the release of several neurotransmitters, including dopamine, serotonin, and norepinephrine, which are associated with mood regulation and stress relief (Benowitz 2010; Ortells and Arias 2010). Nicotine also activates nicotinic acetylcholine receptors in the hypothalamus, specifically in the arcuate nucleus, which regulates feeding behaviour (García et al. 2015; Jo et al. 2002). This activation leads to the release of pro-opiomelanocortin neurons, which suppress appetite by promoting safety signals (García et al. 2015; Jo et al. 2002). In the study by Javed et al. (2008), 8% of the respondents stated that gutka chewing helped them achieve "fullness" and control their appetite. Some chewers have even labelled gutka as a breath freshener (Javed et al. 2008). A summary of reasons for *gutka* chewing is presented in Fig. 3.2.

Key Points

- *Gutka* chewers commonly report using the product to relieve mental/psychological stress.
- Some users report that gutka-chewing helps them control their appetite.
- Some users have even labelled *gutka* as a breath freshener.

3.3 Clinical and Radiographic Periodontal Status Among *Gutka* Chewers

Table 3.1 reports the demographic characteristics of five cross-sectional observational studies in which GC and controls were evaluated (Bhardwaj et al. 2021; Javed et al. 2008, 2013, 2014, 2015a). In these studies (Bhardwaj et al. 2021; Javed et al. 2008, 2013, 2014, 2015a), the numbers of GC and controls ranged between 15 and 36 individuals, respectively. The ages of GC and controls ranged between approximately 20 and 70 years and 20 and 65 years. In these studies, GC were addicted to this form of chewing habit for at least 3 years and were placing this ST product in the mouth for approximately 3–40 min per chew (Bhardwaj et al. 2021; Javed et al. 2008, 2013, 2014, 2015a). Results by Javed et al. (2008) showed that the percentage of sites that demonstrated dental plaque, bleeding on probing (BoP), and probing depths (PD) of 4–6 mm and ≥6 mm were significantly higher among GC than controls (Fig. 3.3).

Table 3.1 An overview of the demographics of studies that assessed the periodontal health status among *gutka* chewers and non-chewers (controls)

Authors et al.	Study location	Participants	Age of participants (years)	Gender (male:female)	Duration of *gutka* chewing habit (years)	Duration of *gutka* placement in the mouth (per chew, min)
Javed et al. (2008)	Pakistan	36 gutka chewers 42 non-chewers	51.4 ± 6.2 50.7 ± 5.7	17:19 22:20	8.4 ± 2.7	20 ± 3.4
Javed et al. (2013)	Pakistan	27 gutka chewers 17 non-chewers	36.2 ± 4.1 36.4 ± 2.2	22:5 14:3	5.4 ± 1.5	32.5 ± 5.5
Jacob et al. (2014)	India	15 gutka chewers 15 non-chewers	40.8 ± 14.1 28.3 ± 6.4	13:2 11:4	11.3 ± 9.6	32.6 ± 7.9
Javed et al. (2015a)	Pakistan	45 gutka chewers 50 non-chewers	36.1 ± 2.9 38.5 ± 3.1	28:17 29:21	3.5 ± 0.4	15.5 ± 2.6
Bhardwaj et al. (2021)	India	25 gutka chewers 25 non-chewers	27.7 ± 6.9 27.2 ± 7.5	19:6 18:7	4.16 ± 3.09	7.88 ± 4.81

Table 3.2 Odds ratios of percentages of sites with clinical periodontal inflammation among *gutka* chewers and non-chewers (Javed et al. 2013)

Group comparisons	Group mean difference (%)	95% Confidence intervals of group mean differences	*P* value
Plaque index			
Gutka chewers versus controls	38.4 – 12.0 = 26.4	22.3 to 30.5	$P < 0.05$
Bleeding on probing			
Gutka chewers versus controls	44.7 – 13.0 = 31.7	26.6 to 36.8	$P < 0.05$
Probing depth (4–6 mm)			
Gutka chewers versus controls	12.4 – 5.6 = 6.9	3.0 to 10.8	$P < 0.05$
Probing depth (>6 mm)			
Gutka chewers versus controls	3.2 – 0 = 3.2	0.7 to 5.7	$P < 0.05$

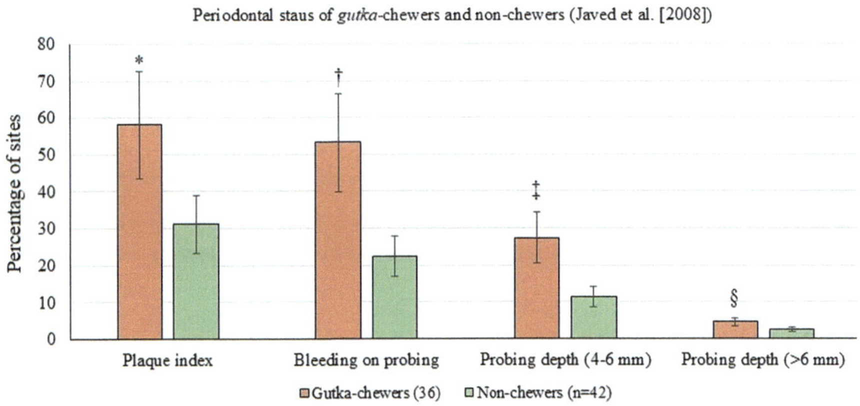

Fig. 3.3 Comparison of clinical periodontal status among gutka chewers and non-chewers assessed in the study by Javed et al. (2008). *Compared with plaque index among non-chewers ($P < 0.01$); †compared with bleeding on probing among non-chewers ($P < 0.001$); ‡compared with probing depth (4–6 mm) among non-chewers ($P < 0.01$); §compared with probing depth (>6 mm) among non-chewers ($P < 0.05$). Similarly, another clinical study evaluated the clinical and radiographic periodontal status among 27 gutka chewers and 17 non-chewers (Javed et al. 2013). In this study (Javed et al. 2013), GC were addicted to this ST chewing habit for approximately 5 years and were placing *gutka* in the mouth for nearly 40 min per chew. The odds ratios for the percentages of sites that demonstrated dental plaque, BOP and PD (4–6 mm and >6 mm) were significantly elevated in GC than controls (Javed et al. 2013) (Table 3.2). In this study (Javed et al. 2013), the mean marginal bone loss on the mesial and distal surfaces was significantly higher among GC than controls (Fig. 3.4). Similar results were reported in the clinical study by Bhardwaj et al. (2021). In summary, Bhardwaj et al. (2021) also reported that scores of plaque index, BoP, PD (4–6 mm and >6 mm), and MBL are significantly elevated among GC than non-chewers

A study performed assessed the PD, gingival recession (GR) and clinical attachment loss (CAL) among 15 GC and 15 controls (Jacob et al. 2014). In this study, GC were placing gutka in the mouth for approximately 32 min/chew and had been chewing gutka for nearly 11 years. According to the results, full-mouth GR and

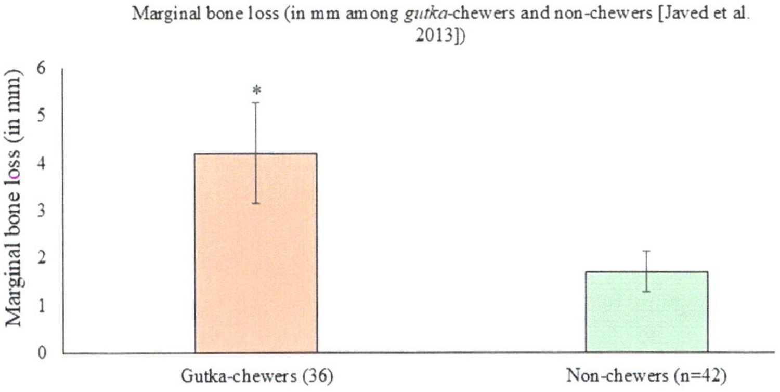

Fig. 3.4 Comparison of marginal bone loss among *gutka* chewers and non-chewers (Javed et al. 2013). *Compared with non-chewers ($P < 0.05$)

CAL were significantly higher in the GC group (2.02 ± 0.31 mm and 4.60 ± 0.56 mm, respectively) than in the controls (1.21 ± 1.15 mm and 3.70 ± 0.32 mm, respectively) ($P < 0.01$). However, there was no difference in PD among GC (2.64 ± 0.28 mm) and controls (1.61 ± 0.55 mm) (Jacob et al. 2014). The authors suggested frictional and/or chemical trauma to the gingival tissues from the components of *gutka*, including AN may have increased scores of GR and CAL in these individuals. It is likely that the high scores of GR and CAL reduced the PD among GC; however, the study did not provide a logical justification for the increased score of PD among controls than GC (Jacob et al. 2014). It is pertinent to note that the study by Jacob et al. (2014) was conducted in the state of Rajnandgaon, India, where a government ban is in place on the sale of *gutka*. Yet, this ST product is illegally purchased and consumed by many users.

Key Points

- Frictional and/or chemical trauma to the gingival tissues from the components of *gutka*, such as areca nut may increase scores of gingival recession and clinical attachment loss.
- Despite a governmental ban, *gutka* is illegally purchased by many consumers in India.

3.3.1 Effect of *Gutka* on Oral Microbiome

There are no studies that have assessed the counts and species of periodontopathogenic bacteria among GC. It is hypothesized that the counts of periodontopathogenic bacteria, such as *Aggregatibacter actinomycetemcomitans*, *Porphyromonas gingivalis*, and *Prevotella intermedia*, are higher in the saliva and the oral biofilm of GC than non-chewers. Further studies are needed to test this hypothesis. Nevertheless, with regard to oral yeasts, it has been reported that there is no significant difference in the oral *Candida* (predominantly *Candida albicans* and *C. tropicalis*) carriage among GC and non-chewers (Javed et al. 2014).

Key Points

- There are no studies that have assessed the counts and species of periodontopathogenic bacteria among *gutka*-chewers.
- There is no significant difference in the oral *Candida* carriage among *gutka*-chewers and non-chewers.

3.4 Potential Mechanisms

The precise mechanism/s through which *gutka* jeopardizes periodontal soft and osseous tissues is uncertain; however, it has been reported that habitual *gutka* consumption is associated with an increased expression of destructive inflammatory cytokines (including interleukin [IL] 1-beta, and IL-6) in the unstimulated whole saliva and gingival crevicular fluid of GC than controls (Jacob et al. 2014; Javed et al. 2015a; Makino et al. 2008). Such cytokines increase vascular permeability and stimulate the expression of adhesion molecules, enabling the extravasation of immune cells into the gingival connective tissue. Once there, neutrophils and macrophages release reactive oxygen species (ROS) and proteolytic enzymes that exacerbate tissue damage (Malkowska et al. 2006). Moreover, pro-inflammatory cytokines such as IL-1β and tumour necrosis factor-alpha (TNF-α) induce the production of matrix metalloproteinases (MMPs) by fibroblasts and immune cells. The MMPs degrade extracellular matrix proteins, including collagen, which weakens periodontal connective tissue (Sapna et al. 2014). Furthermore, proinflammatory cytokines such as IL-1β and TNF-α upregulate the expression of receptor activator of nuclear factor kappa-B ligand (RANKL) and suppress osteoprotegerin (OPG) production. This RANKL/OPG imbalance promotes osteoclast differentiation and activity leading to MBL, a hallmark of periodontitis (Gaffen and Hajishengallis 2008).

Key Points

- Gutka consumption is linked to elevated levels of pro-inflammatory cytokines (e.g., IL-1β, IL-6, and TNF-α) in saliva and gingival crevicular fluid.
- Pro-inflammatory cytokines stimulate fibroblasts and immune cells to produce MMPs, which degrade extracellular matrix components.
- An imbalance in RANKL and OPG expression, induced by inflammatory cytokines, promotes osteoclast activity and bone resorption.

3.5 In Vitro Studies

To date, no in vitro studies have exclusively investigated the effect of *gutka* on periodontal tissues. However, in vitro studies have assessed the detrimental effects of ST on periodontal tissues in general (Johnson et al. 1996; Lallier et al. 2017; Tipton and Dabbous 1995). Lallier et al. (2017) compared the cytotoxic effects of ST extract on human periodontal ligament (PDL) and gingival fibroblasts. Their findings showed that ST extracts reduced cell viability in a dose-dependent manner (Lallier et al. 2017). Likewise, Johnson et al. (1996) assessed the effects of aqueous ST extracts on human gingival keratinocytes. Their results demonstrated that STE exposure led to a significant increase in the production of prostaglandin E2 and IL-1, both of which are mediators involved in inflammatory responses and tissue destruction. Higher concentrations of ST extracts were associated with decreased cell viability, indicating potential cytotoxic effects (Johnson et al. 1996). Collectively, such in vitro studies suggest that ST extracts have an adverse effect on periodontal tissues by inhibiting fibroblast proliferation, altering extracellular matrix production, and promoting the release of inflammatory mediators (Johnson et al. 1996; Lallier et al. 2017; Tipton and Dabbous 1995). These mechanisms may also contribute to the periodontal destruction observed in *gutka*-users; however, there is a need for in vitro studies explicitly on gutka to comprehend its impact on periodontal and peri-implant soft and osseous tissues..

Key Points

- No in vitro studies have specifically examined the effects of *gutka* on periodontal tissues.
- Smokeless tobacco (ST) extracts have demonstrated dose-dependent cytotoxicity on human periodontal ligament and gingival fibroblasts.
- Exposure to ST extracts increase inflammatory mediators such as prostaglandin E2 and IL-1 in gingival keratinocytes.
- Current in vitro evidence suggests that ST impairs fibroblast proliferation, alters extracellular matrix production, and promotes inflammation.

3.6 Efficacy of Non-surgical Periodontal Therapy Among *Gutka* Chewers

Nicotine, a major component of tobacco, is implicated in delayed wound healing due to its multifaceted physiological effects on cellular and molecular processes. Nicotine exerts vasoconstrictive effects by stimulating the release of catecholamines, such as adrenaline, which constricts blood vessels and reduces blood flow to wound sites (Frick and Seals 1994; Qandil et al. 1997). This diminished perfusion compromises oxygen delivery and nutrient supply, essential for cellular proliferation and tissue repair (Ohno et al. 2023; Sansone et al.

2023). Additionally, nicotine inhibits myofibroblast differentiation and induces toxicity and oxidative stress in gingival fibroblasts (Fang and Svoboda 2005; Rinaldi et al. 2023). Furthermore, nicotine promotes the release of pro-inflammatory cytokines and delays the resolution of inflammation, leading to prolonged tissue injury and reduced healing efficiency (Hapidin et al. 2007; Johnson et al. 2010). It is therefore hypothesized that outcomes of periodontal interventions such as scaling and root planing are compromised in GC compared with non-chewers. To date, only one randomized controlled trial in indexed literature has evaluated the efficacy of non-surgical scaling and root planing (SRP) for the management of periodontitis among GC (Al-Rabiah et al. 2020). In this study self-reported GC with periodontitis were divided into two groups. GC in the test group underwent SRP with adjunct photobiomodulation with a 940 nm indium/gallium/arsenide/phosphorous diode laser. The laser was delivered using a fibre tip with a diameter of 1.76 cm^2 at a power and energy fluence of 0.3 W and 3.41 J/cm^2, respectively. In contrast, controls underwent SRP alone. Periodontal parameters (PI, BoP, PD, CAL, and MBL) were assessed at baseline and at 3- and 6-month follow-ups (Al-Rabiah et al. 2020). The follow-up results showed that SRP with adjuvant photobiomodulation is more effective in reducing periodontal soft tissue inflammatory parameters (PI, BoP, and PD) but not CAL among GC (Al-Rabiah et al. 2020). Moreover, there was no significant difference in MBL in both groups throughout the study duration (Al-Rabiah et al. 2020). The authors of the present chapter suggest that the results reported in this RCT (Al-Rabiah et al. 2020) should be interpreted with caution. Firstly, the study was performed solely among GC with periodontitis. In other words, non-chewers with periodontitis were not included and treated in this study. Thus, the severity of periodontitis among *gutka* chewers and non-chewers could not be assessed at baseline and follow-up. Moreover, the follow-up duration was relatively short (180 days), which could potentially explain why marginal bone levels remain unchanged throughout the study. Nevertheless, the efficacy of periodontal interventions towards regenerating osseous tissues among ST product users is a subject that warrants additional long-term follow-up clinical trials. It is hypothesized that the persistence of the *gutka*-chewing habit may potentially counteract the anti-inflammatory benefits of scaling and root planing (SRP), with or without adjunctive photobiomodulation therapy, thereby perpetuating periodontal inflammation. In contrast, discontinuation of this habit before or following periodontal intervention is expected to result in more favourable outcomes. Oral health care providers should adopt a holistic approach to patient care, addressing not only the clinical management of periodontal disease but also educating patients about the detrimental effects of tobacco on both oral and systemic health. Comprehensive patient education and support in cessation of harmful habits, such as gutka chewing, are anticipated to yield more sustained treatment success and contribute to an enhanced quality of life, particularly among vulnerable populations.

Key Points

- Al-Rabiah et al. (2020) evaluated the effect of non-surgical periodontal therapy with and without photobiomodulation outcomes for treating periodontitis among *gutka* chewers and non-chewers.
- This trial compared SRP with and without adjunctive photobiomodulation.
- This trial showed greater improvement in soft tissue inflammatory parameters (PI, BoP, PD) in the laser-assisted than in the control group.
- No significant difference in CAL or MBL was observed between the intervention and control groups during the 6-month follow-up.

3.7 Effect of *Gutka* on Peri-implant Health

A recent systematic review and meta-analysis evaluated studies that assessed peri-implant clinical and radiographic parameters among nicotinic product users (including ST users) and controls (individuals not using any form of nicotinic products) (Vámos et al. 2024). Indexed databases (PubMed, Web of Science, EMBASE, and CENTRAL) were searched until April 2023 for potentially relevant articles published solely in the English language. A total of 3296 dental implants were evaluated in 18 studies. The results showed that peri-implant crestal bone loss (CBL), BoP, and PI were significantly higher among ST users compared with controls and individuals using waterpipe, electronic nicotine delivery systems, and cigarettes (Vámos et al. 2024). However, peri-implant PD was significantly higher among ST, waterpipe users, and cigarette smokers compared with controls (Vámos et al. 2024). It has been reported that ST users and cigarette smokers are more susceptible to peri-implant soft tissue inflammation and CBL as compared to controls, and there is no difference in the severity of peri-implant diseases in the former groups (Akram et al. 2018). This study also showed that the peri-implant sulcular fluid in cigarette smokers and ST users contains proinflammatory cytokines (IL-1β and MMP-9) in high concentrations in contrast to controls (Akram et al. 2018). However, the type of ST being used by the study participants remained undocumented in the study by Akram et al. (2018).

Although there is a paucity of research specifically examining the effects of *gutka* on peri-implant tissues, this should not be interpreted as evidence suggesting that *gutka* chewing is non-hazardous to peri-implant soft and osseous tissues. In fact, *gutka* consumption is well-documented to have deleterious effects on periodontal tissues (Baig et al. 2018; Jacob et al. 2014; Javed et al. 2008, 2010, 2015a). Therefore, it is highly plausible that this form of ST similarly compromises the health of peri-implant tissues. It is reasonable to hypothesize that *gutka* chewing may adversely affect the stability of dental implants by inducing a state of oxidative stress in peri-implant tissues and augmenting the accumulation of osteoclasts, pathogenic bacteria, and pro-inflammatory cytokines thereby exposing patients to peri-implant diseases, peri-implant mucositis, and peri-implantitis. Additionally, the hard and fibrous nature of certain *gutka* components, such as AN, promotes occlusal abrasions on tooth surfaces and can lead to the formation of cracks in the crown, which may extend into the roots (Anand et al. 2014; Gao et al. 2001). In the latter scenario, tooth extraction becomes the only therapeutic option in many, if not all cases. In addition, ceramic chipping and fracture of dental prostheses (such as ceramic crowns) are potential complications encountered in habitual AN chewers (Jamal et al. 2020). It is highly plausible that GC are more prone to occlusal chipping, cracks, and/or fractures of implant-retained prostheses compared to non-chewers, given the mechanical stresses exerted by ingredients in *gutka* such as AN. Further studies are warranted to explore this relationship and provide conclusive evidence, but the existing knowledge underscores the need for caution and proactive measures to mitigate potential risks associated with *gutka* use.

Key Points

- There is a paucity of research specifically examining the effects of *gutka* on peri-implant tissues.
- It is hypothesized that *gutka* chewing may adversely affect the stability of dental implants.
- Since gutka-chewing is a risk-factor of periodontitis, it is likely a potential risk-factor of peri-implant diseases as well.
- It is hypothesized that gutka chewing increases the risk of occlusal chipping, cracks, and/or fractures of implant-retained prostheses compared to non-chewers.

3.8 Conclusion

Habitual *gutka* chewing is a risk factor for periodontitis and potentially peri-implant diseases (peri-implant mucositis and peri-implantitis). The mechanism of action is uncertain.

References

Abdullah SM, Huque R, Siddiqi K, Kanaan M, Huque S, Ullah S, Garg S et al (2024) Non-compliant packaging and illicit smokeless tobacco in Bangladesh, India and Pakistan: findings of a pack analysis. Tob Control 33:333–340

Akram Z, Vohra F, Bukhari IA, Sheikh SA, Javed F (2018) Clinical and radiographic peri-implant parameters and proinflammatory cytokine levels among cigarette smokers, smokeless tobacco users, and nontobacco users. Clin Implant Dent Relat Res 20:76–81

Al-Rabiah M, Al-Hamoudi N, Al-Aali KA, Slapar L, AlHelal A, Al Deeb M, Mokeem SA et al (2020) Efficacy of scaling and root planing with photobiomodulation for treating periodontitis in gutka chewers: a randomized controlled trial. Photobiomodul Photomed Laser Surg 38:545–551

Anand R, Dhingra C, Prasad S, Menon I (2014) Betel nut chewing and its deleterious effects on oral cavity. J Cancer Res Ther 10:499–505

Baig S, Rubab Z, Farooq W (2018) Molecular pathogenesis of chewable tobacco. J Coll Physicians Surg Pak 28:381–385

Benowitz NL (2010) Nicotine addiction. N Engl J Med 362:2295–2303

Bhardwaj P, Chowdhary Z, Sharma V, Ladani R, Modi SK, Bhardwaj S, Hundal KD (2021) Comparative evaluation of periodontal inflammatory conditions among gutka-chewers with and without prediabetes. Indian J Dent Res 32:15–22

Changrani J, Gany F (2005) Paan and gutka in the United States: an emerging threat. J Immigr Health 7:103–108

Chugh A, Arora M, Jain N, Vidyasagaran A, Readshaw A, Sheikh A, Eckhardt J et al (2023) The global impact of tobacco control policies on smokeless tobacco use: a systematic review. Lancet Glob Health 11:e953–e968

Constance J (2018) The use of smokeless tobacco among UK South Asian communities. London Metropolitan University

Fang Y, Svoboda KK (2005) Nicotine inhibits myofibroblast differentiation in human gingival fibroblasts. J Cell Biochem 95:1108–1119

Frick WG, Seals RR Jr (1994) Smoking and wound healing: a review. Tex Dent J 111:21–23

Gaffen SL, Hajishengallis G (2008) A new inflammatory cytokine on the block: re-thinking periodontal disease and the Th1/Th2 paradigm in the context of Th17 cells and IL-17. J Dent Res 87:817–828

Gao YJ, Yin XM, Wu HJ (2001) Relationship between vertical root fracture and the habits of chewing betel nut. Hunan Yi Ke Da Xue Xue Bao 26:161–162

García AP, Aitta-aho T, Schaaf L, Heeley N, Heuschmid L, Bai Y, Barrantes FJ et al (2015) Nicotinic α4 receptor-mediated cholinergic influences on food intake and activity patterns in hypothalamic circuits. PLoS One 10:e0133327

Hapidin H, Othman F, Soelaiman IN, Shuid AN, Luke DA, Mohamed N (2007) Negative effects of nicotine on bone-resorbing cytokines and bone histomorphometric parameters in male rats. J Bone Miner Metab 25:93–98

Jacob PS, Nath S, Patel RP (2014) Evaluation of interleukin-1β and 8 in gutka chewers with periodontitis among a rural Indian population. J Periodontal Implant Sci 44:126–133

Jamal S, Ghafoor R, Khan FR, Zafar K (2020) Five year evaluation of the complications observed in porcelain fused to metal (PFM) crowns placed at a university hospital. J Pak Med Assoc 70:845–850

Javed F, Altamash M, Klinge B, Engström PE (2008) Periodontal conditions and oral symptoms in gutka-chewers with and without type 2 diabetes. Acta Odontol Scand 66:268–273

Javed F, Chotai M, Mehmood A, Almas K (2010) Oral mucosal disorders associated with habitual gutka usage: a review. Oral Surg Oral Med Oral Pathol Oral Radiol Endod 109:857–864

Javed F, Tenenbaum HC, Nogueira-Filho G, Nooh N, O'Bello Correa F, Warnakulasuriya S, Dasanayake AP et al (2013) Periodontal inflammatory conditions among gutka chewers and non-chewers with and without prediabetes. J Periodontol 84:1158–1164

Javed F, Tenenbaum HC, Nogueira-Filho G, Nooh N, Taiyeb Ali TB, Samaranayake LP, Al-Hezaimi K (2014) Oral Candida carriage and species prevalence amongst habitual gutka-chewers and non-chewers. Int Wound J 11:79–84

Javed F, Al-Kheraif AA, Al Amri MD, Mikami T, Vohra F, Warnakulasuriya S, Romanos GE (2015a) Periodontal parameters and whole salivary cytokine profiles among habitual gutka chewers and non-chewers. J Periodontol 86:689–695

Javed F, Vohra F, Al-Kheraif AA, Malmstrom H, Romanos GE (2015b) Comparison of periodontal inflammatory conditions among habitual gutka chewers and betel quid chewers. Oral Dis 21:437–442

Jo YH, Talmage DA, Role LW (2002) Nicotinic receptor-mediated effects on appetite and food intake. J Neurobiol 53:618–632
Johnson GK, Poore TK, Payne JB, Organ CC (1996) Effect of smokeless tobacco extract on human gingival keratinocyte levels of prostaglandin E2 and interleukin-1. J Periodontol 67:116–124
Johnson GK, Guthmiller JM, Joly S, Organ CC, Dawson DV (2010) Interleukin-1 and interleukin-8 in nicotine- and lipopolysaccharide-exposed gingival keratinocyte cultures. J Periodontal Res 45:583–588
Khabir M (2024) Exploring gutka consumption: healthcare risks on maternal and child health in Karachi, Pakistan. Addiction 119:2221–2222
Lallier TE, Moylan JT, Maturin E (2017) Greater sensitivity of oral fibroblasts to smoked versus smokeless tobacco. J Periodontol 88:1356–1365
Makino A, Yamada S, Okuda K, Kato T (2008) Nicotine involved in periodontal disease through influence on cytokine levels. FEMS Immunol Med Microbiol 52:282–286
Malkowska A, Kasprzak A, Stopa J (2006) Proinflammatory cytokines in pathogenesis of periodontal disease. Pol Merkur Lekarski 20:93–98
Muthukrishnan A, Warnakulasuriya S (2018) Oral health consequences of smokeless tobacco use. Indian J Med Res 148:35–40
Ohno Y, Taura D, Okamoto K, Fujita H, Honda-Kohmo K, Matsuo K, Sone M (2023) Nicotine reduces reactive oxygen species and enhances cell proliferation via the α4 nicotinic acetylcholine receptor subunit in human induced pluripotent stem cells. Stem Cells Dev 32:237–245
Ortells MO, Arias HR (2010) Neuronal networks of nicotine addiction. Int J Biochem Cell Biol 42:1931–1935
Qandil R, Sandhu HS, Matthews DC (1997) Tobacco smoking and periodontal diseases. J Can Dent Assoc 63:187–192, 185–194
Rinaldi S, Pieper E, Schulz T, Zimmermann R, Luch A, Laux P, Mallock-Ohnesorg N (2023) Oral nicotine pouches with an aftertaste? Part 2: in vitro toxicity in human gingival fibroblasts. Arch Toxicol 97:2343–2356
Sansone L, Milani F, Fabrizi R, Belli M, Cristina M, Zagà V, de Iure A et al (2023) Nicotine: from discovery to biological effects. Int J Mol Sci 24:14570
Sapna G, Gokul S, Bagri-Manjrekar K (2014) Matrix metalloproteinases and periodontal diseases. Oral Dis 20:538–550
Sinha DN, Rizwan SA, Aryal KK, Karki KB, Zaman MM, Gupta PC (2015) Trends of smokeless tobacco use among adults (aged 15-49 years) in Bangladesh, India and Nepal. Asian Pac J Cancer Prev 16:6561–6568
Tipton DA, Dabbous MK (1995) Effects of nicotine on proliferation and extracellular matrix production of human gingival fibroblasts in vitro. J Periodontol 66:1056–1064
Vámos O, Komora P, Gede N, Hegyi P, Kelemen K, Varga G, Mikulás K et al (2024) The effect of nicotine-containing products on peri-implant tissues: a systematic review and network meta-analysis. Nicotine Tob Res 26:1276–1285

Effect of Betel-Quid Chewing on Periodontal and Peri-implant Health

4

Zain Uddin Ahmed and Fawad Javed

Abbreviations

AN	Areca nut
BoP	Bleeding on probing
BQ	Betel quid
CBL	Crestal bone loss
CPI	Community periodontal index
MBL	Marginal bone loss
PCR	Polymerase chain reaction
PD	Probing depth
PI	Plaque index

Learning Goals

- Understand the composition and regional variations of betel quid (BQ).
- Recognize the cultural and traditional significance of BQ use in different parts of the world.
- Identify the biologically active ingredients in BQ and their potential effects on oral tissues.
- Analyse the impact of BQ use on periodontal health based on current scientific literature.

Z. U. Ahmed (✉)
Department of Community Dentistry and Oral Disease Prevention, Eastman Institute of Oral Health, University of Rochester, Rochester, NY, USA

F. Javed
Department of Orthodontics and Dentofacial Orthopedics, Eastman Institute for Oral Health, University of Rochester, Rochester, NY, USA

F. Javed, S. Warnakulasuriya (eds.), *Smokeless Tobacco and its Effects on Periodontal Health*, https://doi.org/10.1007/978-3-032-16409-4_4

- Explore the mechanisms through which BQ components may contribute to periodontal disease.
- Evaluate the clinical presentation and oral manifestations associated with chronic BQ chewing.
- Assess the role of public health policies and education in addressing BQ-related oral health issues.

4.1 Introduction

Betel quid (BQ), widely known as *paan*, is a traditional chewable preparation that plays a significant role in the cultural, religious, and social fabric of many South Asian communities, including Bangladesh, India, Nepal, and Pakistan. Over the years, consumption of BQ has transcended geographical boundaries, primarily due to migration patterns that have brought this practice to various parts of the world including the United Kingdom, Italy and the United States (Auluck et al. 2009; Changrani et al. 2006; Petti and Warnakulasuriya 2018). Globally, it is estimated that approximately 10%–25% of the world's population engages in betel quid chewing (Agustina et al. 2024; Chen et al. 2017; Gupta and Jain 2024; Kloee Titu Eki and Ngadilah 2023). This practice ranks fourth in addictiveness after nicotine, ethanol, and caffeine, with an estimated 600 million users worldwide (Zdrojewicz et al. 2015). Betel quid chewing has deep historical and cultural roots, especially in South Asia, where it serves various purposes, ranging from religious rituals and social bonding to simply acting as a digestive aid (de la Monte et al. 2020; Franke et al. 2014; Singh et al. 2020). In many traditional settings, offering BQ is considered a gesture of respect and hospitality, particularly during religious ceremonies, weddings, and festivals, where it is commonly referred to as "thamboolam" in the Sanskrit language (RoseBazaar 2024). Historically, BQ chewing symbolized wealth and beauty, with elaborate betel sets made from precious materials like silver, gold, and porcelain signifying the owner's social rank as shown in Fig. 4.1 (Toprani and Patel 2013).

The preparation typically involves wrapping slices of areca nut (AN) and a pinch of slaked lime in a betel leaf, often with tobacco and flavour-enhancing sweeteners like cardamom or fennel seeds (Fig. 4.2a–h). These additives may improve the taste but can also alter the oral environment, promoting bacterial growth and exacerbating periodontal damage (Uehara et al. 2021). A BQ, after placement in the vestibule, is gently chewed and sucked intermittently. It is then held against the buccal sulcus for prolonged durations and continued to be sucked and chewed upon intermittently. This process increases the salivary flow and BQ-chewers usually expectorate reddish-brown serous saliva (due to *Catechu* paste) during each cycle of BQ consumption. The quid is ultimately spat out with some of the constituents being ingested. The purpose of this chapter is to provide a comprehensive review of the betel quid, its consumption patterns, and its impact on periodontal health.

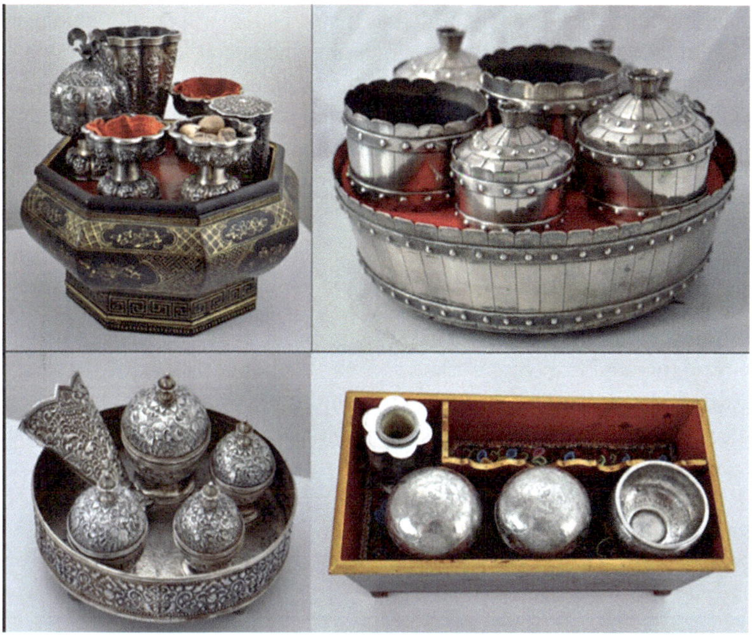

Fig. 4.1 Different types of betel-quid preparing sets (Micheal Blackman Ltd., UK)

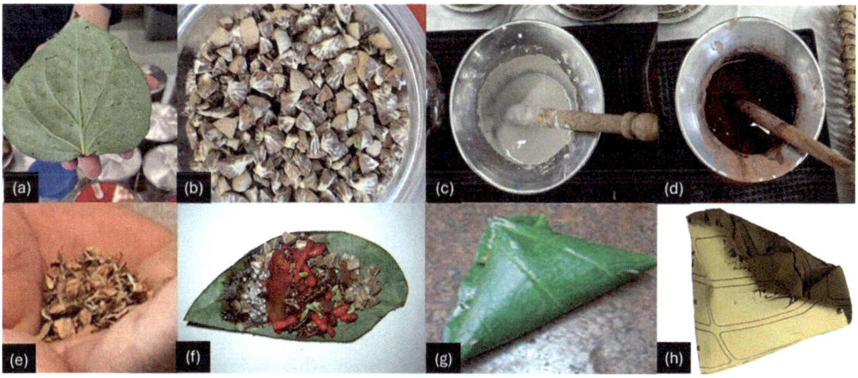

Fig. 4.2 (**a**) *Piper betle* leaf; (**b**) shopped areca nut (*chaalia*); (**c**) slaked lime; (**d**) *Catechu* paste; (**e**) powdered dry tobacco leaves; (**f**) betel-quid; (**g**) betel quid with contents wrapped inside; and (**h**) betel-quid being sold in non-branded paper pouches

4.1.1 Reasons for Chewing Betel-Quid

The BQ is often consumed during social gatherings, festivals, and religious ceremonies as a symbol of hospitality and respect (Gupta and Warnakulasuriya 2002). Moreover, it has been reported that stress relief is another key factor that influence this widespread habit (Iqbal and Yakub 2013). In Taiwan, peer influence, alertness, and social bonding have been identified as major factors, especially among adolescents (Lee et al. 2012). Similarly, peer pressure and social influence play a crucial role, particularly among younger populations, such as university students in India (Ray et al. 2003). Additionally, indigenous communities associate betel-quid chewing with spiritual beliefs and traditional medicinal practices (Ma et al. 2017). While these reasons differ across populations and contexts, they collectively demonstrate the deeply embedded nature of BQ chewing in various cultural and social structures.

Key Points

- BQ is commonly used in social, festive, and religious settings as a sign of hospitality and respect.
- Stress relief is a significant factor driving BQ consumption.
- Peer pressure and social influence significantly affect BQ use among university students.
- Reasons for BQ use vary by region but reflect its deep cultural and social integration.

4.2 Effect of Betel-Quid Chewing on Periodontal Health

Chronic BQ chewing induces a complex cascade of harmful effects on periodontal health, characterized by chronic inflammation, tissue destruction, microbial dysbiosis, and mechanical trauma (Agustina et al. 2024). The combination of powdered tobacco, slaked lime, and physical abrasion induced by constituents such as areca nut jeopardizes the periodontium leading to gingival inflammation and recession. Table 4.1 provides an overview of clinical studies that investigated the effect of habitual BQ chewing on periodontal health (Giovannoni et al. 2018; Hsiao et al. 2014; Javed et al. 2013, 2015). In a study from Taiwan, Hsiao et al. (2014) assessed the effect of BQ chewing on periodontal health. In this study periodontal statuses of 78 BQ-chewers and 36 non-chewers with ages ranging between 30 and 60 years were evaluated (Hsiao et al. 2014). Nearly 75% of the BQ chewers were chewing quids throughout the week whereas 11.3% and 12.9% of the individuals reported that they chewed BQ four to six times/week and one to three times/week, respectively. Nearly 44% of the BQ chewers had a chewing history of at least 20 years and 27.7% had a chewing history of at least a decade (Hsiao et al. 2014). The remaining (nearly 28%) were chewing BQ for less than a decade. At least 85% of the BQ-chewers were chewing BQ containing additives such as AN, slaked lime, *catechu* paste, and artificial fragrances (Hsiao et al. 2014). Scores of full-mouth plaque index (PI) and marginal bone loss (MBL) were significantly higher among BQ-chewers than non-chewers. Moreover, regression analysis showed a statistically significant association between age, PI, and daily frequency of BQ-chewing (Hsiao et al. 2014).

Table 4.1 Overview of clinical studies that investigated the effect of habitual betel-quid (BQ) chewing on periodontal health

Authors et al. and location	Study design	Participants	Gender	Age (years)	Periodontal parameter/s assessed	Periodontal parameters
Hsiao et al. (2014) Taiwan	Case-control	78 BQ-chewers 36 Non-chewers	41 Males; 37 Females 11 Males; 25 Females	30–60	MBL	MBL was significantly higher in BQ-chewers than non-chewers
Javed et al. (2013) Pakistan	Case-control	70 BQ-chewers[a] 50 Non-chewers	49 Males; 21 Females 29 Males; 21 Females	36–52	PI BoP PD MBL	PI, BoP, PD, and MBL were significantly higher in BQ-chewers than non-chewers PI, BoP, PD, and MBL were significantly higher in individuals chewing BQ with than without tobacco
Javed et al. (2015) Pakistan	Case-control	45 BQ-chewers 50 Non-chewers	30 Males; 15 Females 29 Males; 21 Females	23–43	PI BoP PD MBL	PI, BoP, PD, and MBL were significantly higher in BQ-chewers than non-chewers
Giovannoni et al. (2018) Spain	Case-control	430 BQ chewers	240 Males; 190 Females	20–65	CPI	BQ chewing habit increased the likelihood of a higher CPI by 6.76-fold

BoP bleeding on probing, *BQ* betel-quid, *CPI* community periodontal index, *MBL* marginal bone loss, *PD* probing depth, *PI* plaque index

[a]35 individuals were chewing BQ with and 35 without tobacco

Javed et al. (2013) compared the periodontal status among individuals chewing BQ (with and without tobacco) and non-chewers. In this study (Javed et al. 2013), individuals were chewing BQ for approximately 13 years and were consuming five to six quids daily. Periodontal inflammatory parameters, PI, bleeding on probing (BoP), probing depth (PD), and MBL were significantly higher among BQ-chewers than non-chewers; however, these parameters were significantly higher among individuals who chewed BQ with than without tobacco (Javed et al. 2013). A graphic

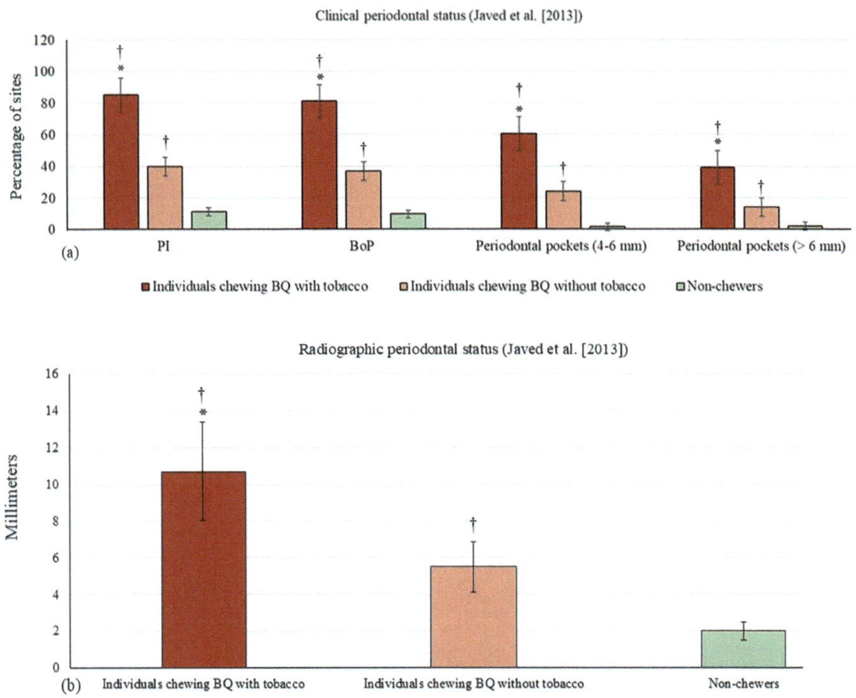

Fig. 4.3 (**a**) Clinical periodontal status of betel-quid (BQ) chewers and non-chewed assessed in the study by Javed et al. (2013). *Compared with individuals chewing BQ without tobacco ($P < 0.01$); †compared with non-chewers ($P < 0.01$); (**b**) Radiographic periodontal status of betel-BQ chewers and non-chewed assessed in the study by Javed et al. (2013). *Compared with individuals chewing BQ without tobacco ($P < 0.01$); †compared with non-chewers ($P < 0.01$)

summary of the periodontal parameters among BQ-chewers and non-chewers presented in the study by Javed et al. (2013) is shown in Fig. 4.3a, b. It is postulated that nicotine in the presence of additives such as arecoline (from AN) and slaked lime further augments a state of oxidative stress in periodontal tissues, thereby worsening periodontal inflammation in individuals chewing BQ with than without tobacco. In this study (Javed et al. 2013), individuals chewing BQ with tobacco held the BQ in the right buccal vestibule and chewed it for a longer duration (approximately 2 h) in contrast to individuals chewing BQ without tobacco (approximately 20 min). Nevertheless, chewing BQ without tobacco is by no means harmless to periodontal tissues as it still contains hazardous constituents such as AN and slaked lime. In this context, it is also pertinent to mention that individuals who chew BQ, whether with or without tobacco, expose their oral tissues to various aryl hydrocarbons, including benzo[a]pyrene and dimethylbenzanthracene (Liu et al. 2021; Rao 1984). These compounds are known to promote inflammatory responses, which may contribute to the heightened prevalence and severity of oral diseases observed in BQ users (Warnakulasuriya 2009). Results from another study, which compared the clinicoradiographic status among BQ-chewers and non-chewers reported that the percentage of sites demonstrating BoP ($P < 0.01$), supragingival plaque accumulation ($P < 0.01$), PD (4–6 mm and >6 mm) ($P < 0.01$), and MBL ($P < 0.01$) are significantly higher among BQ-chewers than non-chewers (Javed et al. 2015). In this study (Javed et al. 2015), the mean duration of BQ chewing (approximately 4 years) and duration of placement in the mouth (nearly 20 min) was relatively short; however, BQ-chewers displayed worse periodontal status than non-chewers. It has been reported that conventional ingredients in a BQ such as AN, dried powdered tobacco, and slaked lime accelerate the production of pro-inflammatory cytokines in periodontal tissues such as interleukin 1-beta and tumour necrosis factor-alpha that contribute towards periodontal inflammation (Chang et al. 2009). Nevertheless, in the study by Javed et al. (2015), BQ-chewers were not vigilant towards routine domestic oral hygiene maintenance (OHM) protocols such as toothbrushing and flossing of interproximal spaces. It is speculated that poor OHM may also have contributed to the compromised periodontal status in BQ-chewers in contrast to on-chewers (Javed et al. 2015). Results from a study from Spain reported that BQ-chewers exhibited a community periodontal index (CPI) score of 3–4 compared to non-chewers that have CPI scores of less than 3 in all jaw sextants (Giovannoni et al. 2018). In this study, higher prevalences of CPI 3–4 scores were associated with the mandibular teeth in BQ-chewers and non-chewers (Giovannoni et al. 2018).

Key Points

- Chronic BQ chewing causes severe periodontal damage through mechanisms like chronic inflammation, microbial imbalance, tissue destruction, and physical trauma.
- BQ with tobacco is more harmful than BQ without tobacco, significantly increasing plaque, bleeding on probing, probing depth, and marginal bone loss.
- Hazardous chemicals in BQ (e.g., benzo[a]pyrene, dimethylbenzanthracene) and conventional ingredients like slaked lime and areca nut stimulate the production of pro-inflammatory cytokines, intensifying periodontal inflammation.
- Poor oral hygiene among BQ users may exacerbate periodontal damage.

4.3 Alteration of Oral Flora in Betel-Quid Chewers

A limited number of studies have assessed the impact of BQ chewing on oral microbiome (Bahuguna et al. 2023; Fernando et al. 2009; Hernandez et al. 2017; Ling et al. 2001; Uehara et al. 2021). In a comparative analysis study from Sri Lanka, Uehara et al. (2021) assessed the effect of BQ chewing on oral microflora. Nineteen BQ-chewers and 23 non-chewers (controls) with mean ages of 37.9 ± 6.19 and 34.6 ± 10.7 years, respectively. The BQ chewers were addicted to the chewing habit for an average duration of 11.8 ± 9.37 years. Samples were collected using buccal swabs and 16S rRNA gene sequencing was performed to identify and compare the bacterial communities present among the groups (Uehara et al. 2021). A total of 111 different bacterial genera were detected in BQ-chewers and non-chewers. The most abundant bacterial species among all samples was Streptococcus (32.41 ± 23.51%), followed by *Neisseria* (9.35 ± 9.45%), *Veillonella* (6.61 ± 5.60%), and *Prevotella* (6.39 ± 6.57%) (Uehara et al. 2021). Data analysis of all the abundant genera revealed a lower abundance of *Streptococcus*, *Lautropia*, and *Actinobacillus* among BQ-chewers than non-chewers ($P < 0.05$) (Uehara et al. 2021). Moreover, bacteria belonging to the genera *Actinomyces*, *Bifidobacterium*, *Atopobium*, *Tannerella*, *Prevotella*, *Moryella*, *Filifactor*, *Dialister*, *Megasphaera*, *Schwartzia*, *Selenomonas*, *Veillonella*, *Bulleidia*, *Leptotrichia*, *Campylo-bacter*, and *Treponema* were more abundant among BQ-chewers than non-chewers. Briefly, the study showed a higher proportion of periodonto-pathogenic bacteria including *Actinomyces*, *Tannerella*, and *Prevotella* species in the oral cavities of BQ-chewers than non-chewers ($P < 0.05$) (Uehara et al. 2021). The study concluded that chronic BQ-chewing significantly alters oral flora (Uehara et al. 2021). Similarly, results from another study on BQ-chewers and non-chewers aged between 21 and 30 years showed that BQ-chewers exhibit higher levels of *Prevotella* (29%) and *Bacteroides* (11%); whereas non-chewers had higher abundances of *Bacteroides* (14.56%) and *Streptococcus* (14%) species (Bahuguna et al. 2023). Furthermore, the proportion of *Helicobacter pylori* is higher in the oral cavity of BQ-chewers than non-chewers (Fernando et al. 2009) (Table 4.2).

Table 4.2 Overview of studies comparing the oral microbiota between betel quid chewers and non-chewers

Authors et al. (year) and location	Bacterial sampling	Study sample	Bacterial identification	Main results
Bahuguna et al. (2023) India	Tongue dorsum, hard and soft palate, subgingival region, cheeks, and buccal mucosa	11 BQ-chewers 11 NC	16S sequencing	Significant differences in alpha diversity between BQ chewers and NC Higher abundance of *Prevotella* (29%) and *Bacteroides* (11%) in BQ chewers; higher abundance of *Bacteroides* (14.56%) and *Streptococcus* (14%) in NC Altered microbiota in BQ chewers with 0–10 years of exposure than those with over 10 years
Hernandez et al. (2017) Papua New Guinea		66 Current BQ-chewers 25 Former BQ-chewers 49 NC	454 pyrosequencing	Elevated levels of *Streptococcus anginosus* (16-fold) in BQ-chewers with precancerous and cancerous oral lesions than those without lesions Oral human papillomavirus was more often identified among BQ-chewers with oral precancerous and cancerous oral lesions than those without lesions
Ling et al. (2001) China	Subgingival plaque	34 BQ-chewers 32 NC	PCR	BQ chewers may harbour higher levels of *Aggregatibacter actinomycetemcomitans* and *Porphyromonas gingivalis* than NC
Uehara et al. (2021) Sri Lanka	Buccal swab sample	19 BQ-chewers 19 NC	Next-generation sequencing	*Actinomyces*, *Bifidobacterium*, *Atopobium*, *Tannerella*, *Prevotella*, *Moryella*, *Filifactor*, *Dialister*, *Megasphaera*, *Schwartzia*, *Selenomonas*, *Veillonella*, *Bulleidia*, *Leptotrichia*, *Campylobacter*, and *Treponema* were abundant among BQ-chewers than NC
Fernando et al. (2009) Sri Lanka	Biopsies and serological methods	60 BQ-chewers 60 NC	Assessment of IgG antibody	Proportions of *Helicobacter pylori* were higher in BQ-chewers than NC.

BQ betel-quid, *IgG* immunoglobulin G, *NC* non-chewers, *PCR* polymerase chain reaction

Key Points

- BQ chewing significantly alters the oral microbiome, leading to a distinct bacterial profile compared to non-chewers.
- Periodontopathogenic bacteria such as *Actinomyces*, *Tannerella*, and *Prevotella* are more abundant in BQ-chewers than non-chewers.
- Beneficial bacteria like *Streptococcus*, *Lautropia*, and *Actinobacillus* are significantly reduced in BQ-chewers than non-chewers.
- *Helicobacter pylori*, a known gastrointestinal pathogen, is more prevalent in the oral cavities of BQ-chewers than non-chewers.

4.4 Betel-Quid Chewing and Peri-implant Diseases

The association between BQ chewing and peri-implant diseases (peri-implant mucositis and peri-implantitis) remains largely uninvestigated. To date, one case-control study (Alqutub et al. 2022) compared the peri-implant soft tissue and osseous inflammatory status among BQ-chewers and non-chewers. It found no significant correlation between the duration, daily frequency, or placement time of betel quid in the mouth and the occurrence of peri-implant inflammatory conditions, suggesting that there is no threshold of betel quid consumption that can be considered safe with regard to the progression of periodontal and peri-implant diseases. In this study (Alqutub et al. 2022), participants were divided into three groups as follows: Group-1: Individuals chewing BQ with tobacco ($n = 30$); Group-2: Individuals chewing BQ without tobacco ($n = 30$); and Group-3: Non-chewers ($n = 30$). In groups 1 and 2, individuals were chewing betel-quid for 14.5 ± 3.8 and 11.6 ± 1.3 years, were placing BQ in the right buccal vestibule and were consuming 9.2 ± 0.5 and 8.9 ± 0.2 quids/day. In groups 1 and 2, each BQ was placed in the mouth for a mean duration of 32.6 ± 5.6 and 23.5 ± 0.7 min, respectively. A total of 31, 33, and 32 dental implants were in function among patients in groups 1, 2, and 3 and were in function for approximately 3 years in each group. All implants were replacing missing first or second molars in both arches. Regardless of whether BQ was chewed with or without tobacco, scores of modified plaque index, modified gingival index, peri-implant PD, and crestal bone loss (CBL) were significantly higher among all BQ-chewers compared with non-chewers (Table 4.3). However, there was no statistically significant correlation between duration of betel-quid chewing habit, daily frequency of betel-quid consumption and duration of betel-quid placement in the mouth with periodontal and peri-implant clinical-radiographic parameters among patients who chewed BQ either with or without tobacco (Alqutub et al. 2022).

Table 4.3 An overview of the results reported in the study by Alqutub et al. (2022)

Parameters	Individuals chewing BQ with tobacco	Individuals chewing BQ without tobacco	Non-chewers
Demographics			
Participants	30	30	30
Number of implants	31	33	32
Male:female	21:9	22:8	20:10
Age in years	47.4 ± 5.2 years	45.1 ± 2.2 years	44.2 ± 1.3 years
Betel-quids chewed daily (*n*)	9.2 ± 0.5 quids/day	8.9 ± 0.2 quids/day	NA
Duration of betel-quid chewing habit (in years)	14.5 ± 3.8 years	11.6 ± 1.3 years	NA
Daily toothbrushing (twice)	23.3%	33.3%	73.3%
Peri-implant parameters			
Modified plaque index	2.5 ± 0.08[a]	2.3 ± 0.1[a]	0.4 ± 0.06
Modified gingival index	3.1 ± 0.04[b]	2.7 ± 0.07[b]	0.2 ± 0.005
Peri-implant probing depth	4.6 ± 0.2 mm[c]	4.4 ± 0.3 mm[c]	1.5 ± 0.008 mm
Crestal bone loss (mesial surface)	3.7 ± 0.06 mm[d]	3.7 ± 0.06 mm[d]	0.4 ± 0.005 mm
Crestal bone loss (distal surface)	3.5 ± 0.08 mm[e]	3.4 ± 0.04 mm[e]	0.3 ± 0.007 mm

NA not applicable, *mm* millimetres
[a]Compared with controls ($P < 0.05$)
[b]Compared with controls ($P < 0.05$)
[c]Compared with controls ($P < 0.05$)
[d]Compared with controls ($P < 0.05$)
[e]Compared with controls ($P < 0.05$)

Key Points

- *Limited research*: The link between BQ chewing and peri-implant diseases like peri-implant mucositis and peri-implantitis remains largely unexplored.
- *One study in indexed literature* showed that BQ-chewers may be at an increased risk of developing peri-implant diseases than non-chewers.
- Ingredients in a BQ, such as areca-nut, powdered tobacco, and slaked lime paste may contribute to peri-implant soft tissue inflammation and crestal bone loss.
- It is hypothesized that the peri-implant sulci of BQ-chewers harbour increased levels of periodontopathogenic microbes compared with non-chewers.

There is a notable scarcity of studies investigating the impact of BQ chewing on peri-implant health. However, the existing evidence (Alqutub et al. 2022) suggests that habitual BQ chewers may be at an increased risk of developing peri-implant diseases. The chief ingredients in a BQ such as AN, powdered tobacco, and slaked lime paste possess various biochemical and physiological properties that may potentially contribute to peri-implant soft tissue inflammation and CBL. In summary, AN and powdered tobacco, key components of BQ, contain alkaloids such as arecoline, which has been shown to induce fibroblast dysfunction, impair collagen synthesis, induce irreparable DNA damage, and promote pro-inflammatory cytokine release (Adil et al. 2021; Chang et al. 2013; Jeng et al. 2001; Rehman et al. 2016). Similarly, slaked lime paste creates an alkaline microenvironment that can cause mucosal irritation and chemical burns (Gupta and Ray 2004; Reichart and Phillipsen 1998), potentially leading to ulceration and chronic inflammation around dental implants. It is known that habitual BQ chewing alters the subgingival microbiota and facilitates the growth of periodontopathogenic microbes including *Porphyromonas gingivalis* and *Aggregatibacter actinomycetemcomitans* (Ling et al. 2001). It is, therefore, hypothesized that the peri-implant sulci of BQ-chewers harbour increased levels of periodontopathogenic microbes compared with non-chewers. Such microbial dysbiosis could exacerbate inflammatory conditions around implants, further accelerating peri-implant tissue destruction. To date, there are no studies that have confirmed that habitual BQ chewing is a risk factor for implant failure; however, it is speculated that chronic BQ chewing predisposes peri-implant tissues to inflammatory insults which, if not diagnosed and addressed in a timely manner, may result in loss of implant stability and even implant failure. Further longitudinal and microbiological studies are needed to elucidate the precise effects of BQ constituents on peri-implant soft tissue health, crestal bone stability, and the peri-implant microbiome. Understanding these relationships is crucial for developing targeted preventive and therapeutic strategies for individuals with dental implants who engage in BQ chewing.

4.5 Public Health Concerns and Recommendations

4.5.1 Awareness and Education

Despite the documented risks, awareness of the harmful effects of BQ chewing remains limited among certain populations. There is a dire need for targeted educational campaigns, especially in communities where BQ chewing is a cultural norm and starts at a young age. Highlighting the associations with oral diseases such as periodontal and potentially peri-implant diseases and oral precancer and cancer are crucial for effective prevention.

4.5.2 Healthcare Provider Training

Workshops and training programmes that enhance cultural competency among healthcare professionals can improve communication with patients who chew betel quid. Such training would enable providers to ask relevant questions about BQ use during routine check-ups, leading to early identification of oral health issues. Healthcare providers should also be equipped with cessation strategies tailored towards BQ-chewers. Behavioural counselling, motivational interviewing, and culturally sensitive cessation protocols can significantly improve patient outcomes (Akers et al. 2020; Gordon et al. 2006; Loken et al. 2021; Spangler and Salisbury 1995). Dental practitioners should be encouraged to incorporate BQ-related questions into standard health assessments to facilitate comprehensive care.

4.5.3 Screening and Early Detection

Regular oral screenings are vital in regions or communities with a high prevalence of BQ use. Such screenings can help detect not only periodontal and possibly peri-implant diseases but also oral premalignant (such as oral submucous fibrosis) and malignant diseases including oral squamous cell carcinoma. It is recommended that healthcare facilities integrate BQ-chewing as a risk assessment into routine dental and medical check-ups and community health programmes. This may help facilitate early detection of oral diseases associated with BQ use and promote targeted preventive strategies.

Key Points

- *Limited awareness*: Many individuals in BQ-prevalent communities remain unaware of its serious oral health risks.
- *Early-onset habit*: Betel quid chewing often begins at a young age in certain cultures, increasing the long-term risk for periodontal disease, peri-implant disease, and oral cancers.
- *Proactive screening*: Regular oral health screenings in high-risk populations can lead to early detection of oral diseases particularly among BQ-chewers.
- *Integrative risk assessment*: Including BQ-chewing habits in standard health assessments can help clinicians provide more comprehensive, preventive oral healthcare.

4.6 Conclusion

Habitual BQ chewing is a risk factor for periodontal diseases. There is a lack of evidence regarding the impact of BQ-chewing on peri-implant tissues; however, it is speculated that BQ may increase the risk of peri-implant diseases in susceptible individuals.

References

Adil N, Ali H, Siddiqui AJ, Ali A, Ahmed A, El-Seedi HR, Musharraf SG (2021) Evaluation of cytotoxicity of areca nut and its commercial products on normal human gingival fibroblast and oral squamous cell carcinoma cell lines. J Hazard Mater 403:123872

Agustina R, Mujahidah A, Berniyanti T (2024) Betel nut chewing effects on the incidence of periodontitis. World J Adv Res Rev 23:540–543

Akers L, Andrews JA, Lichtenstein E, Severson HH, Gordon JS (2020) Effect of a responsiveness-based support intervention on smokeless tobacco cessation: the UCare-ChewFree randomized clinical trial. Nicotine Tob Res 22:381–389

Alqutub MN, Alali Y, Tulbah HI, Javed F, Vohra F, Abduljabbar T (2022) Peri-implant clinicoradiographic status among betel-quid chewers and controls. Braz Dent J 33:87–96

Auluck A, Hislop G, Poh C, Zhang L, Rosin MP (2009) Areca nut and betel quid chewing among south Asian immigrants to Western countries and its implications for oral cancer screening. Rural Remote Health 9:1118

Bahuguna M, Hooda S, Mohan L, Gupta RK, Diwan P (2023) Identifying oral microbiome alterations in adult betel quid chewing population of Delhi, India. PLoS One 18:e0278221

Chang LY, Wan HC, Lai YL, Kuo YF, Liu TY, Chen YT, Hung SL (2009) Areca nut extracts increased expression of inflammatory cytokines, tumor necrosis factor-alpha, interleukin-1beta, interleukin-6 and interleukin-8, in peripheral blood mononuclear cells. J Periodontal Res 44:175–183

Chang MC, Lin LD, Wu HL, Ho YS, Hsien HC, Wang TM, Jeng PY et al (2013) Areca nut-induced buccal mucosa fibroblast contraction and its signaling: a potential role in oral submucous fibrosis—a precancer condition. Carcinogenesis 34:1096–1104

Changrani J, Gany FM, Cruz G, Kerr R, Katz R (2006) Paan and gutka use in the United States: a pilot study in Bangladeshi and Indian-Gujarati immigrants in new York City. J Immigr Refug Stud 4:99–110

Chen PH, Mahmood Q, Mariottini GL, Chiang TA, Lee KW (2017) Adverse health effects of betel quid and the risk of oral and pharyngeal cancers. Biomed Res Int 2017:3904098

de la Monte SM, Moriel N, Lin A, Abdullah Tanoukhy N, Homans C, Gallucci G, Tong M et al (2020) Betel quid health risks of insulin resistance diseases in poor young south Asian native and immigrant populations. Int J Environ Res Public Health 17:6690

Fernando N, Jayakumar G, Perera N, Amarasingha I, Meedin F, Holton J (2009) Presence of helicobacter pylori in betel chewers and non betel chewers with and without oral cancers. BMC Oral Health 9:23

Franke AA, Lai JF, Kawamoto CT, Pokhrel P, Herzog TA (2014) University of Hawai'i cancer Center connection: areca (betel) nut consumption: an underappreciated cause of cancer. Hawaii J Med Public Health 73:400–403

Giovannoni ML, Valdivia-Gandur I, Lozano de Luaces V, Varela Véliz H, Balasubbaiah Y, Chimenos-Küstner E (2018) Betel and tobacco chewing habit and its relation to risk factors for periodontal disease. Oral Dis 24:829–839

Gordon JS, Lichtenstein E, Severson HH, Andrews JA (2006) Tobacco cessation in dental settings: research findings and future directions. Drug Alcohol Rev 25:27–37

Gupta J, Jain V (2024) Knowledge, attitude, and practices of areca nut and betel quid chewing among the adult population—a questionnaire-based cross-sectional study. SRM J Res Dent Sci 15:15–21

Gupta PC, Ray CS (2004) Epidemiology of betel quid usage. Ann Acad Med Singap 33:31–36

Gupta PC, Warnakulasuriya S (2002) Global epidemiology of areca nut usage. Addict Biol 7:77–83

Hernandez BY, Zhu X, Goodman MT, Gatewood R, Mendiola P, Quinata K, Paulino YC (2017) Betel nut chewing, oral premalignant lesions, and the oral microbiome. PLoS One 12:e0172196

Hsiao CN, Ting CC, Shieh TY, Ko EC (2014) Relationship between betel quid chewing and radiographic alveolar bone loss among Taiwanese aboriginals: a retrospective study. BMC Oral Health 14:133

Iqbal MP, Yakub M (2013) Smokeless tobacco use: a risk factor for hyperhomocysteinemia in a Pakistani population. PLoS One 8:e83826

Javed F, Tenenbaum HC, Nogueira-Filho G, Qayyum F, Correa FO, Al-Hezaimi K, Samaranayake LP (2013) Severity of periodontal disease in individuals chewing betel quid with and without tobacco. Am J Med Sci 346:273–278

Javed F, Vohra F, Al-Kheraif AA, Malmstrom H, Romanos GE (2015) Comparison of periodontal inflammatory conditions among habitual gutka chewers and betel quid chewers. Oral Dis 21:437–442

Jeng JH, Chang MC, Hahn LJ (2001) Role of areca nut in betel quid-associated chemical carcinogenesis: current awareness and future perspectives. Oral Oncol 37:477–492

Kloee Titu Eki A, Ngadilah C (2023) Excessive deadly addiction chewing betel quid as a double burden, for poverty community Kupang regency, West Timor. Eduvest 3:2107–2118

Lee CH, Ko AM, Yen CF, Chu KS, Gao YJ, Warnakulasuriya S, Sunarjo et al (2012) Betel-quid dependence and oral potentially malignant disorders in six Asian countries. Br J Psychiatry 201:383–391

Ling LJ, Hung SL, Tseng SC, Chen YT, Chi LY, Wu KM, Lai YL (2001) Association between betel quid chewing, periodontal status and periodontal pathogens. Oral Microbiol Immunol 16:364–369

Liu M, Wen C, Pan S (2021) Modulator effect of mangiferin on biochemical characterization in 7,12-dimethylbenz[a]anthracene induced oral cancer in experimental hamsters. Vet Med Sci 7:2015–2025

Loken B, Borgida E, Wang T, Madzelan MK, Williams AL, Hatsukami D, Stepanov I (2021) Can the public be educated about constituents in smokeless tobacco? A three-wave randomized controlled trial. Nicotine Tob Res 23:161–170

Ma W-F, Li C-I, Gritz ER, Tamí-Maury I, Lam C, Lin C-C (2017) A symbol of connectedness between the self and the tribal home: betel quid in the lives of indigenous Taiwanese. Hu Li Za Zhi 64:65

Petti S, Warnakulasuriya S (2018) Betel quid chewing among adult male immigrants from the Indian subcontinent to Italy. Oral Dis 24:44–48

Rao AR (1984) Modifying influences of betel quid ingredients on B(a)P-induced carcinogenesis in the buccal pouch of hamster. Int J Cancer 33:581–586

Ray CS, Gupta P, de Beyer J (2003) Research on tobacco in India (including betel quid and areca nut). UCSF: Center for Tobacco Control Research and Education

Rehman A, Ali S, Lone MA, Atif M, Hassona Y, Prime SS, Pitiyage GN et al (2016) Areca nut alkaloids induce irreparable DNA damage and senescence in fibroblasts and may create a favourable environment for tumour progression. J Oral Pathol Med 45:365–372

Reichart PA, Phillipsen HP (1998) Betel chewer's mucosa—a review. J Oral Pathol Med 27:239–242

RoseBazaar (2024) Significance of thamboolam. Retrieved from https://hoovufresh.com/blogs/news/significance-of-thamboolam-rosebazaar. Accessed 25 Dec 2024

Singh A, Dikshit R, Chaturvedi P (2020) Betel nut use: the south Asian story. Subst Use Misuse 55:1545–1551

Spangler JG, Salisbury PL 3rd (1995) Smokeless tobacco: epidemiology, health effects and cessation strategies. Am Fam Physician 52:1421–1430, 1433–1424

Toprani R, Patel D (2013) Betel leaf: revisiting the benefits of an ancient Indian herb. South Asian J Cancer 2:140–141

Uehara O, Hiraki D, Kuramitsu Y, Matsuoka H, Takai R, Fujita M, Harada F et al (2021) Alteration of oral flora in betel quid chewers in Sri Lanka. J Microbiol Immunol Infect 54:1159–1166

Warnakulasuriya S (2009) Causes of oral cancer—an appraisal of controversies. Br Dent J 207:471–475

Zdrojewicz Z, Kosowski W, Królikowska N, Stebnicki M, Stebnicki MR (2015) Betel—the fourth most popular substance in the world. Pol Merkur Lekarski 39:181–185

Effect of *Shammah* on Periodontal and Peri-implant Tissues

5

Mansour Al-Askar and Asma Saleh Almeslet

Abbreviations

BoP	Bleeding on probing
CAL	Clinical attachment loss
CBL	Crestal bone loss
GR	Gingival recession
MBL	Marginal bone loss
OC	Oral cancer
PDs	Periodontal diseases
PI	Plaque index
PPD	Periodontal probing depth
PT	Probiotic therapy
RCT	Randomized controlled trial
RF	Risk factors
SRP	Scaling and root planing
ST	Smokeless tobacco

M. Al-Askar (✉)
Department of Periodontics and Community Dentistry, College of Dentistry, King Saud University, Riyadh, Saudi Arabia
e-mail: MAlAskar@ksu.edu.sa

A. S. Almeslet
Department of Oral Maxillofacial Surgery and Diagnostic Sciences, College of Medicine and Dentistry, Riyadh Elm University, Riyadh, Saudi Arabia
e-mail: Asma.Almeslet@riyadh.edu.sa

F. Javed, S. Warnakulasuriya (eds.), *Smokeless Tobacco and its Effects on Periodontal Health*, https://doi.org/10.1007/978-3-032-16409-4_5

Learning Goals

- Define *Shammah* and describe its composition, cultural usage, and prevalence in regions such as Saudi Arabia and Yemen.
- Recognize the placement practices and frequency of *Shammah* use, including typical user demographics and behaviours.
- Evaluate the findings of key observational studies that have assessed periodontal status among *Shammah* users and non-users.
- Interpret self-perceived oral symptoms reported by habitual *Shammah* users, and understand how these symptoms correlate with clinical findings.
- Compare the periodontal outcomes of non-surgical periodontal therapy (scaling and root planing) with and without adjunct probiotic therapy among *Shammah* users.
- Assess the hypothesized impact of *Shammah* use on peri-implant health, and recognize the need for further research in this area.
- Discuss the mechanisms by which *Shammah* may impair periodontal and peri-implant wound healing, including the potential role of nicotine and aldehydes.
- Summarize the limitations of existing literature and identify gaps that warrant further longitudinal and interventional studies.
- Develop public health strategies and clinical recommendations for managing oral health in populations with habitual *Shammah* use.

5.1 What Is *Shammah*?

Shammah (also known as *shamma* and Yemeni snuff) is a traditional form of ST predominantly used in the Arabian peninsula, particularly in Saudi Arabia (most commonly in the southwestern Jazan province), Yemen, and surrounding regions. It is composed of powdered tobacco blended with ingredients such as lime carbonate, ash, spices (black pepper), and occasionally aromatic oils (Alsanosy 2014; Scheifele et al. 2007; Hazarey and Desai 2025) (Fig. 5.1). Despite being officially banned in Saudi Arabia (Bakdash 2017), its sale and usage persist covertly, with users often refraining from openly acknowledging its consumption (Alsanosy 2014). *Shammah* is placed in the oral cavity as a quid (Allard et al. 1999; Alsanosy 2014); and the reported placement sites include the vestibule of the mouth, the gingivobuccal sulcus, and the lower labial or buccal vestibules, where it is often retained for extended periods (Alsanosy 2014). The insoluble components are ultimately spat out. Habitual *shammah* usage causes extrinsic staining of teeth (Fig. 5.2). Users as young as 10–13 years of age have been reported to use *shammah* habitually (Alsanosy 2014). It is surprising yet concerning that *shammah* has also been used in infants to minimize pain associated with tooth eruption (Alsanosy 2014).

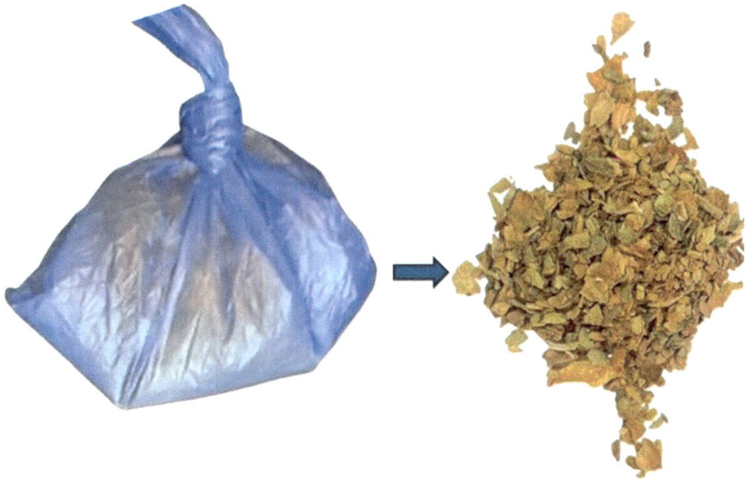

Fig. 5.1 Shammah is sold in non-branded plastic pouches

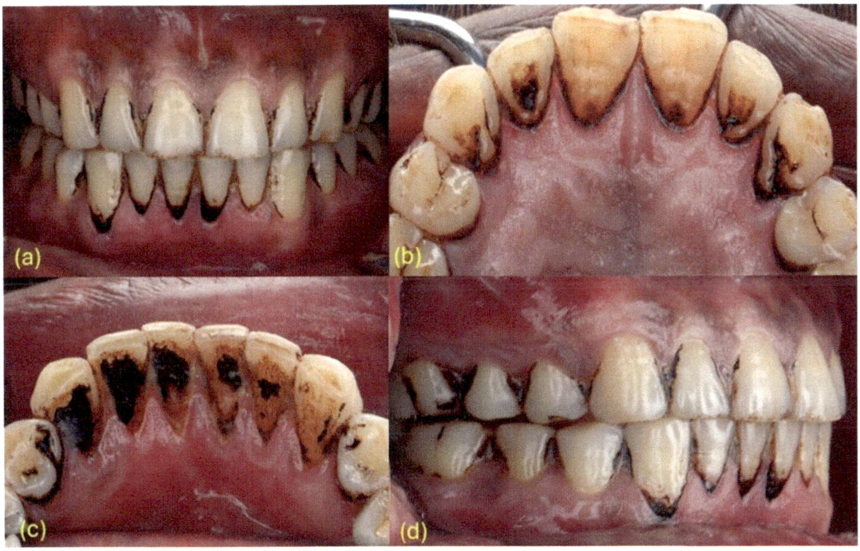

Fig. 5.2 Intra-oral images of a 22-year-old male habitual *shammah*-chewer. (**a**) Frontal view; (**b**) palatal view; (**c**) lingual view; and (**d**) buccal view

Key Points

- *Shammah* is a traditional form of smokeless tobacco (ST) made from powdered tobacco mixed with lime carbonate, ash, spices, and sometimes aromatic oils.
- It is predominantly used in the Arabian Peninsula, especially in southwestern Saudi Arabia and Yemen.
- Although officially banned in Saudi Arabia, *Shammah* is still used covertly.
- Habitual use of *Shammah* has been reported in children as young as 10–13 years old.
- Alarmingly, *Shammah* has even been used in infants to alleviate teething pain.

5.2 *Shammah* and Periodontal Diseases

We reviewed indexed scientific databases (PubMed, EMBASE, Scopus, and Web of Knowledge) to identify studies that assessed the periodontal status in self-reported *shammah* users. A review of pertinent indexed literature showed that, to date, there are only two clinical investigations that have compared the periodontal health status among *shammah* users and controls (individuals not using tobacco in any form) (Al-Askar et al. 2017; Al Agili and Park 2013).

5.2.1 An Overview of the Methodology and Results Reported in the Study by Al-Askar et al. (2017)

In a cross-sectional observational study, Al-Askar et al. (2017) evaluated clinical and radiographic periodontal inflammatory parameters and self-perceived oral symptoms among 47 male *shammah* users and 41 male controls (individuals not using tobacco in any form). The authors used a structured questionnaire to record demographics (age, gender, family history of tobacco use, daily frequency of *shammah* chewing, and duration of its use in years) and self-rated oral symptoms (pain in teeth, pain on chewing, bleeding gums, and burning sensation in mouth) (Al-Askar et al. 2017). The study measured the following periodontal parameters among *shammah* users and compared them with controls: plaque index (PI), bleeding on probing (BoP), PPD, and clinical attachment loss (CAL). Full mouth mesial and distal marginal bone loss (MBL) was also radiographically measured on all teeth (excluding supernumerary teeth, third molars, and grossly carious teeth). A summary of the demographics of *shammah*-chewers and controls is shown in Table 5.1.

The results showed that the percentage of tooth surfaces that visually demonstrated the presence of dental plaque and BoP were significantly higher among *shammah* users than controls (Fig. 5.3a). Moreover, sites with PPD (4–6 mm and >6 mm) and CAL were more often manifested among *shammah* users than controls.

Table 5.1 Demographics of the *shammah*-chewers and controls

Parameters	*Shammah*-chewers	Controls
Participants (*n*)	47	41
Male gender	47	41
Mean age	42.1 ± 5.4 years	45.7 ± 3.9 years
Duration of *shammah*-chewing habit	21.5 ± 2.5 years	NA
Family history of tobacco usage	61.7%	14.6%
Daily frequency of *shammah* chewing	7.6 ± 0.8 times	NA
Duration for which *shammah* was held in the oral cavity	27.7 ± 4.2 min	NA

From Al-Askar et al. (2017)
NA not applicable

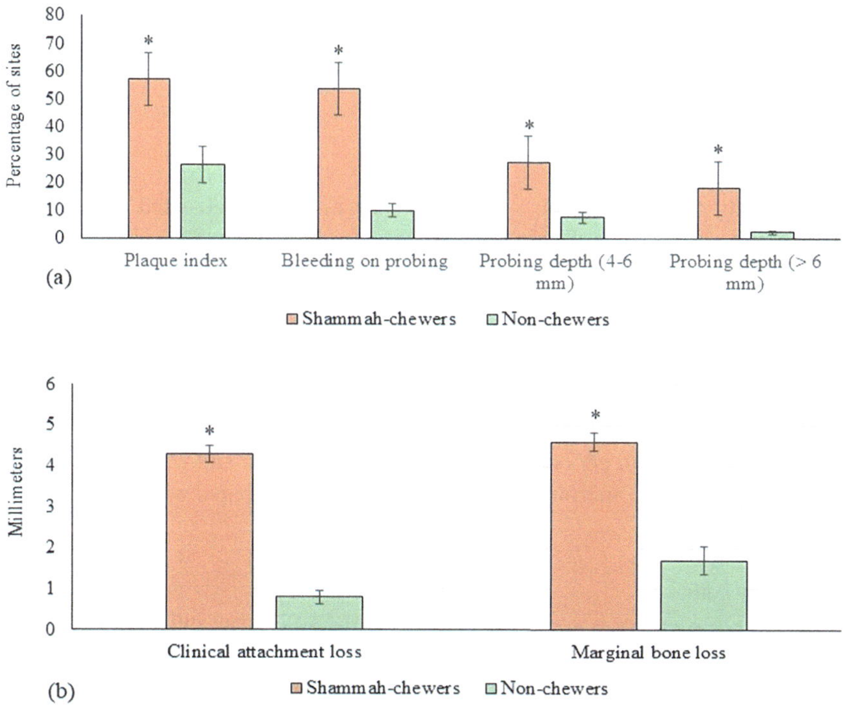

Fig. 5.3 (a) Percentage of sites comparing visible plaque, bleeding on probing, and periodontal pockets (4–6 mm and >6 mm) among self-reported *shammah*-chewers and non-chewers. *Comparison with non-chewers in the same group ($P < 0.01$). (**b**) Comparison of clinical attachment loss and marginal bone loss (in millimetres) among self-reported *shammah*-chewers and non-chewers. *Comparison with non-chewers in the same group ($P < 0.01$). (These results were modified from the study by Al-Askar et al. (2017))

The overall MBL was significantly higher among *shammah* users than controls (Fig. 5.3b). In this study (Al-Askar et al. 2017), *shammah* users chewed this ST product approximately eight times daily and continued to hold it in the buccal sulcus for an average duration of 27.7 min (range 10–50 min) during each chewing session. Moreover, a family history of tobacco use was more often reported by *shammah* users than controls.

Key Points

- Percentages of sites that demonstrate plaque and gingival bleeding are higher in *shammah* users than non-users.
- Sites with probing depths (4–6 mm and >6 mm) and clinical attachment loss are higher among *shammah* users than non-users.
- In the study by Al-Askar et al. (2017), *shammah* users chewed this ST product approximately eight times daily and continued to hold it in the buccal sulcus for an approximately 27.7 min.

5.2.2 Self-Perceived Oral Symptoms

In this study (Al-Askar et al. 2017), the odds ratios for self-rated pain in teeth ($P < 0.001$), pain during chewing ($P < 0.01$), bleeding gums (BG) ($P < 0.05$), and burning sensation in the mouth ($P < 0.01$) were significantly higher in *shammah*-chewers than controls. It has been reported that placing smokeless tobacco (ST) for at least 5 min significantly increases PPD compared to individuals who chew ST products for shorter durations. This seems to be a reason for the higher odds of self-perceived pain in teeth and pain while chewing among *shammah*-chewers in the study by Al-Askar et al. (2017). Al-Askar et al. (2017) concluded that habitual use of *shammah* is associated with periodontal soft tissue inflammation and MBL, and self-perceived oral health is compromised in these individuals compared with controls.

Key Points

- *Shammah* use is associated with periodontal soft tissue inflammation and loss of alveolar bone.
- Self-perceived oral symptoms such as burning sensation in mouth and pain on chewing are worse in *shammah* users than non-users.

5.2.3 An Overview of the Methodology and Results Reported in the Study by Al Agili and Park (2013)

In a cross-sectional observational study, Al Agili and Park (2013) compared the periodontal status and self-perceived oral symptoms among *shammah* users and controls using a convenience sampling method. Middle-school students habitually

Table 5.2 Demographics and behaviour related to *shammah* use by adolescents in Jeddah, Saudi Arabia

Variables	Value
Total number of participants	270
Mean age of participants	15.7 ± 1.5 years
Gender (male)	270 adolescents
Age at starting *shammah* use	12.6 ± 2.4 years
Number of times *shammah* was chewed daily	5.6 ± 4.8 times
Number of minutes for which *shammah* was held in the mouth	11 ± 10.9 min
Placing *shammah* in the mouth before going to sleep	6.4%
Placing *shammah* in the mouth before breakfast	33.5%
Use of *shammah* during studies/exams	51.3%
Awareness about the content of *shammah*	17.8%

Modified from the study by Al Agili and Park (2013)

chewing *shammah* and residents of the city of Jeddah, Saudi Arabia were included (Al Agili and Park 2013). From a clinical perspective, full mouth PI, BoP, PD, gingival recession (GR), CAL and were assessed. Two hundred and seventy male *shammah*-chewers with a mean age of 15.7 ± 1.5 years were included. The demographics of the study population are shown in Table 5.2.

In this study, *shammah*-chewers reported that they started chewing this form of ST at approximately 12 years of age (Al Agili and Park 2013), and the majority of the participants (87%) placed *Shammah* in the upper labial sulcus. They used *shammah* approximately six times daily and kept it in their mouths for nearly 11 min before spitting it out. Nearly 6% adolescents were placing *shammah* in the mouth before going to sleep and approximately 33% individuals reported that they chewed *shammah* every morning before breakfast. Nearly half of the patient population (~51%) stated that they consumed *shammah* during studying and academic examinations as it helped them to concentrate on studies (Table 5.2).

5.2.4 Self-Rated Oral Symptoms of Participants Assessed in the Study by Al Agili and Park (2013)

In contrast to the study by Al-Askar et al. (2017), most of the participants reported no self-perceived symptoms (pain in teeth, pain in gums, and bad breath) (Table 5.3). The authors of this chapter suggest interpreting the outcomes presented in Table 5.3 with caution, as the results may be biased due to factors such as age and duration of *shammah* use. In the study by Al-Askar et al. (2017), participants were in their mid-40s, whereas in the study by Al Agili and Park (2013), participants were approximately 15 years old (Tables 5.1 and 5.3). Furthermore, in the former study, participants had been chewing *shammah* for at least two decades, whereas in the

Table 5.3 Self-perceived oral symptoms among *shammah*-chewers

Self-perceived oral symptoms	Number of participants	Percentage
Pain in teeth		
Yes	88	32.6
No	182	67.4
Pain in gums		
Yes	36	13.3
No	234	86.7
Bad breath		
Yes	62	23
No	208	77

Modified from Al Agili and Park (2013)

Table 5.4 Periodontal status of patients evaluated in the study by Al Agili and Park (2013)

Variables	Score
Dental plaque (% of individuals)	92%
Gingival inflammation (% of individuals)	39%
Mean PPD in mm	2.03 ± 0.39 mm
Gingival recession (% of individuals)	1%
Mean gingival recession in mm	1 mm ± NA
Mean CAL in mm	1.06 ± 0.38 mm

CAL clinical attachment loss, *PPD* probing pocket depth, *NA* not available, *mm* millimetres

latter study, the history of *shammah* use was significantly shorter, approximately 3 years (Tables 5.1 and 5.3). It is hypothesized that as these adolescents included in the study by Al Agili and Park (2013) age and their duration of *shammah* use increases, they may face a heightened risk of developing adverse self-rated oral symptoms such as those referenced above). Further longitudinal studies are needed to test this hypothesis.

5.2.5 Periodontal Status of Participants Assessed in the Study by Al Agili and Park (2013)

Ninety-six percent of the students had plaque deposits on their teeth and the mean plaque index score was 1.66 ± 0.51. Although 39% of individuals demonstrated signs of gingival inflammation (gingival redness and bleeding), the mean CAL was 1.06 ± 0.38 mm, 1% had GR, and the mean PPD ranged from 1.1 to 3.4 mm. None of the *shammah*-chewers had periodontal disease (Table 5.4). Al Agili and Park (2013) stated that due to the age of the participants (~15 years) and short duration of *shammah*-chewing habit (approximately 3 years), their study was unable to detect a relationship between habitual *shammah*-chewing and periodontal disease. Nevertheless, by no means does this statement suggest that habitual *shammah*-chewing does not jeopardize periodontal health.

5.3 Effect of Non-surgical Interventions for Managing Periodontitis Among *Shammah*-Chewers and Non-chewers

It is well-documented that non-surgical scaling and root planing (SRP) is commonly performed for the management of periodontitis and yields satisfactory outcomes (Cobb and Sottosanti 2021; Kwon et al. 2021; Smiley et al. 2015). To date, there is only one randomized controlled trial (RCT) in indexed databases that has assessed the efficacy of non-surgical SRP with and without adjunct probiotic therapy (PT) for managing periodontitis among *shammah*-chewers and non-chewers (Vohra et al. 2020). In this RCT (Vohra et al. 2020), *shammah*-chewers and non-chewers were randomly divided into two groups: (a) individuals that underwent SRP alone; and (b) individuals that underwent SRP with adjunct PT. Periodontal parameters (plaque index, BOP, PPD, CAL, and mesial and distal MBL) were measured on all teeth except third molars at baseline and at 6-month follow-up. Results from the study by Vohra et al. (2020) do not demonstrate that *shammah* is a risk factor for periodontitis; however, the findings are interesting from a therapeutic perspective. However, the 6-month follow-up results showed that regardless of whether SRP is done alone or in combination with adjunct therapies such as PT, the outcomes (in terms of reduction in periodontal inflammation) are compromised in *shammah* users compared to non-chewers with periodontitis. Regardless of the limited scientific evidence available, it is evident that *shammah* use predisposes individuals to oral inflammatory conditions, including periodontitis. However, a particularly concerning aspect is that managing periodontitis in this population may pose significant challenges, likely due to compromised wound healing associated with habitual *shammah* use. Table 5.1 provides an overview of studies (Al-Askar et al. 2017; Al Agili and Park 2013; Vohra et al. 2020) that assessed the relationship between periodontal health and habitual *shamma* use.

Key Points

- To date, one randomized controlled trial has evaluated the effectiveness of SRP with and without probiotic therapy in *shammah* users.
- Regardless of the treatment modality (SRP alone or with probiotics), *shammah* users show less improvement in periodontal inflammation compared to non-users.
- The reduced efficacy of periodontal treatment in *shammah* users may be due to impaired wound healing associated with habitual use.

5.3.1 Peri-implant Health Status Among *Shammah*-Chewers

Dental implants are a modern substitute for traditional fixed and removable dental prostheses, such as bridges and dentures, respectively. Studies (Chiapasco et al. 2020; Howe et al. 2019; Lacarbonara et al. 2022) have shown that dental implants can osseointegrate and remain functionally and aesthetically stable for prolonged durations in partially as well as completely edentulous individuals. However, in a manner similar to natural teeth, peri-implant soft and osseous tissues are vulnerable to inflammatory insults. Periodontal and peri-implant diseases (peri-implant mucositis and peri-implantitis) share significant similarities in their aetiology, pathogenesis, and risk factors, highlighting a strong correlation between the two conditions (Ivanovski and Lee 2018; Robitaille et al. 2016). Habitual use of tobacco products is a well-known risk factor for periodontal and peri-implant diseases (Javed et al. 2019). Several studies have shown that tobacco smoking increases the risk of periodontitis as well as peri-implantitis in susceptible patient populations (Caggiano et al. 2022; Ford and Rich 2021; Jepsen et al. 2018; Ramôa et al. 2017; Sgolastra et al. 2015). According to a cross-sectional observational study (Akram et al. 2018), habitual use of ST products increases the risk of peri-implant soft tissue inflammation thereby increasing peri-implant probing depths and gingival redness. This condition is called "peri-implant mucositis", which is comparable to gingivitis in natural dentition. If left untreated in a timely manner, peri-implant inflammation augments to compromise peri-implant osseous tissues causing crestal bone loss (CBL). To date, there is only one study published in indexed databases that has shown that habitual use of ST products enhances the risk of peri-implant diseases in vulnerable populations (Akram et al. 2018). Moreover, results by Akram et al. (2018) showed that the scores of peri-implant inflammatory parameters (modified plaque and bleeding indices, peri-implant PD and CBL) are significantly higher in individuals using combustible and non-combustible nicotinic products compared to individuals not using any form of tobacco product (Table 5.5). Since *shammah* use is a risk factor of periodontitis, it is hypothesized that the risk of peri-implant diseases (peri-implant mucositis and peri-implantitis) is higher among patients using

Table 5.5 Comparison of peri-implant clinical and radiographic status among smokeless tobacco-chewers, cigarette-smokers, and controls

Implant-related parameters	Smokeless-tobacco-chewers	Cigarette-smokers	Controls
Participants (*n*)	44 Males	42 Males	45 Males
Number of implants (*n*)	56 Implants	51 Implants	66 Implants
Mean age in years	44.6 ± 4.9 years	47.8 ± 6.1 years	46.2 ± 5.7 years
Modified plaque index (% of sites)	61.7%*	64.2%*	32.6%
Modified bleeding index (% of sites)	54.7%*	22.8%*	39.9%
Probing depth > 4 mm (% of sites)	6.2%*	5.9%*	4.8%
Crestal bone loss (mesial) (in mm)	4.8 ± 0.6 mm*	4.1 ± 0.3 mm*	2.4 ± 0.5 mm
Crestal bone loss (distal) (in mm)	5.3 ± 1.1 mm*	4.6 ± 0.4 mm*	2.3 ± 0.3 mm

Modified from the study by Akram et al. (2018)
Controls: Individuals not using any form of nicotinic product
*Compared with controls ($P < 0.05$)

this form of ST product. Moreover, it is also hypothesized that the outcome of peri-implant therapeutic interventions, such as mechanical debridement of infected peri-implant tissues, is compromised in shammah users, possibly due to the detrimental effects of nicotine and its related aldehydes on wound healing. Further well-designed and power-adjusted studies are needed to test these hypotheses.

Key Points

- Peri-implant tissues are vulnerable to inflammation, much like periodontal tissues around natural teeth, with peri-implant mucositis and peri-implantitis sharing similar causes and risk factors.
- Tobacco use, including ST such as *shammah*, is a significant risk factor for both periodontal and peri-implant diseases, increasing inflammation, probing depths, and bone loss.
- It is hypothesized that *shammah* users may experience poorer therapeutic outcomes for peri-implant disease due to nicotine's negative effects on wound healing, highlighting the need for more focused research in this area.

5.4 Recommendations

Despite its health risks, *shammah* remains culturally ingrained in many communities, often used socially or as a habit-forming practice. Public health efforts in regions where *shammah* is prevalent aim to raise awareness of its dangers and promote cessation programmes to reduce its usage. Given the challenges in managing periodontal and possibly peri-implant inflammatory conditions among *shammah* users, it is crucial to implement targeted public health interventions. These should include raising awareness about the detrimental effects of *shammah* use on oral health and promoting cessation programmes tailored to this population. *Shammah* users should be taught effective oral hygiene measures. Additionally, healthcare providers should adopt specialized periodontal treatment protocols to address the unique needs of *shammah* users, focusing on enhancing wound healing and improving overall periodontal outcomes. Further research is essential to explore innovative therapeutic strategies for managing periodontitis effectively in these individuals.

Key Points

- Despite known health risks, *shammah* use remains widespread due to cultural and social practices.
- Regions with high *shammah* usage need focused public health campaigns to raise awareness and encourage cessation.
- Tailored cessation programmes and oral hygiene education are essential for managing the oral health of *shammah* users.
- Healthcare providers should implement customized periodontal treatment strategies to improve outcomes in this population.

References

Akram Z, Vohra F, Bukhari IA, Sheikh SA, Javed F (2018) Clinical and radiographic peri-implant parameters and proinflammatory cytokine levels among cigarette smokers, smokeless tobacco users, and nontobacco users. Clin Implant Dent Relat Res 20:76–81

Al Agili DE, Park HK (2013) Oral health status of male adolescent smokeless tobacco users in Saudi Arabia. East Mediterr Health J 19:711–719

Al-Askar M, Abduljabbar T, Vohra F, Pasumarthy S, Gholamiazizi E, Yunker M, Romanos GE et al (2017) Comparison of self-perceived oral symptoms and periodontal parameters among habitual shamma-chewers, gutka-chewers, and non-chewers. Quintessence Int 48:251–260

Allard WF, DeVol EB, Te OB (1999) Smokeless tobacco (shamma) and oral cancer in Saudi Arabia. Community Dent Oral Epidemiol 27:398–405

Alsanosy RM (2014) Smokeless tobacco (shammah) in Saudi Arabia: a review of its pattern of use, prevalence, and potential role in oral cancer. Asian Pac J Cancer Prev 15:6477–6483

Bakdash A (2017) Shammah (smokeless tobacco) and public health. Asian Pac J Cancer Prev 18:1183–1190

Caggiano M, Gasparro R, D'Ambrosio F, Pisano M, Di Palo MP, Contaldo M (2022) Smoking cessation on periodontal and peri-implant health status: a systematic review. Dent J (Basel) 10:162

Chiapasco M, Tommasato G, Palombo D, Del Fabbro M (2020) A retrospective 10-year mean follow-up of implants placed in ridges grafted using autogenous mandibular blocks covered with bovine bone mineral and collagen membrane. Clin Oral Implants Res 31:328–340

Cobb CM, Sottosanti JS (2021) A re-evaluation of scaling and root planing. J Periodontol 92:1370–1378

Ford PJ, Rich AM (2021) Tobacco use and Oral health. Addiction 116:3531–3540

Hazarey V, Desai K (2025) Description of smokeless tobacco products, their chemical composition and practices. In: Javed F, Warnakulasuriya S (eds) Smokeless tobacco and its effects on periodontal health. Springer, Cham

Howe MS, Keys W, Richards D (2019) Long-term (10-year) dental implant survival: a systematic review and sensitivity meta-analysis. J Dent 84:9–21

Ivanovski S, Lee R (2018) Comparison of peri-implant and periodontal marginal soft tissues in health and disease. Periodontology 2000 76:116–130

Javed F, Rahman I, Romanos GE (2019) Tobacco-product usage as a risk factor for dental implants. Periodontology 2000 81:48–56

Jepsen S, Caton JG, Albandar JM, Bissada NF, Bouchard P, Cortellini P, Demirel K et al (2018) Periodontal manifestations of systemic diseases and developmental and acquired conditions: consensus report of workgroup 3 of the 2017 world workshop on the classification of periodontal and peri-implant diseases and conditions. J Periodontol 89(Suppl 1):S237–s248

Kwon T, Lamster IB, Levin L (2021) Current concepts in the management of periodontitis. Int Dent J 71:462–476

Lacarbonara M, Cazzolla AP, Lacarbonara V, Lo Muzio L, Ciavarella D, Testa NF, Crincoli V et al (2022) Prosthetic rehabilitation of maxillary lateral incisors agenesis using dental mini-implants: a multicenter 10-year follow-up. Clin Oral Investig 26:1963–1974

Ramôa CP, Eissenberg T, Sahingur SE (2017) Increasing popularity of waterpipe tobacco smoking and electronic cigarette use: implications for oral healthcare. J Periodontal Res 52:813–823

Robitaille N, Reed DN, Walters JD, Kumar PS (2016) Periodontal and peri-implant diseases: identical or fraternal infections? Mol Oral Microbiol 31:285–301

Scheifele C, Nassar A, Reichart PA (2007) Prevalence of oral cancer and potentially malignant lesions among shammah users in Yemen. Oral Oncol 43:42–50

Sgolastra F, Petrucci A, Severino M, Gatto R, Monaco A (2015) Smoking and the risk of peri-implantitis. A systematic review and meta-analysis. Clin Oral Implants Res 26:e62–e67

Smiley CJ, Tracy SL, Abt E, Michalowicz BS, John MT, Gunsolley J, Cobb CM et al (2015) Systematic review and meta-analysis on the nonsurgical treatment of chronic periodontitis by means of scaling and root planing with or without adjuncts. J Am Dent Assoc 146:508–524.e505

Vohra F, Bukhari IA, Sheikh SA, Albaijan R, Naseem M, Hussain M (2020) Effectiveness of scaling and root planing with and without adjunct probiotic therapy in the treatment of chronic periodontitis among shamma users and non-users: a randomized controlled trial. J Periodontol 91:1177–1185

Effect of Naswar on Periodontal Health

6

Muhammad Saad Shaikh and Fawad Javed

Abbreviations

BoP	Bleeding on probing
CAL	Clinical attachment loss
CTX	C-terminal telopeptide of type I collagen
ELISA	Enzyme-linked immunosorbent assay
GCF	Gingival crevicular fluid
ICTP	Carboxyterminal telopeptide of type I collagen
IL	Interleukin
MBL	Marginal bone loss
PD	Probing depth
PI	Plaque index
ROS	Reactive oxygen species
ST	Smokeless tobacco
TAC	Total antioxidant capacity
TOS	Total oxidant status
TNF-α	Tumour necrosis factor-alpha
UWS	Unstimulated whole saliva

M. S. Shaikh
Department of Oral Biology, Sindh Institute of Oral Health Sciences, Jinnah Sindh Medical University, Karachi, Pakistan

F. Javed (✉)
Department of Orthodontics and Dentofacial Orthopedics, Eastman Institute for Oral Health, University of Rochester, Rochester, NY, USA
e-mail: fawad_javed@urmc.rochester.edu

F. Javed, S. Warnakulasuriya (eds.), *Smokeless Tobacco and its Effects on Periodontal Health*, https://doi.org/10.1007/978-3-032-16409-4_6

Learning Goals

- Understand the composition and common usage patterns of naswar.
- Differentiate naswar from other forms of smokeless tobacco products.
- Describe the chemical properties of naswar, including its pH and nicotine content, and their biological implications.
- Describe the clinical effects of naswar on periodontal tissues.
- Interpret evidence from cross-sectional studies on naswar and periodontal health.
- Explain the role of collagen degradation biomarkers (CTX and ICTP) as indicators of periodontal tissue destruction in naswar users.
- Analyze salivary inflammatory biomarkers linked to naswar use.
- Recognize socio-behavioural contributors to periodontal disease among naswar users.
- Evaluate the potential impact of naswar on peri-implant health.
- Understand the regulatory gaps related to naswar sales and usage.
- Analyse sociodemographic and behavioural factors (e.g., education, hygiene practices, stress) that influence naswar use and periodontal health.
- Assess the need for public health interventions.
- Comprehend the role of oxidative stress in periodontal destruction.
- Identify regulatory gaps in naswar control policies, including packaging, labelling, taxation, and vendor compliance.
- Promote the concept of naswar as a modifiable risk factor for periodontal and potentially peri-implant diseases, advocating for clinical screening and patient education.
- Propose future research directions, such as microbiome studies and longitudinal clinical trials, to further understand the effects of naswar on oral health.

6.1 Introduction

In contrast to conventional combustible tobacco products such as cigarettes, pipes, cigars, and waterpipes, smokeless tobacco (ST) encompasses a broad category of non-combusted tobacco products that are commonly chewed and less often inhaled (Tomar et al. 2019). It is estimated that approximately 356 million individuals worldwide habitually use ST products (Gupta et al. 2011; Mehrotra et al. 2019; Rumgay et al. 2024). Habitual ST use poses a significant global public health concern due to its significant association with oral and systemic diseases, including periodontitis, oral precancer and cancer, and gastrointestinal carcinoma (Chaturvedi et al. 2013; Javed et al. 2010; Vaishnav et al. 2025).

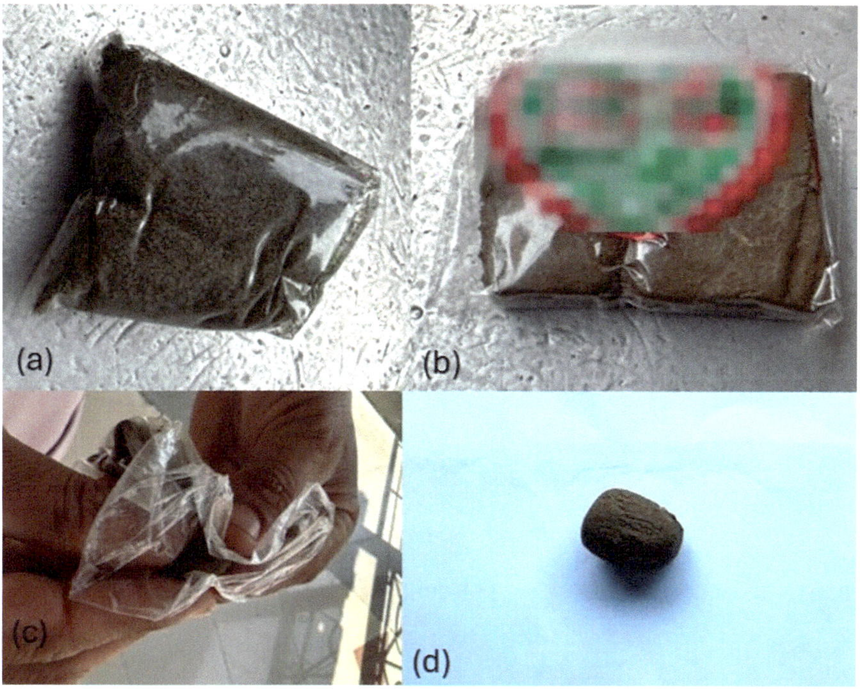

Fig. 6.1 (**a**) Non-branded green naswar; (**b**) branded brown naswar; (**c**) user shaping naswar into a small "ball shape" using the thumb and index fingers. (**d**) A prepared small ball of naswar ready for oral use (commonly placed in the mandibular labial sulcus or the labial sulcus opposing mandibular premolars)

Naswar (also known as niswaar and niswar) is a form of a moist non-chewable ST product commonly used in South and Central Asia, particularly in countries such as Afghanistan, Iran, Pakistan, and parts of India (Amirzada et al. 2024; Jayant and Deo 1986; Khan et al. 2019; Mehra et al. 2020). Naswar typically consists of sun-dried, powdered tobacco mixed with slaked lime, wood ash, and various flavouring agents such as cardamom or menthol (Saeed et al. 2024). Naswar use is more common in males than females (Abbasi et al. 2019; Rahim et al. 2022). Naswar is commercially sold in branded and non-branded plastic bags or sachets with each packet weighing around 45 g on average (Khan et al. 2017; Saeed et al. 2012). Naswar is extracted from its pouch and rolled into a "ball-shape" and is commonly placed inside the lower labial sulcus and sometimes on the floor of the mouth and held for prolonged durations (15–30 min) (Fig. 6.1a–d) (Akram et al. 2018). This allows nicotine and other chemicals to be absorbed through the oral mucosa into the bloodstream (Akram et al. 2018; Saeed et al. 2012). Table 6.1 summarizes the general characteristics of various naswar types commercially available across Pakistan (Saeed et al. 2024).

Table 6.1 General characteristics of various naswar brands commercially available in Pakistan

Brand[a]	City in Pakistan	Brand in use since the year	Estimated price in PKR[b]	Chief ingredients	pH	Ash (%)
Brand 1	Kohat	1995	PKR 20.00	Tobacco leaves Wood ash Slaked lime Flavourings such as cardamom and menthol	8.14	10.9
Brand 2	Kohat	1997	PKR 20.00	Tobacco leaves Wood ash Slaked lime Flavourings such as cardamom and menthol	8.73	16
Brand 3	Peshawar	1997	PKR 20.00	Tobacco leaves Wood ash Slaked lime	8.7	16.4
Brand 4	Mardan	1998	PKR 20.00	Tobacco leaves Wood ash Slaked lime Flavourings such as cardamom and menthol	8.7	32.4
Brand 5	Bannu	1999	PKR 20.00	Tobacco leaves Wood ash Slaked lime Flavourings such as cardamom and menthol	8.3	16.2
Brand 6	Swat	2000	PKR 10.00	Tobacco leaves Wood ash Slaked lime Flavourings such as cardamom and menthol	8.8	10.5
Brand 7	Mansehra	2000	PKR 10.00	Tobacco leaves Wood ash Slaked lime Flavourings such as cardamom and menthol	8.9	21.1
Brand 8	Dera Ismail Khan	2003	PKR 10.00	Tobacco leaves Wood ash Slaked lime Flavourings such as cardamom and menthol	8.5	26.4

Modified from Saeed et al. (2024)

[a]To maintain objectivity, the exact brand name of the naswar product has been anonymized

[b]As of April 18, 2025, one Pakistani Rupee (PKR) is equivalent to 0.0036 US Dollars (Source: www.exchange-rates.org)

Key Points

- Naswar is a moist, non-chewable form of smokeless tobacco (ST), predominantly used in South and Central Asia, particularly in countries like Pakistan, Afghanistan, and Iran.
- Chemical composition of naswar includes sun-dried powdered tobacco, slaked lime, wood ash, and flavourings like cardamom or menthol, contributing to its cytotoxic potential.
- Naswar is commonly placed in the lower labial sulcus for 15–30 min, facilitating the absorption of nicotine and other harmful substances through the oral mucosa into the bloodstream.
- Naswar use is more prevalent among males and is sold in branded or non-branded plastic sachets, each typically weighing around 45 g.

6.1.1 Composition of Naswar

The chief chemical in naswar (pH ranging from 8.5 to 9) is nicotine (approximately 15 mg/g) (Saeed et al. 2024). Other chemicals identified in naswar include carboxylic (cotinine, norcotinine, 1,3-Diethylurea) and polyaromatic (benzoic acid, 2-ethylhexyl ester, Benzene, 4-ethyl-1,2-dimethyl-), naphthalene, undecane, and tridecane (Saeed et al. 2024). It has also been reported that naswar contains traces of metals, including lead, arsenic, nickel, cobalt, chromium, cadmium, and nitrate, which are linked to oral inflammatory conditions, including periodontitis and cancer (Foulds et al. 2003; Saeed et al. 2012, 2024; Ullah et al. 2017).

Key Points

- The chief component in Naswar is nicotine.
- Naswar contains traces of metals, including lead, arsenic, nickel, cobalt, chromium, cadmium, and nitrate.
- Constituents of naswar are linked to oral inflammatory conditions, including periodontitis and cancer.

6.2 Objective

The objective of this chapter is to provide an overview of studies that assessed the effect of naswar on periodontal health.

6.3 Effects of Naswar on Periodontal Health

6.3.1 Effect on Clinical Status of Periodontal Soft and Osseous Tissues

A limited number of studies published in indexed databases have assessed the effects of naswar on periodontal soft and osseous tissues (Abbasi et al. 2019; Akram et al. 2018; Al-Hamoudi et al. 2018; Daood et al. 2018; Muhammad et al. 2021; Rahim et al. 2022). In a cross-sectional observational study, Rahim et al. (2022) assessed the severity of periodontal clinical parameters (plaque index [PI], bleeding on probing [BoP], probing depth [PD], and clinical attachment loss [CAL]) among 100 naswar users and 100 non-users (controls). All participants were male with a mean age of 38.4 ± 8.2 years. Sixty-eight percent of individuals reported that they had been using naswar for the past decade, 22% had been using this ST product for 11–21 years, and the remaining 10% had been using naswar for over 21 years. Scores of PI and percentages of sites that demonstrated BoP were significantly higher among naswar-dippers than controls ($P < 0.001$) (Rahim et al. 2022). Scores of CAL and PD were higher among naswar users than controls ($P < 0.001$) (Rahim et al. 2022) (Table 6.2). The study also found a significant association between the severity of periodontal parameters and the amount of naswar consumed daily (Fig. 6.2). Likewise, results from another cross-sectional analytical investigation on 84 male participants (42 naswar users and 42 non-users) showed that sites demonstrating PD of 4 and 5–6 mm and CAL were significantly higher among naswar users than non-users ($P < 0.05$) (Abbasi et al. 2019). However, this study showed no significant difference in scores of PI, BoP, and number of missing teeth among naswar users and non-users (Abbasi et al. 2019). The mean age of participants was not reported in the study by Abbasi et al. (2019); however, their age ranged between 18 and 50 years. Similar results were reported in another study (Daood et al. 2018) (Table 6.2).

Key Points

- Multiple studies have shown that naswar users exhibit significantly higher scores of probing depth and clinical attachment loss compared to non-users, indicating more severe periodontal breakdown.
- Rahim et al. (2022) reported significantly elevated plaque index and bleeding on probing in naswar users versus controls, reflecting poor oral hygiene and ongoing inflammation.
- The severity of periodontal damage was positively correlated with the duration and daily frequency of naswar use, suggesting a dose-dependent effect on periodontal health (Rahim et al. 2022).
- Abbasi et al. (2019) found no significant differences in plaque index and bleeding on probing scores between naswar users and non-users, indicating variability in clinical outcomes across studies.
- Despite methodological differences, findings from Daood et al. (2018) and others consistently support the association between naswar use and worsened periodontal clinical parameters.

Table 6.2 Overview of cross-sectional observational studies that assessed the effect of naswar use on periodontal soft and osseous tissues

Authors et al. (year)	Mean age	Gender	Study groups	Duration of ST use (in years)	Daily frequency of ST use	Results
Rahim et al. (2022)	38.4 ± 8.2 years	200 Males	100 Naswar users 100 Non-users/ controls	≤10 years: 68% of users 11–21 years: 22% of users ≥21 years: 10% of users	5–10 times/day: 15% of users 11–20 times/day: 65% of users 21–30 times/day: 20% of users	PI was higher in naswar users (2.35 ± 0.45) than in controls (1.78 ± 0.38) ($P < 0.001$) BoP was higher in naswar users (62.5%) than in controls (38.2%) ($P < 0.001$) CAL was higher in naswar-dippers (3.9 ± 0.7 mm) than in controls (2.5 ± 0.5 mm) ($P < 0.001$) PD was higher in naswar-dippers (4.1 ± 0.8 mm) than in controls (2.9 ± 0.6 mm) ($P < 0.001$)
Abbasi et al. (2019)	Naswar users: 33.7 ± 10.8 years Non-users: 36.4 ± 4.9 years	84 Males	42 Naswar users 42 Non-users/ controls	12.8 ± 8.1 years	20.3 ± 10.6 times per day	No difference in the percentages of sites that displayed plaque among naswar users (3.1%) and non-users (2.6%) Sites displaying BoP were higher in naswar users (56.6 ± 9.3%) than in controls (28.5 ± 5.7%) ($P < 0.001$) Mean CAL was higher among naswar users (2.9 mm) than controls (2.1 mm) ($P < 0.001$)
Al-Hamoudi et al. (2018)	Naswar users: 34.9 years (28–42 years) Non-users: 35.2 years (25–43 years)	142 Males	72 Naswar users 70 Non-users/ controls	16.1 years (8–29 years)	7.3 times daily (2–12 times)	Percentages of sites that displayed plaque were higher in naswar users (54.2%) than in controls (22.4%) ($P < 0.01$) Percentages of sites that displayed BoP were higher in naswar users (57.8%) than in controls (8.2%) ($P < 0.01$) Percentages of sites that displayed PD of 4–6 mm were higher in naswar users (29.7%) than in controls (6.3%) ($P < 0.01$) Percentages of sites that displayed PD > 6 mm were higher in naswar users (20.4%) than in controls (2.7%) ($P < 0.01$) Mean CAL was higher in naswar users (4.2 mm) than in controls (0.9 mm) ($P < 0.01$) Mean MBL was higher in naswar users (4.9 mm) than controls (1.85 mm) ($P < 0.01$)

(continued)

Table 6.2 (continued)

Authors et al. (year)	Mean age	Gender	Study groups	Duration of ST use (in years)	Daily frequency of ST use	Results
Daood et al. (2018)	Naswar users: 34.9 years Non-users: 35.2 years	87 Males	42 Naswar users 45 Non-users/ controls	12.3 ± 3.4 years	8.5 times/day	Percentages of sites that displayed plaque were higher in naswar users (54.2%) than in controls (22.4%) ($P < 0.01$) Percentages of sites that displayed BoP were higher in naswar users (57.8%) than in controls (8.2%) ($P < 0.01$) Percentages of sites that displayed PD of 4–6 mm were higher in naswar users (29.7%) than in controls (6.3%) ($P < 0.01$) Percentages of sites that displayed PD of >6 mm were higher in naswar users (20.4%) than in controls (2.7%) ($P < 0.01$) Mean CAL was higher in naswar users (4.2 mm) than controls (0.9 mm) ($P < 0.01$) Mean MBL was higher in naswar users (4.9 mm) than controls (1.8 mm) ($P < 0.01$)

BoP bleeding on probing, *CAL* clinical attachment loss, *MBL* marginal bone loss, *NR* not reported, *PD* probing depth, *PI* plaque index, *ST* smokeless tobacco

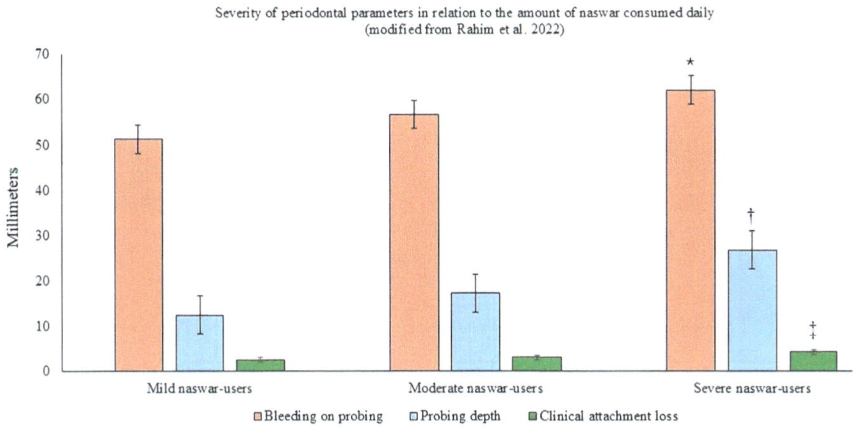

Fig. 6.2 Severity of periodontal parameters in relation to the amount of naswar consumed daily (Modified from the study by Rahim et al. (2022)). *Compared with moderate naswar users ($P < 0.001$) and mild-naswar users ($P < 0.001$); †compared with moderate naswar users ($P < 0.001$) and mild-naswar users ($P < 0.001$); ‡compared with moderate naswar users ($P < 0.001$) and mild-naswar users ($P < 0.001$). Mild users: up to half a packet per day (approx. <23 g); moderate users: up to one packet per day (up to 45 g); and severe users: one to two packets per day (45–90 g)

A split-mouth cross-sectional study (Akram et al. 2018) assessed the clinical and radiographic periodontal inflammatory parameters among 72 self-reported naswar users and 75 individuals chewing a different type of ST product (gutka). There were no controls (individuals not using any nicotinic product) in this study (Akram et al. 2018). The mean ages of naswar users and gutka-chewers were 47.3 ± 2.8 and 45.2 ± 0.8 years, respectively. In this study (Akram et al. 2018), scores of PI, BoP, PD, CAL, and marginal bone loss (MBL) were compared among the test-side (side where the ST product was placed) and the opposing control-side (sites where naswar or gutka were never placed). The results showed that scores of PI ($P < 0.05$), BoP ($P < 0.05$), PD ($P < 0.05$), CAL ($P < 0.05$), and MBL ($P < 0.05$) were significantly higher in the test compared with the control sides among naswar users and gutka-chewers. There was no difference in the severity of clinical and radiographic periodontal inflammatory parameters among naswar users and gutka-chewers (Akram et al. 2018) (Fig. 6.3a, b). This implies that both types of ST products (naswar and gutka) are similarly detrimental to periodontal health when placed habitually in the oral vestibule. This indicates localized periodontal inflammation and tissue destruction is closely associated with the habitual placement of ST products in the oral cavity.

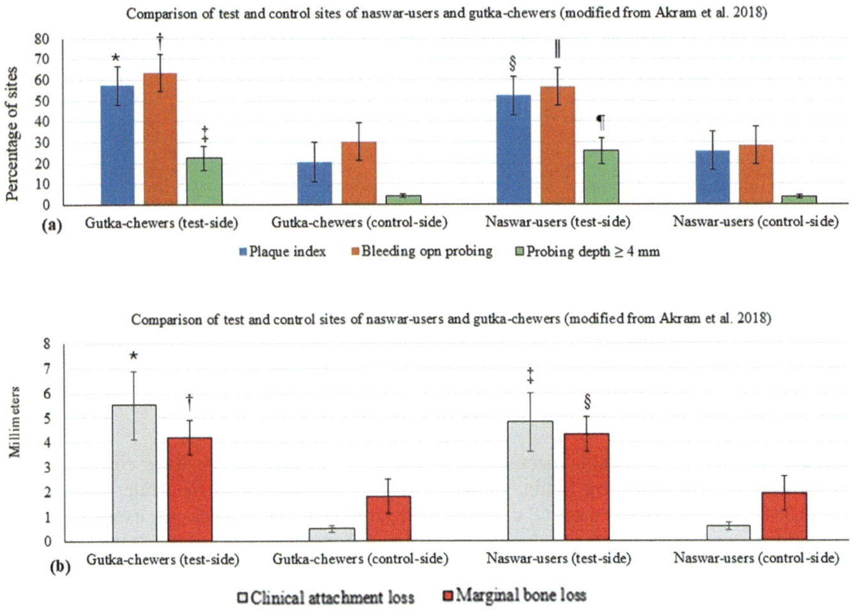

Fig. 6.3 Comparison of clinical periodontal parameters among the test and control-sides among gutka-chewers and naswar users (Modified from the study by Akram et al. (2018)). Test-side: buccal/labial sulcus in which gutka/naswar was placed; control-side: opposing buccal/labial sulcus in which gutka/naswar was never placed. (**a**) *Compared with plaque index on the control-side among gutka-chewers ($P < 0.05$); †compared with bleeding on probing on the control-side among gutka-chewers ($P < 0.05$); ‡compared with the percentage of sites that had probing depths of at least 4 mm on the control side among gutka-chewers ($P < 0.05$); §compared with plaque index on the control-side among naswar users ($P < 0.05$); ‖compared with bleeding on probing on the control-side among naswar users ($P < 0.05$); ¶compared with the percentage of sites that had probing depths of at least 4 mm on the control side among naswar users ($P < 0.05$). (**b**) *Compared with clinical attachment loss on the control-side among gutka-chewers ($P < 0.05$); †compared with marginal bone loss on the control-side among gutka-chewers ($P < 0.05$); ‡compared with clinical attachment loss on the control-side among naswar users ($P < 0.05$); §compared with marginal bone loss on the control side among naswar users ($P < 0.05$)

Key Points (Akram et al. 2018)

- A split-mouth cross-sectional study was conducted on 72 naswar users and 75 gutka-chewers to assess the localized periodontal effects of ST use.
- Clinical (PI, BoP, PD, CAL) and radiographic (MBL) parameters were compared between the test-side (where the ST product was placed) and the contralateral control-side (not exposed to ST) within the same individual.
- All periodontal parameters—plaque index, bleeding on probing, probing depth, clinical attachment loss, and marginal bone loss—were significantly higher on the test-side compared to the control-side ($P < 0.05$) in both user groups.

- No significant difference in periodontal destruction was observed between naswar users and gutka-chewers, indicating both products are equally harmful.
- Habitual placement of ST products in the oral vestibule leads to localized periodontal inflammation and tissue destruction, regardless of the ST type.

6.3.2 Overview of Laboratory-Based Investigations That Assessed the Inflammatory Effect of Naswar

6.3.2.1 Expression of Proinflammatory Cytokines in Unstimulated Whole Saliva

Unstimulated whole saliva (UWS) is a complex biological fluid that has been labelled as a "valuable tool" for assessing the oral inflammatory response, particularly among individuals using nicotinic products (Javed et al. 2014, 2015a, b). A limited number of studies have investigated the whole salivary immunoinflammatory response among naswar users and non-users (Abbasi et al. 2019; Sohail et al. 2020).

Interleukin 1-beta (IL-1β) is a proinflammatory cytokine produced primarily by activated macrophages and neutrophils in response to microbial stimuli. It plays a central role in the host immune response by promoting inflammation, tissue destruction, and bone resorption. Studies have linked whole salivary IL-1β expression with the aetiopathogenesis of periodontal diseases such as periodontitis (Gomes et al. 2023; Isaza-Guzmán et al. 2016; Javed et al. 2015b). In the study by Abbasi et al. (2019), whole salivary IL-1β levels were assessed among naswar users and non-users using enzyme-linked immunosorbent assay (ELISA). The results showed that whole salivary IL-1β levels were significantly elevated among naswar users (8.3 ± 3.1 ng/mL) compared with non-users (2.3 ± 1.1 ng/mL) ($P < 0.05$). Moreover, results based on linear regression analysis showed a statistically significant correlation between IL-1β levels and clinical periodontal parameters (PD [4 mm and 4-6 mm], CAL, PI, and BoP) ($P < 0.01$) (Abbasi et al. 2019). The authors proposed that prolonged exposure to the hazardous constituents of naswar increases gingival inflammation (clinically manifested as increased PD and CAL), which increases the expression of destructive inflammatory cytokines (such as IL-1β), thereby worsening periodontal inflammation in vulnerable individuals (Abbasi et al. 2019).

Interleukin-8 (IL-8) is a chemokine produced by various cells, including gingival epithelial cells, fibroblasts, and macrophages, in response to microbial stimulation and tissue injury (Dongari-Bagtzoglou and Ebersole 1998). It plays a pivotal role in the innate immune response by acting as a potent chemoattractant and activator of neutrophils, guiding their migration to sites of infection and inflammation (Fredriksson et al. 2002). In the context of periodontal disease, IL-8 is significantly upregulated in response to bacterial pathogens such as *Porphyromonas gingivalis* and *Aggregatibacter actinomycetemcomitans* (Ahlstrand et al. 2019; Gasmi Benahmed et al. 2022). Sohail et al. (2020) assessed the whole salivary IL-8 levels among 30 naswar users and controls (n = 30) using the ELISA technique. The results showed that whole salivary IL-8 levels were significantly higher among naswar users (73.48 ± 46.52 pg/mL) than controls (33.39 ± 22.44 pg/mL) ($P < 0.001$) (Sohail et al. 2020). These results demonstrate that habitual naswar use is associated with an elevated inflammatory response in the oral cavity, specifically linked to periodontal disease.

Tumour necrosis factor-alpha (TNF-α) is a proinflammatory cytokine that has been reported to exhibit elevated levels in the whole saliva of naswar users and has been associated with the early detection of oral cancer in these individuals (Muhammad et al. 2021). However, to date, no studies have specifically investigated salivary or gingival crevicular fluid (GCF) levels of TNF-α in relation to periodontal diseases among naswar users and non-users. It is hypothesized that naswar users exhibit higher concentrations of TNF-α in both saliva and GCF compared to non-users. Further well-designed and power-adjusted studies are warranted to evaluate this hypothesis and to elucidate the potential role of TNF-α as a biomarker for periodontal inflammation in individuals who use naswar.

Key Points

- Unstimulated whole saliva (UWS) is a valuable diagnostic tool for assessing periodontal disease.
- Studies have shown significantly higher levels of IL-1β in the UWS of naswar users than non-users.
- Elevated salivary IL-1β levels in naswar users significantly correlate with clinical signs of periodontal disease, such as probing depth, clinical attachment loss, plaque index, and bleeding on probing.
- IL-8, a neutrophil chemoattractant, is significantly upregulated in naswar users, suggesting a strong innate immune response contributing to periodontal disease.
- While elevated salivary TNF-α levels have been reported in naswar users, their specific association with periodontal disease remains under-investigated.

6.3.2.2 Collagen Degradation

Collagen plays a fundamental role in the structural integrity and maintenance of periodontal tissues, particularly within the gingival connective tissue and periodontal ligament. During the progression of periodontal disease, the degradation of type I collagen, a principal component of the extracellular matrix, serves as a hallmark of active tissue destruction. Two key biomarkers indicative of collagen breakdown are the C-terminal telopeptide of type I collagen (CTX) and the cross-linked carboxyterminal telopeptide of type I collagen (ICTP). These degradation products, when detected in oral fluids such as UWS and GCF reflect ongoing collagenolytic activity and have been used as biochemical indicators of periodontal tissue destruction. Daood et al. (2018) assessed the whole salivary levels of CTX and ICTP among 42 habitual naswar users and 45 systemically healthy non-users. The results demonstrated that naswar users exhibited significantly higher levels of both CTX (176.34 ± 63.22 pg/mL) and ICTP (6.48 ± 2.89 ng/mL) in whole saliva compared to non-users, who presented with CTX levels of 109.83 ± 51.39 pg/mL and ICTP levels of 3.44 ± 1.61 ng/mL ($P < 0.001$) (Daood et al. 2018). The micro-Raman-spectroscopy-based results showed that the rates of CTX and ICTP release were significantly higher among naswar users than non-users ($P < 0.05$) (Daood et al. 2018). These elevated biomarker levels among naswar users were correlated with significantly worse clinical (CAL and PD) and radiographic periodontal outcomes (MBL). These findings suggest that habitual naswar use is associated with heightened collagen degradation activity, indicating more extensive periodontal tissue destruction and highlighting the potential of CTX and ICTP as non-invasive salivary biomarkers for monitoring periodontal disease in smokeless tobacco users.

Key Points

- Degradation of type I collagen is a hallmark of active periodontal tissue destruction.
- CTX (C-terminal telopeptide of type I collagen) and ICTP (cross-linked carboxyterminal telopeptide of type I collagen) are key biochemical markers that indicate collagen degradation and periodontal destruction.
- Habitual naswar users show significantly higher salivary levels of CTX and ICTP compared to non-users.
- Elevated levels of CTX and ICTP among naswar users correlate with worse periodontal clinical and radiographic outcomes.

6.3.2.3 Oxidative Stress Imbalance

Oxidative stress (OS) plays a pivotal role in the pathogenesis of periodontal disease, characterized by an imbalance between the production of reactive oxygen species (ROS) and the body's antioxidant defences (Chen et al. 2019; Levy 2015). This imbalance leads to tissue damage, inflammation, and the progression of periodontal disease (Chen et al. 2019). A case control study from Pakistan investigated the impact of habitual naswar use on salivary OS markers and antioxidant capacity (Ahmad et al. 2023). This study was performed on 84 individuals (42 naswar users and 42 age-matched healthy non-users) (Ahmad et al. 2023). The results showed that naswar users had significantly higher mean salivary pH and flow rate than non-users, with values of 7.7 and 0.71 mL/min, respectively, versus 6.95 and 0.52 mL/min in non-users ($P < 0.001$). While the differences in total oxidant status (TOS) and total antioxidant capacity (TAC) among the two groups were not statistically significant, naswar users tended to exhibit a higher mean TOS (51.6 ± 42 μmol/L) and a slightly lower TAC (0.55 ± 0.18 mmol/L) than non-users (TOS: 45.5 ± 38.2 μmol/L; TAC: 0.57 ± 0.17 mmol/L). Moreover, correlation analysis demonstrated a strong positive association between decayed-missing-and-filled teeth scores and the duration of naswar use ($r = 0.796$, $P < 0.001$), as well as a moderate correlation with the daily frequency of use ($r = 0.515$, $P < 0.001$). These results suggest that naswar use enhances OS while diminishing the antioxidant defence system in the oral cavity, potentially contributing to the development and progression of periodontal disease.

Key Points

- Habitual naswar users exhibit significantly higher salivary pH and flow rate compared to non-users.
- Naswar users tend to have higher total oxidant status (TOS) and slightly lower total antioxidant capacity (TAC), suggesting a trend towards increased oxidative stress.
- Naswar use may contribute to periodontal disease by promoting oxidative stress and weakening the oral antioxidant defence system.

6.3.2.4 Sociodemographic Factors

Besides the biological factors contributing to the increased risk of periodontal disease among naswar users than non-users, psychosocial and behavioural determinants, including patient education, oral hygiene maintenance practices, and socioeconomic status also play critical roles in influencing the use of nicotinic products including naswar (Al-Hamoudi et al. 2018; Javed et al. 2007). Individuals with an underprivileged education status (including health literacy) are more likely to engage in high-risk behaviours, such as ST use, due to a lack of awareness about its detrimental effects on oral and systemic health (Jain et al. 2021; Petersen and Kwan 2011). Naswar is often perceived as a coping mechanism for psychological stress and anxiety, especially among populations facing social and economic hardship. In these settings, naswar is frequently marketed or believed to reduce stress and improve mood, making it an attractive option for individuals with few psychosocial support systems (Aslam et al. 2021; Kakde et al. 2012). It is worth mentioning that in the study by Akram et al. (2018), 75% of the naswar users reported that they used this ST product to manage "psychological stress", whereas the remaining provided no reason for using naswar.

In the study by Rahim et al. (2022), nearly 70% of the naswar users reported that they brushed their teeth once daily and 10% reported that they brushed teeth three times in 1 week. Similarly, in another study, nearly 80% of the naswar users reported that they brushed teeth once daily (Al-Hamoudi et al. 2018). In the study by Abbasi et al. (2019), nearly 60% of the naswar users were uneducated, and in the study by Al-Hamoudi et al. (2018), 15% of the naswar users had graduated from an institution. It is possible that disadvantaged educational and socioeconomic circumstances compel individuals to prioritize the acquisition of fundamental necessities, such as food, shelter, and income generation, over the maintenance of oral health. In the context of limited resources and competing daily survival demands, oral hygiene practices and routine dental care may be perceived not as essential components of general health, but rather as non-essential or privileged services, accessible primarily to those with economic stability and higher health literacy. This perspective reflects a broader systemic inequity wherein individuals from lower socioeconomic strata may lack both the knowledge and the means to engage in preventive oral health behaviours or seek timely dental interventions. Consequently, oral health is often relegated to a lower priority, increasing vulnerability to conditions such as periodontal disease, particularly in populations that also engage in high-risk habits like naswar use. Addressing these disparities requires a multifaceted public health approach that repositions oral healthcare as a basic human right and integrates it into primary health strategies targeting underserved communities.

Key Points

- Psychosocial and behavioural determinants, such as education, oral hygiene practices, and socioeconomic status significantly influence the higher prevalence of periodontal disease among naswar users.
- Individuals with limited education or health literacy are more likely to use ST products, including naswar, due to a lack of awareness about its harmful effects on oral and systemic health.
- Naswar is often used to cope with psychological stress and anxiety, particularly in economically disadvantaged populations lacking adequate psychosocial support.
- Naswar users generally maintain poor oral hygiene, with most brushing only once a day or even less frequently, which may contribute to periodontal issues.
- A significant proportion of naswar users are uneducated or undereducated, suggesting that limited access to education and economic hardship leads to deprioritizing oral health in favour of basic survival needs.
- Comprehensive public health strategies promoting oral health among underserved communities are required.

6.3.2.5 Alteration in Oral Microbiota

There is a notable lack of research specifically examining the composition and dynamics of the oral microbiota in naswar users, particularly in relation to subgingival biofilm samples collected from both users and non-users. Given the established role of the subgingival microbiome (such as the red complex bacteria) in periodontal disease pathogenesis, this represents a significant gap in the literature. Based on current evidence, it is hypothesized that the chronic inflammatory burden, when combined with poor oral hygiene practices and limited literacy commonly observed among naswar users, may contribute to the overgrowth of pathogenic bacterial species within the subgingival environment. It is further conjectured that these pathogenic microorganisms may be more prevalent in the periodontal pockets on the side of habitual naswar placement, likely due to prolonged local exposure to naswar constituents and mechanical irritation/trauma. However, these assumptions remain speculative, as empirical data from well-designed microbiome studies are currently unavailable. Thus, there is a compelling need for future investigations utilizing high-throughput sequencing technologies to characterize the oral microbiome profiles of naswar users compared to non-users, which may elucidate microbial pathways contributing to tobacco-related periodontal disease.

Key Points

- Chronic inflammation, poor oral hygiene, and limited literacy among naswar users may contribute to the proliferation of pathogenic subgingival bacteria.
- Pathogenic bacteria may be more prevalent in periodontal pockets on the side of habitual naswar placement, likely due to localized exposure and trauma.
- Existing hypotheses lack empirical support, as there are currently no well-designed microbiome studies addressing this issue in naswar users.

6.3.3 Hypothetical Effects of Habitual Naswar Use on Peri-implant Health

A vigilant review of indexed literature revealed no studies that investigated the effect of naswar on peri-implant tissues. Chronic exposure to naswar constituents, such as nicotine, slaked lime, heavy metals (e.g., arsenic, lead, cadmium), and ROS have been consistently associated with increased PD, CAL, BoP, MBL, and elevated inflammatory cytokine levels (such as IL-1β, IL-8, and TNF-α) in the periodontal sulci and tissues indicating a heightened local inflammatory state. Such proinflammatory cytokines are also contributors to peri-implant soft tissue inflammation (peri-implant mucositis) and crestal bone loss (peri-implantitis) (Javed et al. 2011). Moreover, an increased oxidative stress in periodontal tissues of naswar users has been linked with the aetiopathogenesis of periodontitis in these individuals (Ahmad et al. 2023). Similarly, it has been reported that OS in peri-implant tissues is a risk-factor for peri-implantitis (Sánchez-Siles et al. 2016). Such observations are compelling to suggest a connection between naswar use and peri-implant disease initiation/progression. Furthermore, as indicated in the literature, naswar users frequently demonstrate compromised oral hygiene practices and reduced access to dental care, often due to limited health literacy and socioeconomic constraints (Abbasi et al. 2019; Al-Hamoudi et al. 2018). These behavioural and social factors may compound the biological risks by enabling plaque accumulation and delaying the detection and management of peri-implant inflammation. Although there are currently no published studies specifically assessing the effects of naswar on peri-implant tissues, the overlapping pathological mechanisms observed in periodontal and peri-implant diseases suggest a rationale to suspect a similar detrimental effect of naswar on dental implants. Therefore, longitudinal and mechanistic clinical studies and laboratory-based investigations are warranted to evaluate the impact of naswar on peri-implant health and to confirm its role as a modifiable risk factor for peri-implant diseases.

Key Points

- Increased oxidative stress linked to naswar use may contribute to both periodontitis and peri-implantitis, indicating a potential shared aetiopathogenesis.
- Naswar users often exhibit poor oral hygiene and limited access to dental care due to lower health literacy and socioeconomic barriers, which can exacerbate peri-implant disease risk.
- No indexed studies have specifically investigated the impact of naswar use on peri-implant tissues.

6.3.4 Regulatory Gaps and Policy Recommendations for Naswar Control

Current tobacco control regulations in countries such as Pakistan are frequently not adhered to by ST (including naswar) vendors. Despite a general awareness among merchants regarding the harmful health effects associated with naswar use, many continue to violate laws that prohibit sales to minors and restrict promotional activities (Ahmad et al. 2020, 2022). Enhancing enforcement mechanisms and imposing stricter penalties for non-compliance may improve adherence to these regulatory frameworks. Moreover, naswar packaging often lacks adequate content disclosures and mandated health warnings, elements that are essential for informing consumers about the potential health hazards of product use. In alignment with the guidelines set forth by the World Health Organization's Framework Convention on Tobacco Control (FCTC), the inclusion of prominent and graphic health warnings on naswar packaging could serve to enhance public awareness and potentially deter its use (Ahmad et al. 2020; Saeed et al. 2012). It is notable that naswars' low market price (Table 6.1) also seems to contribute to its widespread accessibility, particularly among economically disadvantaged populations and minors. Adopting a taxation strategy similar to those implemented for other tobacco products such as cigarettes could decrease affordability and, in turn, reduce consumption (Khan et al. 2019; Ochani et al. 2022). Notably, several naswar vendors have expressed a willingness to transition to alternative forms of employment, provided that feasible and sustainable options are made available. Thus, government-led initiatives aimed at offering alternative livelihoods and economic incentives could play a pivotal role in curbing naswar production and distribution (Ahmad et al. 2021).

Key Points

- Many ST vendors, including those selling naswar, often violate regulations, especially those restricting sales to minors and promotional practices.
- Naswar products frequently lack proper content labelling and health warnings, which undermines consumer awareness.
- Implementing graphic health warnings, as recommended by the WHO FCTC, could help deter use.

6.3.4.1 Community-Based Anti-tobacco and Oral Health Promotion Campaigns

Cultural perceptions regarding the naswar consumption can be transformed by involving community leaders and influencers in awareness campaigns. It is critical to launch and promote public awareness campaigns on the detrimental effects of ST products (including naswar) on oral and systemic health. It has been reported that many ST product users are either uninformed or underinformed of these hazards. Consequently, routine and continuous educational initiatives in the form of health awareness campaigns may help lower the consumption of naswar in vulnerable populations (Kamal et al. 2023; Ochani et al. 2022). Targeted interventions in educational institutions and communities are required since naswar usage is more common among young people. These must highlight the probability of addiction and the long-term hazards of naswar (Ahmad et al. 2021; Basharat et al. 2012) on overall health. Programs for rehabilitation are yet another crucial element of these efforts. It is essential to establish detoxification centres for addiction treatment (Alam 2023, 2024). Such initiatives could also comprise support mechanisms for people trying to leave naswar consumption (Kamal et al. 2023).

Key Points

- Many users are unaware of the health risks of ST products including naswar.
- Involving community leaders and influencers in awareness campaigns can help shift cultural perceptions and reduce naswar consumption.
- Targeted programmes in educational institutions and communities are necessary to emphasize its addictive nature and long-term health risks associated with naswar use.
- Establishing detoxification centres and providing support mechanisms are essential for individuals seeking to overcome naswar addiction.

6.3.4.2 Role of the State

One of the most direct and potentially effective strategies to curtail naswar consumption is the implementation of a comprehensive governmental ban on its manufacture, distribution, and sale. By eliminating naswar from the commercial supply chain, such a ban would drastically limit public access to the product. However, realistically, enforcing such a ban presents significant challenges in countries such as Afghanistan and Pakistan, where naswar use is deeply embedded within cultural practices and daily routines, especially among adult males. Additionally, the economic dependency of local communities on naswar production and sales poses a critical barrier; for many individuals and small-scale vendors, naswar serves as a primary source of income. Thus, the abrupt removal of this commodity from the marketplace could lead to economic displacement and potential resistance from affected stakeholders. Moreover, weak regulatory infrastructure, limited law enforcement capacity, and the absence of alternative livelihood programmes further complicate the feasibility of a successful ban.

Key Points

- A government ban on naswar could help reduce public access.
- Weak regulatory systems and a lack of alternative income opportunities in countries such as Afghanistan and Pakistan hinder the successful implementation and sustainability of a naswar ban.

6.4 Conclusion

The habitual use of naswar presents significant challenges to periodontal health due to its chemical composition, method of consumption, and direct contact with oral tissues. Evidence suggests a strong association between naswar use and periodontitis. These effects are likely compounded by poor oral hygiene practices, underprivileged education, and deprived living standards among naswar users.

References

Abbasi ZA, Hadi NI, Zubairi AM, Hosein M (2019) Salivary interleukin 1-beta levels and clinical periodontal parameters in habitual naswar users and non-users. Pak J Med Sci 35:674–679

Ahlstrand T, Kovesjoki L, Maula T, Oscarsson J, Ihalin R (2019) Aggregatibacter actinomycetemcomitans LPS binds human interleukin-8. J Oral Microbiol 11:1549931

Ahmad F, Khan Z, Siddiqi K, Khan MN, Boeckman M, Dregger S, Bauld L et al (2020) Compliance of oral snuff (Naswar) packaging and sales practices with national tobacco control laws and the relevant articles of framework convention on tobacco control in Khyber Pakhtunkhwa Pakistan. Nicotine Tob Res 22:2224–2230

Ahmad F, Boeckmann M, Khan Z, Zeeb H, Khan MN, Ullah S, Dreger S et al (2021) Implementing smokeless tobacco control policy in Pakistan: a qualitative study among Naswar supply chain actors. Tob Control 30:548–552

Ahmad F, Khan Z, Siddiqi K, Khan MN, Kibria Z, Forberger S, Bauld L et al (2022) Awareness, perceptions of and compliance with tobacco control policies among naswar vendors in Khyber Pakhtunkhwa Pakistan. Tob Control 31:e111–e117

Ahmad I, Binmadi N, Afridi SG, Aljohani S, Shah I, Saidal A, Shahzad M (2023) Salivary oxidative stress and antioxidant capacity in smokeless tobacco (Naswar) users. Clin Cosmet Investig Dent 15:121–132

Akram Z, Abduljabbar T, Hosain M, Al-Sowygh ZH, Al-Hamoudi N, Vohra F, Javed F (2018) Comparison of periodontal inflammatory parameters among habitual gutka-chewers and naswar-dippers: a split-mouth retrospective clinical study. Acta Odontol Scand 76:141–147

Alam F (2023) Addiction to naswar: a growing threat to public health. https://www.app.com.pk/features/addiction-to-naswar-a-growing-threat-to-public-health/. Accessed 6 Apr 2025

Alam F (2024) Addiction to naswar: a growing threat to public health. https://www.nation.com.pk/02-Sep-2024/addiction-to-naswar-a-growing-threat-to-public-health. Accessed 7 Apr 2025

Al-Hamoudi N, Mokeem S, Jabbar TA, FahimVohra AZ (2018) Self-perceived oral symptoms and periodontal inflammatory conditions in habitual naswar dippers. Pak J Med Sci 34:1272–1277

Amirzada MZ, Sahrai MS, Hayat MS, Ishaq N, Yasin AG, Ahadi AN, Fazli N et al (2024) Associations of tobacco use, physical activity and diet with hypertension in the city of Kandahar, Afghanistan: a community-based cross-sectional study. BMC Res Notes 17:385

Aslam S, Javed A, Usman H, Naz L, Mushtaq S (2021) Behavioral and Psychological attributes of the smokeless tobacco consumers in Karachi. Ann Psychophysiol 8:34–42

Basharat S, Kassim S, Croucher R (2012) Availability and use of Naswar: an exploratory study. J Public Health 34:60–64

Chaturvedi P, Vaishampayan SS, Nair S, Nair D, Agarwal JP, Kane SV, Pawar P et al (2013) Oral squamous cell carcinoma arising in background of oral submucous fibrosis: a clinicopathologically distinct disease. Head Neck 35:1404–1409

Chen M, Cai W, Zhao S, Shi L, Chen Y, Li X, Sun X et al (2019) Oxidative stress-related biomarkers in saliva and gingival crevicular fluid associated with chronic periodontitis: a systematic review and meta-analysis. J Clin Periodontol 46:608–622

Daood U, Abduljabbar T, Al-Hamoudi N, Akram Z (2018) Clinical and radiographic periodontal parameters and release of collagen degradation biomarkers in naswar dippers. J Periodontal Res 53:123–130

Dongari-Bagtzoglou AI, Ebersole JL (1998) Increased presence of interleukin-6 (IL-6) and IL-8 secreting fibroblast subpopulations in adult periodontitis. J Periodontol 69:899–910

Foulds J, Ramstrom L, Burke M, Fagerström K (2003) Effect of smokeless tobacco (snus) on smoking and public health in Sweden. Tob Control 12:349–359

Fredriksson M, Bergström K, Asman B (2002) IL-8 and TNF-alpha from peripheral neutrophils and acute-phase proteins in periodontitis. J Clin Periodontol 29:123–128

Gasmi Benahmed A, Kumar Mujawdiya P, Noor S, Gasmi A (2022) *Porphyromonas gingivalis* in the development of periodontitis: impact on dysbiosis and inflammation. Arch Razi Inst 77:1539–1551

Gomes PR, Rocha MD, Lira JA, Coelho FA, Alves EH, Nascimento HM, Oliveira SM et al (2023) Salivary biomarkers present in patients with periodontitis without clinical distinction: findings from a meta-analysis. Med Oral Patol Oral Cir Bucal 28:e457–e466

Gupta PC, Ray CS, Sinha DN, Singh PK (2011) Smokeless tobacco: a major public health problem in the SEA region: a review. Indian J Public Health 55:199–209

Isaza-Guzmán DM, Hernández-Viana M, Bonilla-León DM, Hurtado-Cadavid MC, Tobón-Arroyave SI (2016) Determination of NLRP3 (rs4612666) and IL-1B (rs1143634) genetic polymorphisms in periodontally diseased and healthy subjects. Arch Oral Biol 65:44–51

Jain V, Rifai MA, Naderi S, Barolia R, Iqbal S, Taj M, Jia X et al (2021) Association of smokeless tobacco use with the use of other illicit drugs in the United States. Am J Med 134:e15–e19

Javed F, Näsström K, Benchimol D, Altamash M, Klinge B, Engström PE (2007) Comparison of periodontal and socioeconomic status between subjects with type 2 diabetes mellitus and non-diabetic controls. J Periodontol 78:2112–2119

Javed F, Chotai M, Mehmood A, Almas K (2010) Oral mucosal disorders associated with habitual gutka usage: a review. Oral Surg Oral Med Oral Pathol Oral Radiol Endod 109:857–864
Javed F, Al-Hezaimi K, Salameh Z, Almas K, Romanos GE (2011) Proinflammatory cytokines in the crevicular fluid of patients with peri-implantitis. Cytokine 53:8–12
Javed F, Tenenbaum HC, Nogueira-Filho G, Nooh N, Taiyeb Ali TB, Samaranayake LP, Al-Hezaimi K (2014) Oral Candida carriage and species prevalence amongst habitual gutka-chewers and non-chewers. Int Wound J 11:79–84
Javed F, Al-Kheraif AA, Al Amri MD, Alshehri M, Vohra F, Al-Askar M, Malmstrom H et al (2015a) Periodontal status and whole salivary cytokine profile among smokers and never-smokers with and without prediabetes. J Periodontol 86:890–898
Javed F, Al-Kheraif AA, Al Amri MD, Mikami T, Vohra F, Warnakulasuriya S, Romanos GE (2015b) Periodontal parameters and whole salivary cytokine profiles among habitual gutka chewers and non-chewers. J Periodontol 86:689–695
Jayant K, Deo M (1986) Oral cancer and cultural practices in relation to betel quid and tobacco chewing and smoking. Cancer Detect Prev 9:207–213
Kakde S, Bhopal R, Jones C (2012) A systematic review on the social context of smokeless tobacco use in the south Asian population: implications for public health. Public Health 126:635–645
Kamal Z, Shahzad M, Khan TA, Niaz F, Hayat K (2023) Oral candidal carriage and its correlation with salivary oxidative stress in smokeless tobacco users. Pak J Med Health Sci 17:534–534
Khan Z, Dreger S, Shah SMH, Pohlabeln H, Khan S, Ullah Z, Rehman B et al (2017) Oral cancer via the bargain bin: the risk of oral cancer associated with a smokeless tobacco product (Naswar). PLoS One 12:e0180445
Khan Z, Suliankatchi RA, Heise TL, Dreger S (2019) Naswar (smokeless tobacco) use and the risk of oral cancer in Pakistan: a systematic review with meta-analysis. Nicotine Tob Res 21:32–40
Levy Y (2015) Oxidative stress, antioxidants and periodontal disease. Arch Oral Biol 60:1461–1462
Mehra R, Mohanty VR, Mehra K, Kapoor S (2020) Afghan frontier: understanding tobacco practices among migrant population in India. Asian Pac J Cancer Prev 21:1931–1937
Mehrotra R, Yadav A, Sinha DN, Parascandola M, John RM, Ayo-Yusuf O, Nargis N et al (2019) Smokeless tobacco control in 180 countries across the globe: call to action for full implementation of WHO FCTC measures. Lancet Oncol 20:e208–e217
Muhammad W, Khan MM, Zafar S, Alqutub MN, AlMubarak AM, Mokeem S, Khan ZA et al (2021) Assessment of unstimulated whole salivary tumor necrosis factor alpha (TNF-α) and cellular micronuclei levels in snuff (Naswar) users and non-users for early diagnosis of oral squamous cell carcinoma. Int J Environ Res Public Health 18:7230
Ochani S, Ochani A, Ochani K (2022) Naswar, a smokeless tobacco: awareness and regulation in Pakistan. Asia Pac J Public Health 34:741–742
Petersen PE, Kwan S (2011) Equity, social determinants and public health programmes—the case of oral health. Community Dent Oral Epidemiol 39:481–487
Rahim A, Syed K, Ahad B, Farooq A, Ayub Z, Batool SM (2022) Comparison of severity of periodontal clinical parameters among naswar/snuff users: cross sectional study. PLoS One 17:e0273288
Rumgay H, Nethan ST, Shah R, Vignat J, Ayo-Yusuf O, Chaturvedi P, Guerra ENS et al (2024) Global burden of oral cancer in 2022 attributable to smokeless tobacco and areca nut consumption: a population attributable fraction analysis. Lancet Oncol 25:1413–1423
Saeed M, Muhammad N, Khan SA, Gul F, Khuda F, Humayun M, Khan H (2012) Assessment of potential toxicity of a smokeless tobacco product (naswar) available on the Pakistani market. Tob Control 21:396–401
Saeed M, Asad M, Shahzad M, Akram M, Khan Z (2024) Biochemical composition of a smokeless tobacco product (NASWAR) used in Pakistan. J King Saud Univ Sci 36:103168
Sánchez-Siles M, Lucas-Azorin J, Salazar-Sánchez N, Carbonell-Meseguer L, Camacho-Alonso F (2016) Salivary concentration of oxidative stress biomarkers in a group of patients with peri-Implantitis: a transversal study. Clin Implant Dent Relat Res 18:1015–1022

Sohail K, Siddiqi KM, Baig MZ, Sahibzada HA, Maqbool S (2020) Salivary biomarker interleukin-8 levels in Naswar users and non-users. J Coll Physicians Surg Pak 30:99–101
Tomar S, Hecht S, Jaspers I, Gregory R, Stepanov I (2019) Oral health effects of combusted and smokeless tobacco products. Adv Dent Res 30:4–10
Ullah A, Khan A, Iqbal Z, Khan I (2017) Evaluation of serum copper level in Naswar (smokeless tobacco) addicts using flame atomic absorption spectroscopy. Arch Iran Med 20:649–651
Vaishnav B, Valiyil AS, Anand S, Ghosal A, Pailla R, Nair GR (2025) Effects of smokeless tobacco use on the upper gastrointestinal tract mucosa: gross and histopathological changes. Ann Afr Med 24:450–455

Effect of *Toombak* on Periodontal Health

7

Salah O. Ibrahim

Abbreviations

CAL	Clinical attachment loss
CMV	Cytomegalovirus
EBV	Epstein-Barr virus
GTSS	Global Tobacoo Survillence System
HPV	Human papilloma virus
IARC	International Agency for Research on Cancer
Iso-NNAL	4-(methylnitrosamino)-4-(3-pyridyl)-1-butanol
NAB	N-nitrosoanabasine
NAT	N-nitrosoanatabine
NCSs	non-communicable diseases
NNAL	4-(methylnitrosamino)-1-(3-pyridyl)-1-butanol
NNK	4-(methylnitrosamino)-1-(3-pyridyl)-1-butanone
NNN	N-nitrosonornicotine
OC	Oral cancer
OR	Odds ratios
PD	Periodontal disease
PoS	Point of sale
ST	Smokeless tobacco
TSNA	Tobacco-specific nitrosamines
USSR	Union of Soviet Socialist republics

S. O. Ibrahim (✉)
Voss Dental Specialist Group Center, Vossevangen, Norway

F. Javed, S. Warnakulasuriya (eds.), *Smokeless Tobacco and its Effects on Periodontal Health*, https://doi.org/10.1007/978-3-032-16409-4_7

Learning Goals

- Understand the historical, cultural, and socioeconomic context of *toombak* use in Sudan.
- Identify the chemical and microbial composition of *toombak.*
- Explain the mechanisms through which *toombak* exerts toxic effects on oral tissues, such as cytotoxicity, DNA damage, and inflammation.
- Assess the relationship between *toombak* use and periodontal diseases.
- Examine the overlapping pathogenic mechanisms between periodontal diseases and oral cancers.
- Evaluate the current gaps in research and clinical attention regarding the effects of *toombak* on periodontal health.
- Discuss the recommendations for future research, public health policies, and clinical approaches aimed at reducing the burden of *toombak*-related oral diseases.

7.1 General History and Background of *Toombak* Use

7.1.1 History and Background

Sudan is located in the Middle East and North Africa (MENA) region and is the third-largest country in Africa, with a population of approximately 45.6 million. The country faces significant challenges, including a predominantly rural population and a rapidly evolving demography marked by an increasing burden of non-communicable diseases (NCDs).

In Sudan, the local population widely consumes *Nicotiana rustica*, a tobacco species with high levels of nicotine and nornicotine, to produce a traditional form of snuff known as "*toombak*". While the nasal use of *toombak* is confined to the southernmost regions of the country, oral consumption is prevalent throughout the rest of Sudan. The cultivation of *toombak* primarily takes place in sandy or silty soils that receive substantial rainfall in northwestern Sudan. The crop is sown during November and December at the end of the rainy season (September–October) and is never irrigated. Harvesting begins between February and March, once the leaves turn yellow and develop brownish spots—referred to as the "smallpox stage". After harvesting, the leaves are left in the field to dry uniformly, then bundled, moistened with water, and stored for fermentation for several weeks at temperatures ranging from 30 to 45°C. The bundles are periodically separated to ensure even drying, which typically occurs between April and May. Once dried, the tobacco leaves are ground and stored for a year to undergo ageing (Idris 1992).

The introduction of *toombak* to Sudan has been attributed to an Islamic religious teacher who may have arrived from Egypt, Timbuktu (Mali), or Morocco. Alternative theories suggest that it was introduced from Turkey or the Arabian Peninsula. One of the early names for *toombak*, Sauté, meaning "sniffing" in the local language, indicates that it was initially consumed nasally. Over time, various commercial names have emerged for *toombak*, including El-Sanf (denoting high quality), Wad Amari (named after the individual believed to have introduced it), Sultan El-Kaif (referring to its purported ability to enhance one's mood), and El-Dokh (meaning "state of dizziness") (Idris 1992). *Toombak* is widely available for purchase at numerous market shops and is heavily advertised at points of sale, where vendors often use commercial branding to attract buyers (Idris 1992).

Key Points

- Sudan has a population of around 45.6 million and faces major public health challenges, including a growing burden of non-communicable diseases.
- *Toombak*, a traditional form of smokeless tobacco made from *Nicotiana rustica*, is commonly consumed orally across Sudan, with nasal use limited to southern regions.
- *Toombak* is grown mainly in northwestern Sudan, harvested during the dry season, and undergoes a unique drying, fermentation, and ageing process that can take over a year.
- The origin of *toombak* in Sudan is linked to religious and trade influences from various regions, and it is now widely available and aggressively marketed with various brand names.

7.1.2 Processing of *Toombak*

Processing of *toombak* for sale is usually conducted by *toombak* vendors (Idris 1992). It is performed by preparing four parts of a coarse powder of dried *Nicotiana rustica* leaves (Fig. 7.1a) in a bowl and from another one the concentrate of sodium bicarbonate is added gradually in lesser amounts to the tobacco (Idris 1992). The concentrate is prepared first by adding water to the sodium bicarbonate, mixed thoroughly, and left for about 2–3 h before being used. While adding the solution, the product is mixed vigorously by both hands and concurrently assessed by the sensation of the tips of the fingers until it becomes moist and hardened. The output is then transferred to special airtight tin containers, pressed down by both hands (palms) to get rid of air, which are then covered firmly for about 2 h (to achieve fermentation of the product), thereafter, the product becomes ready for sale or use (Fig. 7.1b). Before buying, users ask for a bit of *toombak* to smell or taste, since the aroma and taste decide the quality rank and grading of the product either as grade one (high quality with quick absorption) or grade two (low quality with slow absorption). Of note, the sodium bicarbonate used in processing of *toombak*, is obtained by digging

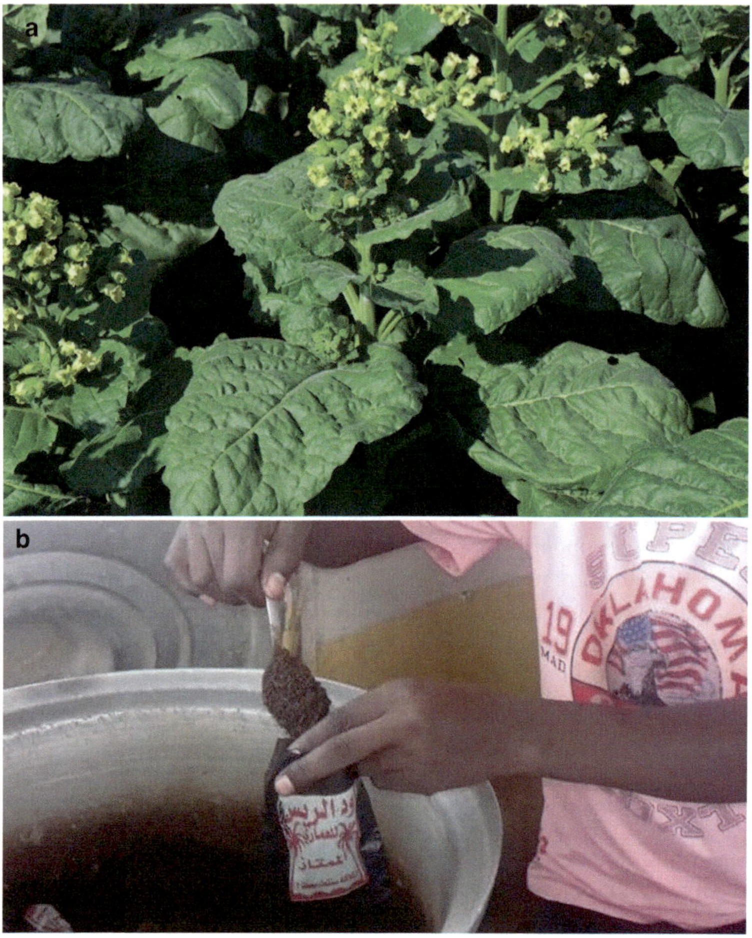

Fig. 7.1 (**a**) *Nicotiana runstica.* (*Curtesy of Dr Amel Sami, APC Microbiome Ireland, School of Microbiology, University College Cork, Cork, Ireland.* Personal iStock account at https://www.istockphoto.com/photos). (**b**) T*oombak* prepared in an airtight tin container ready for sale. Note the commercial advertisement on the plastic bag carrying the name of the shop which reads "*Captain's son for high quality toombak*". Note also direct contact of seller's fingers with product and rusty spoon table. (*Current author photo*). (**c**) *Toombak* sold in small plastic bags each taking about 100 grams. (*Curtesy of Dr Amel Sami, APC Microbiome Ireland, School of Microbiology, University College Cork, Cork, Ireland*). (**d**) A dip of *toombak* "*saffa*" of about 10 grams weight ready to use. (*Current author photo*). (**e**, **f**) *Toombak* dip "saffa" placed either at the gingivo-labial area of the upper (**e**) or lower (**f**) jaw. (*Curtesy of Dr Amel Sami, APC Microbiome Ireland, School of Microbiology, University College Cork, Cork, Ireland*)

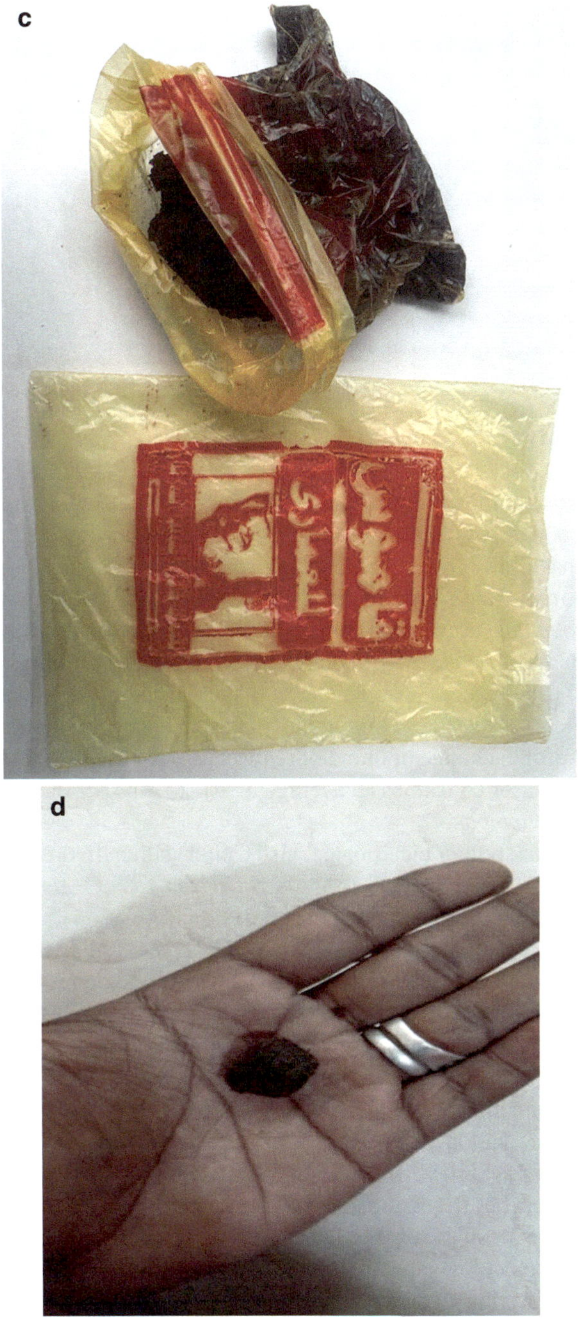

Fig. 7.1 (continued)

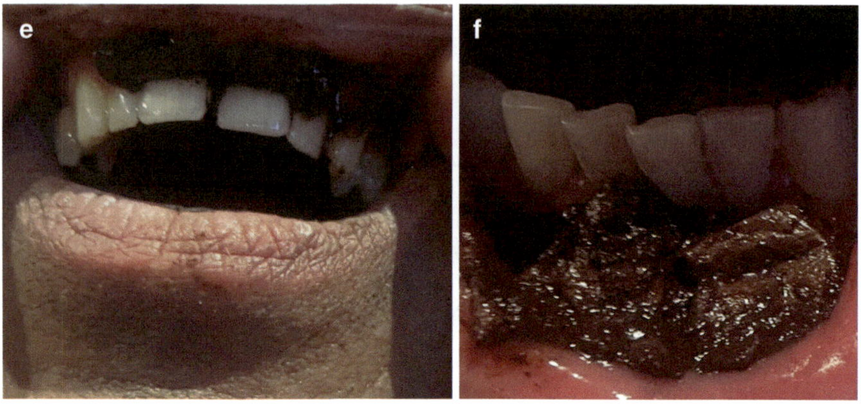

Fig. 7.1 (continued)

the soil of a known mountain in the western part of the Sudan known as natron (sodium bicarbonate) mountain. Adding sodium bicarbonate creates an alkaline environment that allows for high absorption rates of nicotine through the mouth lining. Currently, *toombak* is sold in small plastic bags each taking about 100 grams (Fig. 7.1c). *Toombak* users carry round or box-shaped tin cans in their pocket, named hookah and are like plastic bags, though some people use king-size ones. Hookah is still used by some people, and it makes an indentation in the pocket of a user, thus one can easily guess and identify a user. This helps users communicate with each other for exchange of brand or request of a dip usually in a friendly atmosphere. A regular user consumes an average of 10–20 dips per day, thus requiring a steady supply of *toombak*.

Natron or atron (sodium bicarbonate, also called sodium hydrogen carbonate), is a mineral rock with the chemical formula $Na_2H(CO_3)_22H_2O$. Its colour is grey to yellowish white and is of alkaline pH. There is no information on either the history or reasons behind use of atron as an additive to *toombak*. It may be used to homogenize the leaves to a fine sticky form as atron is used in Sudan to homogenize vegetables during cooking. Atron, opposed to lime used in other parts of the world, is, as mentioned above, added to *toombak* for its alkaline effects. It has been shown that at high pH (11.0–11.8) nicotine is completely protonated and its rate of absorption is increased (Brunnemann and Hoffmann 1974). Studies of nass, a type of snuff used in the former Union of Soviet Socialist Republics (USSR), which contains lime and has high pH (11–11.8), have shown that when the product is placed in the mouth, nicotine reaches the central nervous system very quickly (Brunnemann et al. 1985). Thus, pH value in tobacco products can influence the absorption and thereby the extent of pharmacological activity of nicotine (Brunnemann et al. 1985). Atron quickens the absorption of nicotine from *toombak* through the oral mucosa and rapidly reaches the central nervous system.

Key Points

- *Toombak* is made by mixing coarse powder from dried *Nicotiana rustica* leaves with a sodium bicarbonate solution.
- The moist mixture is pressed into airtight tin containers and sealed for about 2 h to allow fermentation, after which the product is ready for sale or use.
- Consumers judge the quality of *toombak* based on its aroma and taste.
- *Toombak* is typically sold in 100-gram plastic bags.
- The alkaline pH from atron facilitates rapid nicotine absorption into the bloodstream, intensifying its pharmacological effects and leading to quick delivery to the central nervous system.

7.1.3 Contents and Composition of *Toombak*

Using gas chromatography with thermal energy analysis, the tobacco-specific-nitrosamines (TSNAs) types, N-nitrosonornicotine (NNN), 4-(methylnitrosamino)-1-(3-pyridyl)-1-butanone (NNK), N-nitrosoanatabine (NAT) and N-nitrosoanabasine (NAB), were quantified in *toombak* and saliva of *toombak* users (Idris et al. 1991; Idris et al. 1992). Exceptionally high levels (mean; range, mg/g *toombak*/dry wt) of NNN (1.13; 0.50–3.08), NNK (2.31; 0.62–7.87; 31), NAT (0.08; 0.02–0.2), and NAB (0.22; 0.02–2.37) were found (Idris et al. 1991; Idris et al. 1992). Previously, the highest levels of NNN and NNK in any oral tobacco found were 0.154 and 0.014 mg/g dry wt, respectively (Tso 1982). Two additional TSNAs, 4-(methylnitrosamino)-1-(3-pyridyl)-1-butanol (NNAL) and 4-(methylnitrosamino)-4-(3-pyridyl)-1-butanol (iso-NNAL) were found in the saliva of *toombak* users for the first time and were confirmed by gas chromatography mass spectrum (Idris et al. 1992). Exposure to TSNAs has also been assessed by measuring the content in the saliva of 21 *toombak* users, where nine out of ten subjects had detectable levels of TSNAs in their saliva before dipping (total TSNAs: 0.01–1.0 mg/ml). During *toombak* use, TSNAs concentrations have reached g/ml levels (range: number of positive subjects) for NNN (0.6–1.2, 12/12), NAT (0.6–6.7, 2/12), NAB (0.05–1.9, 12/12), NNK (0.06–6.7, 8/12), NNAL (0.05–3.3, 11/12), and iso-NNAL (0.07–0.4, 8/12). These high levels of TSNAs found in *toombak* were partially attributed to the use of tobacco species, *Nicotiana rustica*, fermentation of *toombak* at elevated temperature, prolonged unrefrigerated storage, and contamination during processing (Anderson et al. 1989; Djordjevic et al. 1993; Prokopczyk et al. 1992).

Key Points

- *Toombak* contains significantly higher levels of TSNAs, notably NNN, NNK, NAT, and NAB.
- The elevated TSNA content in *toombak* is attributed to the use of *Nicotiana rustica* tobacco, high-temperature fermentation, prolonged unrefrigerated storage, and contamination during processing.

7.1.4 Habit Description

The habit of *toombak* dipping is practiced by taking a small portion from the plastic bag or hookah with the three forefingers, usually of the right hand, putting it in the palm of the left hand, and manipulating it by the thumb and middle fingers of the right hand until it forms a ball called *saffa* (Fig. 7.1d), which is of about 10 grams in weight (Idris 1992). The *saffa* is not chewed but dipped and retained between gum and lip or cheeks or floor of the mouth and sucked slowly for about 10–15 min. Men prefer dipping between the lower lip and gum, while women prefer dipping between cheeks and gum. The dipping continues for a period ranging from a few minutes to several hours, until the *saffa* becomes bland. Men periodically spit the insoluble debris that is freed from the bullous and the saliva, which is secreted during *toombak* use, whereas women retain the *saffa*, without spiting because of social unacceptability and avoidance of stigma. The mouth is usually rinsed thoroughly with water after the quid is removed. The *toombak* quid is sometimes retained in the mouth during sleep (Idris 1992).

Key Points

- *Toombak* dipping involves forming a ball (called *saffa*) of about 10 grams, which is placed between the gum and lip or cheek and sucked rather than chewed.
- Men typically place the *saffa* between the lower lip and gum and tend to spit during use, while women place it between the cheek and gum and usually avoid spitting due to social stigma.
- The dipping duration varies, sometimes lasting several hours or even continuing during sleep.

7.1.5 Exposure, Knowledge, and Social Influence of *Toombak* Use

Several epidemiological studies have provided data on prevalence, exposure, and knowledge related to *toombak* use in Sudan. Among adults 18 years and older, a house-to-house cross-sectional survey of 4.535 households with 21.648 eligible individuals, when questioned about tobacco use reported high prevalence of *toombak* use among males (34%) with low prevalence among females (2.5%) (Idris et al. 1998). Another survey (El-Amin et al. 2011) in the period 2005–2006, investigated the influence of parents, friends, and teachers on cigarette smoking and *toombak* dipping among school-going adolescents in Sudan reaching 4.277 participants. The study found that 8.1% had ever used *toombak* and 3.5% were current *toombak* users. For *toombak*, parental *toombak* dipping was associated with adolescents' ever (OR 1.77) and current (OR 1.84) *toombak* use. Friends' smoking was also associated with adolescents' ever (OR 1.81) and current (OR 3.33) *toombak* use. Teachers' *toombak* dipping was associated with adolescents' ever smoking (OR 1.50) but not with current smoking or *toombak* use. The study concluded that tobacco habits of parents, friends, and teachers significantly influence adolescents' tobacco use, with friends having the strongest impact. Another study (Almahdi et al. 2020) investigated the association between *toombak* advertisement at PoS and exposure among 1.670 secondary school students (aged 13–13 years). The study reported that 41.8% of adolescents were exposed to *toombak* advertisements at PoS with a significant association between exposure to *toombak* advertisements at PoS and increased *toombak* use. Another investigation (El-Amin 2019) used self-reported questionnaire based on the Global Tobacco Surveillance System (GTSS) with 1.590 third-year health science students from 25 schools across 13 universities in Sudan and examined use of cigarettes, shisha, and *toombak*. The study reported that 40.3% of the students smoked cigarettes, 33.8% used shisha, 16.2% had dipped *toombak* and 8.3% were current smokers, and that 10.5% smoked on school premises.

Using self-administered questionnaires covering *toombak* use, knowledge of health hazards, attitudes towards *toombak* control, and preventive practices, the knowledge, attitudes, and behaviours of school workers regarding *toombak* use as well as the availability and effectiveness of control policies and preventive practices in schools have been reported in a cross-sectional school-based study with 239 school workers (teachers and other staff members) from 28 randomly selected schools in Khartoum (Almahdi et al. 2017a). The study found that 63% of participants were ≤40 years old, and 50% were female, and most were teachers (79.2%). For *toombak* use**,** 9.6% of school workers had ever used *toombak*, 64.7% of ever users were daily users and that all *toombak* users were male, and 76.2% were ≥40 years old. The study found that *toombak* use among school workers was associated with poor knowledge, negative attitudes towards *toombak* control, and poor preventive practices. Using self-administered questionnaire covering socio-demographics, *toombak* use, and socio-cognitive constructs (information received, social image, attitudes, normative social influence, accessibility), a cross-sectional school-based study was conducted in 2013–2014 including 1670 secondary school students aged 13–16 years from 28 randomly selected schools in the Khartoum State (Almahdi et al. 2017b). The work reported that 10.9% of students had ever used *toombak*, 5.3% intended to use *toombak*, 81.6% had a positive attitude towards *toombak* use, and that older students (≥15 years) and males were more likely to have ever used *toombak*. Males reported higher intention to use *toombak* compared to females. The study suggested that prevalence of *toombak* use among secondary school students is low, with higher usage among males and older students and that students' intention to use *toombak* is influenced by experience and the social image attached to its use.

Key Points

- Prevalence of *toombak* use is higher among Sudanese adult males (34%) than females (2.5%).
- Friends, parents, and teachers significantly influence adolescents' *toombak* use, with friends having the strongest impact on both ever and current use.
- Exposure of adolescents to *toombak* advertisements is significantly associated with its increasing use.
- *Toombak* use is linked to poor knowledge and preventive practices.
- Among students, males and those aged ≥15 years are more likely to use *toombak*, often influenced by social image and experience.

7.2 Impact of *Toombak* Use on Oral Health

7.2.1 Toxic Effect of *Toombak* on Oral Mucosa

Using primary normal human oral keratinocytes, fibroblasts, and a dysplastic oral keratinocyte cell line, the specific effects of *toombak* has been studied and compared to Swedish snuff. Aqueous extracts from moist *toombak* and Swedish snuff were prepared and added in serial dilutions to cultured cells (Costea et al. 2010). Cell viability, morphology, growth, DNA double-strand breaks (γH2AX staining), expression of phosphatidylserine (Annexin V staining), and cell cycle were evaluated after various exposure periods. The work reported a significant decrease in cell number, DNA double-strand breaks, and morphological and biochemical signs of programmed cell death (*apoptosis*). Further, the study found G2/M cell cycle blocks in normal oral keratinocytes and fibroblasts. Of note, Swedish snuff showed less adverse effects on oral cells, mainly at non-clinically relevant dilutions. The study indicated that *toombak* has a higher potential to damage human oral keratinocytes in vitro compared to Swedish snuff. Dysplastic oral keratinocytes were less sensitive to *toombak*-induced cytotoxic effects but still prone to DNA damage, which could lead to further malignant progression, and therefore highlighting the significant health risks associated with the use of *toombak* (Costea et al. 2010).

Key Points

- *Toombak* induces significant cytotoxic effects in human oral epithelial cells, including decreased cell viability, DNA double-strand breaks, apoptosis.
- A potential role for *toombak* in promoting malignant transformation in oral tissues has been reported.

7.2.2 Molecular Biology Findings and *Toombak* Use

During the period 1995–2020, the current author and co-workers have conducted an in-depth investigation related to genomic and proteomic analysis of samples of oral mucosa, pre-cancers, and oral cancers (OCs) from Sudanese *toombak* users. Significant findings were reported in relation to expression and mutation of the tumour suppressor gene *p*53 where high level of mutations was found with a novel mutation in exon 6 in relation to *toombak* use. This is in addition to mutations in exons 5 (codon 130), 6 (codons 190 and 216), and 7 (codons 229, 249 and 252); high expression of keratin (K) 13, 14, and 19; and absence of human papillomavirus (HPV) (Ibrahim 1999). Results supported the possibility that p53 protein forms complexes with the cytoplasmic Keratins, suggesting that it is the truncated p53 protein, which might be involved in the formation of these complexes, in particular, because of *toombak*. Another work (Sapkota 2011) examined expression profile of S100 gene family members in OCs/their pair-wised normal controls in relation to *toombak*. The work reported downregulation of S100A4, S100A6, S100A8, and S100A14 indicating their significance in relation to *toombak* use and highlighted the need for testing of these genes as molecular biomarkers for detection of early changes related to *toombak* use. In addition, the current author and co-workers have also reported significant findings related to mutations of the cell cycle arrest gene *p*21WAF1 (Ibrahim et al. 2002), expression of Bax and Bcl-2 (Loro et al. 2000), cDNA microarray gene expression profile (Ibrahim et al. 2003; Dysvik et al. 2006), and genome-wide profile of chromosol aberrations (Roman et al. 2008) in OCs in relation to *toombak*. The studies reported valuable information on candidate genes, chromosomal aberrations, and proteins examined from Sudanese *toombak* users, with specific findings likely to be involved in the pathogenesis of these OCs.

Key Points

- High mutation rates in tumour suppressor and cell cycle regulatory genes have been found in oral cancers from Sudanese *toombak* users.
- Several genes, including members of the S100 gene family are significantly downregulated in toombak-related oral cancers.

7.3 *Toombak* and Periodontal Diseases

Periodontal disease (PD) is defined as inflammation of the dental supporting tissues including gums, bone socket, outer layer of the roots of teeth, and associated connective tissue (Zhang et al. 2024). Plaque formation is a triggering factor for the disease and the common symptoms include bleeding on probing with gingival colour charges, swelling, pain, and in advanced stages, tooth mobility and loss (Kwona et al. 2021; Zhang et al. 2024). Three factors are known to cause plaque-related periodontitis, which are in a vulnerable host, existence of a pathogen, and the low extent or absence of advantageous microbiota (Zhang et al. 2024). PD is caused by specific pathogens, and it is well known that the "red complex" has been proposed as a pathogenic consortium of PD, consisting of *Porphyromonas gingivalis* (*P. gingivalis*), *Tannerella forsythia* (*T. forsythia*), and *Treponema denticola* (*T. denticola*) (Holt and Ebersole 2005). Also, increasing evidence has identified that more bacteria were detected from PD sites as causative periodontal pathogens, namely, *Aggregatibacter actinomycetemcomitans* (*A. actinomycetemcomitans*), *Fusobacterium nucleatum* (*F. nucleatum*), *Prevotella intermedia* (*P. intermedia*), *Streptococcus intermedius* (*S. intermedius*), *Prevotella tannerae* (*P. tannerae*), *Prevotella melaninogenica* (*P. melaninogenica*), *Prevotella intermedia* (*P. intermedia*), *Campylobacter recta* (*C. recta*), *Capnocytophaga gingivalis* (*C. gingivalis*), *Streptococcus mitis* (*S. mitis*), and so on (Nonnenmacher et al. 2001; Colombo et al. 2009). Further, many other microbial pathogens have been detected in periodontal lesions apart from bacteria, namely, human cytomegalovirus (CMV), Epstein-Barr virus (EBV), HPV, and *Candida* (especially *C. albicans*), which all proved to be associated with PD (Slots and Slots 2011; Sardi et al. 2010).

An imbalance between the pathogenic and saprophytic flora of the oral cavity in a vulnerable individual may cause PD. Through scaling and root planning, and deep pocket debridement, which are considered the primary cure, it is possible to reduce invasive periodontal pathogens significantly. Debridement treatment of PD is possible in two ways, surgical or non-surgical (Kwona et al. 2021; Zhang et al. 2024). Sometimes, systemic antimicrobial administration is a necessity. Although plaque removal using mechanical surface instrumentation is an effective treatment method, pocket recolonization is highly unpredictable (Kwona et al. 2021). Globally, approximately 11% of the world's population may have severe PD, affecting 743 million individuals. Robust literature has identified potential associations between PD and certain non-communicable chronic diseases. Other risk factors for PD include smoking, diabetes, while other contributing factors include overhanging/over-contoured restorations, open interproximal contacts, occlusal trauma, mucogingival deformity and anatomical factors (Kwona et al. 2021). Of note, there is limited evidence demonstrating solid relationship between periodontal or gingival diseases and smokeless tobacco (ST) use and other types of snuff (Kallischnigg et al. 2008).

Key Points

- The "red complex" bacteria, *Porphyromonas gingivalis, Tannerella forsythia*, and *Treponema denticola* are strongly associated with periodontal diseases.
- Approximately 11% of the global population is affected by severe periodontal diseases.
- Clinical evidence linking periodontal diseases with ST use remains limited.

How *toombak* use contributes to non-neoplastic oral diseases is unclear. It certainly increases the risk of OC and pre-cancers, but reviewers disagree as to other oral mucosal conditions. The author searched MEDLINE, EMBASE, and SCOPUS with no limitations by period or language. The main search was based on combinations of the terms "*toombak*", *tombak*", "Sudan", and "other countries" for exposure, and "oral diseases", "mouth diseases", "periodontal diseases", "calculus", "dental plaque", "tooth loss", "mucosal lesions", "gingivitis", "gingival recession", and "teeth problems" for outcome. Further articles were also identified by personal contact, inspection of reference lists in individual published and unpublished papers and reviews. Although there are several studies related to use of *toombak*, the endpoint and focus of both researchers and clinicians in Sudan has been limited to OC and oral mucosal conditions like oral leukoplakia and use of *toombak*. Although clinically (Fig. 7.2a–f), we see patients with characteristic periodontal changes including gingival recession, attachment loss, and bone loss, however, it can be some years before we see a focused clinically oriented and well-documented results from Sudan related to that subject among *toombak* users. While lack of data from Sudan may be attributed to the focus of clinicians on treating the disease rather than addressing other cofounders, this can also be attributed to low supporting evidence related to other findings from countries known with high use of ST and snuff as in the case of South-East Asia, Scandinavia, and the United States (Kallischnigg et al. 2008), resulting in less interest among clinicians and researchers to investigate possible relationship between *toombak* use and PD.

PD is a reaction to oral microbiotome related to bone and tooth loss where introduction to inflammatory conditions advances the infiltration of immune cells to the oral mucosa. Inflammation and immune-related mediators have been accepted as the hallmarks of malignant transformation. Various investigations have approved that the inflammatory mediators delivered during PD, for example proteases, microbial poisons and endotoxins get scattered to extraoral sites. These further outcomes in the incitement of monocytes with the discharge of prostaglandins E2, Interleukin-1, 6, 8, and 17, thromboxane B2, collagenases, and tumour necrosis alpha (Hoare et al. 2019). Several studies were also reviewed showing a strong association between aerodigestive cancers, poor oral health, presence of PD associated with bacteria, tooth loss, and clinical signs of PD such as alveolar bone loss and clinical attachment loss (CAL) (Kavarthapu and Gurumoorthy 2021). Recent evidence suggests a link between PD and incidence of various cancers involving the lung, breast,

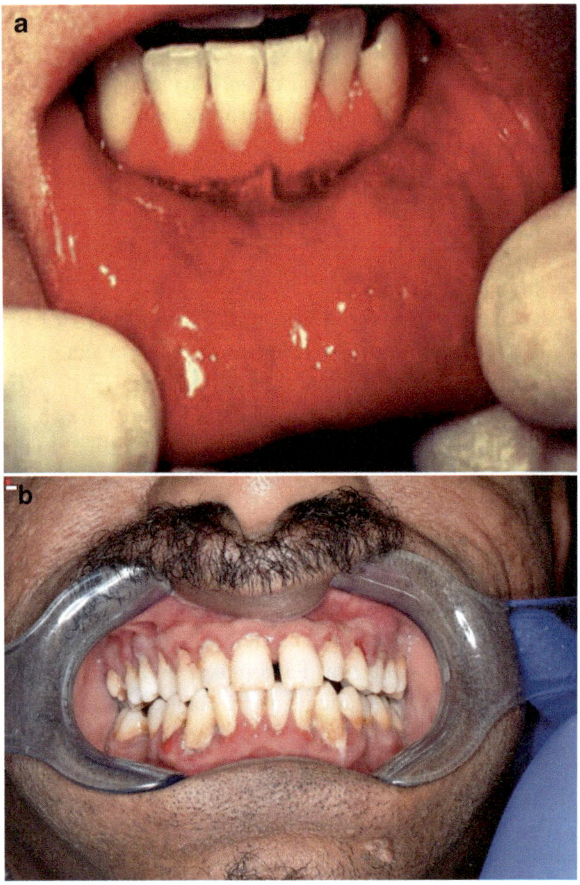

Fig. 7.2 Presence of mild periodontal inflammation and gingival recession at the side where *toombak* is placed (**a**). Presence of inflamed gingiva, bleeding, gingival recession, clinical attachment loss, dental calculus and plaque, presence of pockets, mobile teeth with change in occlusion, and teeth spacing (**b**). Severe periodontal inflammation with swollen gingiva, recession of the gingiva, clinical attachment loss, bleeding on probing, dental plaque and calculus, mobile teeth, missing teeth, and teeth discolouration in *toombak* users (**c**–**f**). (**g**, **h**) Typical clinical case of oral leuokoplakia (**g**) and oral cancer (**h**) in the gingivo-buccal area corresponding to the place where the *toombak* dip is usually placed. Both figures also demonstrate the presence of swollen inflamed gingiva, teeth discolouration, mobile teeth, attrition of teeth, dental calculus, and plaque and gingival recession, which are typical for PD illustrating a possible side-by-side relationship between PD and OCs

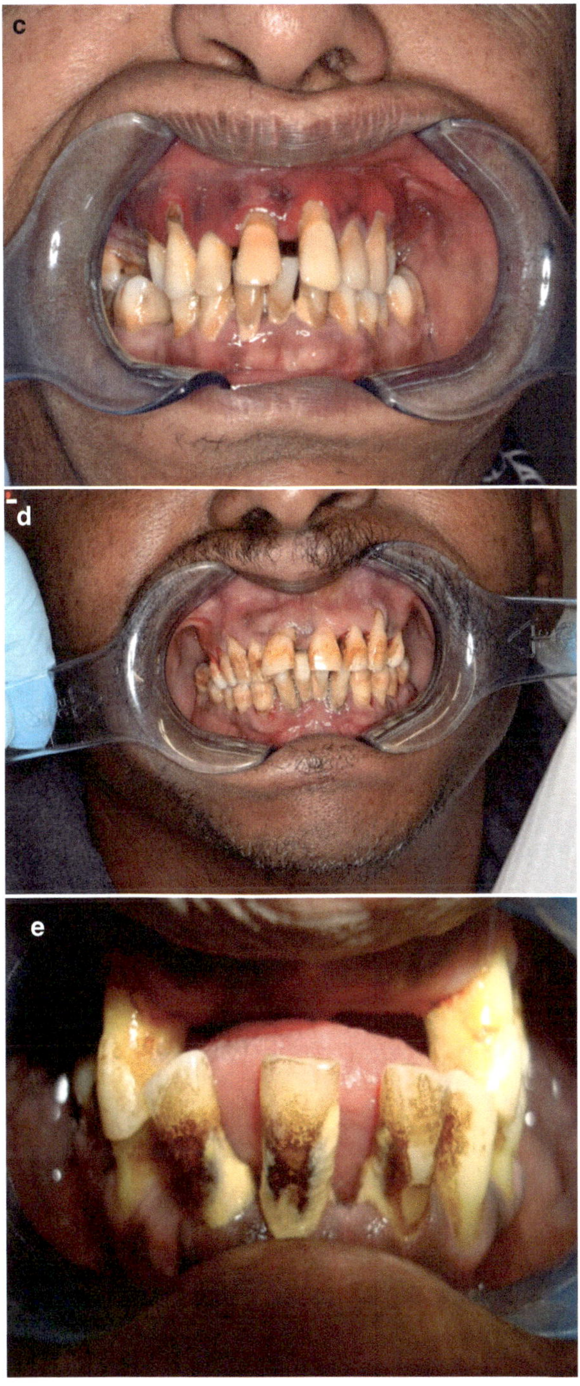

Fig. 7.2 (continued)

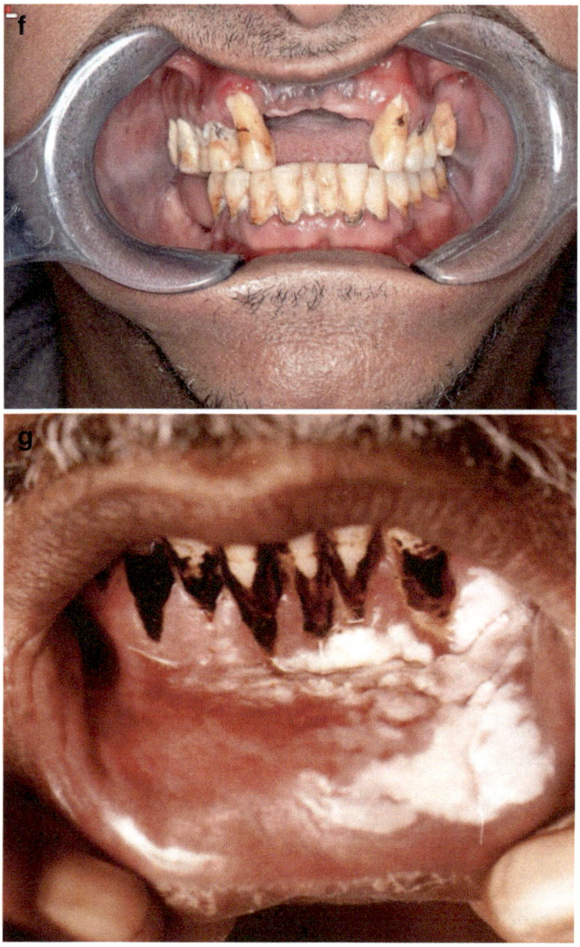

Fig. 7.2 (continued)

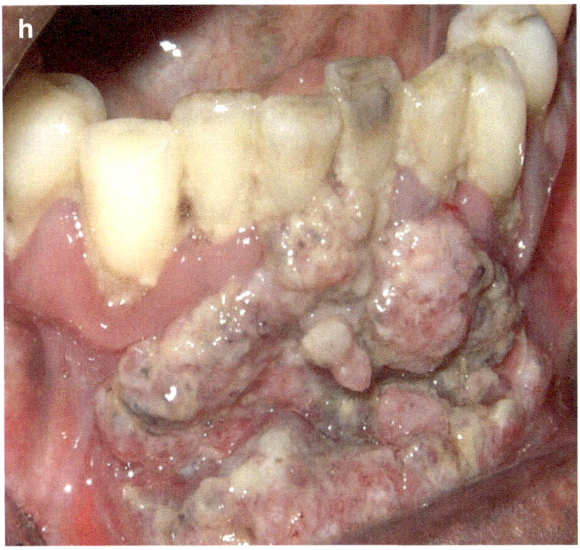

Fig. 7.2 (continued)

gastrointestinal, and head and neck (Baima et al. 2023). Although PD and OCs are two distinct diseases, they share some common pathogenic mechanisms. Current understanding suggests that anaerobic and facultative bacteria implicated in the pathogenesis of PD may colonize and grow within tumours, suggesting their role in tumourigenesis (Baima et al. 2023). Most bacteria in dental plaque are normal flora. However, a few bacteria in the plague associated with diseased periodontal tissues have been identified as putative pathogens. Compared with patients without PD, several studies have reported a two- to fivefold increase in the risk of OCs among those with PD (Javed and Warnakulasuriya 2016; Shin et al. 2019). Studies also suggested that the causal relationship between the extent and severity of chronic PD and the risk of OCs is significant, even after the adjustments for traditional confounding factors, i.e. smoking, alcohol, and Human Papillomavirus (HPV) (Moraes et al. 2016). It has been found that tooth loss because of bone loss in PD is an independent risk factor for head and neck cancer (Shi et al. 2018). Also, high expression of the human telomerase reverse transcription, the expression of which is highly specific to cancer cells, was detected in patients with PD (Katarkar et al. 2015). These findings, when taken together, suggest that there is a striking link between PD and OCs. Moreover, the link was explained by the following: (a) Broken mucosal barrier in PD consequently enhances penetration of carcinogens such as tobacco and alcohol. (b) Immunosuppression leads both to PD and OCs. (c) Viruses such as HPV and *Candida albicans* are found both in PD and OCs. (d) Chronic inflammation in PD contributes to cancer. (e) Dysbacteriosis in PD further leads to carcinogenic effects (Li et al. 2022; Patil et al. 2023).

Key Points

- While *toombak* is strongly associated with oral cancer and pre-cancerous lesions, there is insufficient data linking it to periodontal diseases.
- Periodontal inflammatory conditions among *toombak* users remains under-documented in scientific literature.
- Periodontal diseases and oral cancer share mechanisms such as mucosal barrier breakdown, chronic inflammation, immunosuppression, and microbial dysbiosis.

By in-depth study of clinical cases of OCs and pre-cancers from Sudanese *toombak* users (Fig. 7.2g, h) and with PD being an inflammatory disease caused by oral microbiota resulting in alveolar bone and tooth loss, infiltration of the inflammatory cells into the oral mucosa occurs when there is an exposure to inflammatory conditions. Presence of persistent inflammation and immune mediations may be responsible for the malignant transformation which we see in cases of OCs and pre-cancers from Sudan regarding *toombak* use. Although the focus of clinicians and researchers from Sudan is on OCs and pre-cancers, the author would like to suggest the presence of a contemporaneous relationship between PD and OCs from Sudan about *toomabk* use (Fig. 7.2g, h) taking into consideration the fact that, unfortunately, the focus has always been limited to one side of the clinical problem. The author's observations highlight the need for raising the importance of in-depth clinical examination and regular follow-up of patients with PD, especially among *toombak* users. Here, the current author would like to suggest that PD in *toombak* users might be the triggering indicator for future development of OCs and pre-cancer lesions related to *toombak*.

7.3.1 Oral Microbiome in *Toombak* Users

A recent study (Sami et al. 2021) provided a comprehensive analysis of *toombak's* physical, chemical, and microbial properties. Chemically, *toombak* was found to contain high levels of several heavy metals including chromium, cobalt, copper, and iron, with iron being the most abundant. Some of these metals are classified as carcinogens by the International Agency for Research on Cancer (IARC). In addition, extremely high levels of TSNAs and elevated levels of volatile aldehydes including formaldehyde and acetaldehyde, both known carcinogens, were detected in *toombak*. Microbial analysis and composition of *toombak* revealed that the dominant bacterial phyla were Firmicutes and Actinobacteria. In addition, Genera such as *Corynebacterium*, *Atopococcus*, and *Virgibacillus* were also found abundant. Potentially harmful bacteria like *Staphylococcus gallinarum* and *Oceanobacillus chironomi* were identified, which could contribute to oral infections and carcinogenesis. Metagenomic analysis of *toombak* showed active metal transport and antibiotic resistance pathways, suggesting microbial contributions *to toombak's* toxicity.

Regarding physical structure and pH of *toombak*, scanning electron microscopy analysis revealed the presence of non-homogeneous, irregular particles in *toombak*, which may cause chronic oral abrasions. *Toombak* samples had a highly alkaline pH (above 9) due to the addition of sodium bicarbonate, enhancing nicotine absorption and potentially contributing to mucosal damage. The study suggested that combination of high TSNAs, heavy metals, and pathogenic bacteria in *toombak* increases the risk of OCs, cardiovascular diseases, and other health issues. The abrasive nature of *toombak* particles and its chemical composition may lead to chronic inflammation, as in the case of PD, further elevating cancer risks. The study has also reported differences in chemical and microbial profiles between pre-prepared *toombak* and ready-to-buy samples, which might be influenced by preparation methods and geographical factors (Khartoum North vs. Omdurman). It has been concluded that *toombak* poses significant health risks due to its high content of carcinogenic TSNAs, heavy metals, and harmful microbes, and that product's preparation and storage methods contribute to these risks (Sami et al. 2021). Another work (Smyth et al. 2017) examined the bacterial communities present in ST products, including *toombak*. For bacterial diversity and viability, the work found that dry snuff products exhibited the highest bacterial diversity compared to other ST products like moist snuff, snus, and *toombak*. Total viable bacterial counts ranged from 0 to 9.35×10^7 CFU/g across different products, whereas *toombak* showed the highest viable bacterial counts. For the dominant bacterial phyla, *Actinobacteria* were most abundant in *toombak* products. Regarding manufacturing influence, the study found that heat-treated products, like Swedish snus, had fewer viable bacteria compared to the use of alkalinizing agents (e.g. sodium bicarbonate in *toombak*) which has affected bacterial communities, potentially suppressing certain bacteria while promoting others. Another study (Al-Hebshi et al. 2017) explored how the bacterial composition of ST products varies across different regions, including *toombak*. For bacterial load and diversity, the work reported that *toombak* featured *Facklamia*, *Desemzia*, *Atopostipes*, and *Lysinibacillus*. For predicted functional differences, high carcinogenicity *toombak* showed enrichment in genes encoding cadmium/zinc and nickel transport systems and metals that are linked to cancer development. In another comparative work (Tyx et al. 2016), the bacterial communities present in various ST products, including *toombak* was studied. The work found that *toombak* primarily contained *Actinobacteria* and *Firmicutes*, with families such as Aerococcaceae, Enterococcaceae, and Staphylococcaceae being dominant. *Toombak* contained higher levels of *Corynebacterium*, which may contribute to carcinogen production. Regarding manufacturing influence, products from the same manufacturer tended to have similar microbial communities, and that presence of harmful bacteria and their metabolic by-products, such as nitrosamines, highlights potential health risks for users. For better understanding of the microbial communities and genetic attributes contributing to the high TSNAs content in *toombak*, a recent work (Tyx et al. 2022) investigated the microbiology of *toombak*. The microbiota found was composed of over 99% bacteria. Dominant bacterial phyla included *Actinobacteria* (74.7%) and Firmicutes (19.3%). Key genera included *Enteractinococcus*, *Corynebacterium*, *Staphylococcus*, and *Bacillus*. For genetic attributes, nitrate reduction genes, canonical nitrate reduction genes (e.g. *narG*, *narK*) were found in *Enteractinococcus* and *Corynebacterium*. For antimicrobial resistance genes, various species of *Staphylococcus* exhibited notable antimicrobial resistance genes, while for genetic transference mechanisms, presence of mobile genetic elements, such as the integrating conjugative element ICE6013 in *Staphylococcus aureus* was found. The authors suggested that the high levels of TSNAs in *toombak* are likely due to microbial nitrate reduction, leading to nitrite formation, which reacts with tobacco alkaloids.

Key Points

- *Toombak* exhibits the highest viable bacterial counts among ST products, and shows distinct bacterial diversity.
- Dominant bacterial phyla in *toombak* include *Actinobacteria* and Firmicutes, with harmful genera such as Corynebacterium and Staphylococcus.
- *Toombak* has an alkaline pH (above 9) and contains non-uniform, abrasive particles, potentially causing chronic oral abrasions, inflammation, and enhanced nicotine absorption.
- Differences in microbial and chemical profiles are observed between pre-prepared and retail *toombak*, influenced by preparation methods and geographic origin.

In summary, microbiome of *toombak* predominantly consists of the phyla, Firmicutes and *Actinobacteria* with abundant species including *Corynebacterium casei*, *Atopostipes suicloacalis*, and *Oceanobacillus chironomi*. Genera such as *Corynebacterium*, *Atopococcus*, and *Virgibacillus* were also found, in addition to potentially harmful bacteria like *Staphylococcus gallinarum* and *Oceanobacillus chironomi*. *Toombak* featured *Facklamia*, *Desemzia*, *Atopostipes*, *Lysinibacillus*, *Actinobacteria* and *Firmicutes*, with families such as Aerococcaceae, Enterococcaceae, and Staphylococcaceae being dominant, and higher levels of *Corynebacterium*. Key genera found in *toombak* included *Enteractinococcus*, *Corynebacterium*, *Staphylococcus*, and *Bacillus*. For genetic attributes, nitrate reduction genes and canonical nitrate reduction genes (e.g. *narG*, *narK*) were found in *Enteractinococcus* and *Corynebacterium*. For antimicrobial resistance genes, various species of *Staphylococcus* exhibited notable antimicrobial resistance genes, while for genetic transference mechanisms, presence of mobile genetic elements, such as the integrating conjugative element ICE6013 in *Staphylococcus aureus* was found.

7.4 Recommendations

In Sudan, the oral health sector has encountered considerable multiple challenges and disruptions due to endemic national socioeconomic vulnerabilities, conflicts, economic meltdown, political unrest, and civil strife resulting in disruption of all medical and dental services in many parts of the country. Further, the oral health sector suffers lack of essential medical and dental instruments, materials, and supplies, a shortage of health workers, and poor infection control practices, which present major threats to dental care in the region. Moreover, the frequent closure of dental hospitals and clinics has limited accessibility and utilization of oral health services. Hindrances and disparities impede the oral health system advancement, resulting in fragmented and underdeveloped oral healthcare provision.

There is a high prevalence of oral diseases in Sudan and the consequences illustrate substantial public health problems including pain, impairment of function, and reduced quality of life. Decision makers and health planners in Sudan need information about risk factors for oral diseases to help identify individuals who are at risk of developing oral diseases and to target population-level interventions. There is a serious need to collect data on social and medical status, health behaviours, and demographic data in addition to clinical data related to *toombak* use and oral diseases, in particular PD. Only a few studies exist considering PD in Sudan, but there is no data on PD and use of *toombak*. Most of the studies focused on *toombak* use and OCs and pre-cancers. There is a need to assess periodontal status among *toombak* users. Given the limited infrastructure for oral health services delivery, many people in Sudan do not receive regular dental care and have acute problems when seen by a dentist. In Sudan, the dentist-to-patient ratio is 1:33,000 compared with approximately 1:2000 in most industrialized countries. Relative to the size of the Sudanese population, there are very few dentists, and this restricts access to regular dental care. Other factors which influence dental attendance in Sudan include the lack of public funding for oral healthcare and dental insurance schemes to ameliorate the cost of care. In Sudan, as in many other developing countries, dental treatment is limited to pain relief or emergency care where tooth extraction dominates the services. There are even more barriers to the provision of treatment of oral diseases like PD, which is multifactorial in origin and worthy of further investigations with many visits related to treatment phase, and further regular follow-ups. This, however, indicates a very high cost, which will affect patients' part, or prevailing attitude of dentists towards management of PD in a proper clinical approach. Containment of oral disease could be done by simple, minimally invasive, and affordable dentistry. Wider access to public dental care facilities could be helped by provision of sufficient manpower and continuing education of dentists to ensure that oral healthcare providers have sufficient skills and depth of understanding of aspects of oral healthcare. Clinically, advanced PD, OCs, and pre-cancers from *toombak* users, especially gingival cancer, which are always seen at a late stage of the disease, share some signs and symptoms such as swelling, bleeding, deep periodontal pockets, bone destruction, and tooth mobility. Similarities in the clinical presentations among patients with PD and OCs and pre-cancers from Sudan, in relation to *toombak* use, encourage the clinicians to find more reliable and non-aggressive tools for early detection of OCs/pre-cancers and, at the same time, encourage in-depth research among *toombak* users. To conclude, the author would like to call international researchers and clinicians to participate in highlighting and addressing the problem of PD among Sudanese *toombak* users. The author has not mentioned the possible association between *toombak* use and peri-implantitis, which is due to the fact that implant therapy is illusive and beyond the reach for *toombak* users, and the treatment is solely for patients belonging to high-income group and most of them don't use *toombak*.

Key Points

- The dentist-to-patient ratio in Sudan is alarmingly low (1:33,000).
- There is a critical need for epidemiological data on periodontal disease, especially among *toombak* users.
- Current research is sparse and mostly focused on *toombak*-related oral cancers and pre-cancers, not periodontal diseases.
- There is a strong appeal for international researchers and clinicians to investigate periodontal diseases among *toombak* users.

Acknowledgements The author would like to acknowledge Dr. Amel Sami, APC Microbiome Ireland, School of Microbiology, University College Cork, Cork, Ireland for providing and permitting use of Fig. 7.1a, c, e, and f. The author would also like to express in-depth gratitude and sincere thanks to Professor Ali M Idris and to Professor Saman Warnakulasuriya for their solid rock contribution and collaboration with the author on all aspects related to research on *toombak* addressing and highlighting the problem from the clinical to laboratory findings.

References

Al-Hebshi NN, Alharbi FA, Mahri M, Tsute C (2017) Differences in the Bacteriome of smokeless tobacco products with different oral carcinogenicity: compositional and predicted functional analysis. Genes 8(4):106. https://doi.org/10.3390/genes8040106

Almahdi HM, Åstrøm AN, Ali RW, Nasir EF (2017a) School workers' knowledge, attitude and behaviour related to use of Toombak: a cross sectional study from Khartoum state, Sudan. BMC Oral Health:160. https://doi.org/10.1186/s12903-017-0460-8

Almahdi HM, Ali RW, Nasir EF, Åstrøm AN (2017b) Socio-cognitive correlates of intention to use Toombak: a cross-sectional study among students (13–16 years) in Khartoum State, Sudan. BMC Public Health 88. https://doi.org/10.1186/s12889-017-4606-z

Almahdi HM, Ali RW, Nasir EF (2020) Exposure to the advertisement of toombak at the point-of-sale among adolescents in Khartoum State, Sudan: a cross-sectional study. Tob Prev Cessat 13(6):19. https://doi.org/10.18332/tpc/115800. eCollection 2020

Anderson RA, Burton HR, Fleming PD, Hamilton-Kamp TR (1989) Effect of storage conditions on nitrosated, acylated, and oxidizedpyridine alkaloid derivatives in smokeless tobacco products. Cancer Res 49:5895–5900

Baima G, Minoli M, Michaud DS, Aimetti M, Sanz M, Loos BG, Romandini M (2023) periodontitis and risk of cancer: mechanistic evidence. Periodontol 2000 96(1):83–94. https://doi.org/10.1111/prd.12540

Brunnemann KD, Hoffmann D (1974) The pH of tobacco smoke. Food Cosmetic Toxicol 12:115–124. https://doi.org/10.1016/0015-6264(74)90327-7

Brunnemann KD, Genoble I, Hoffmann D (1985) N-nitrosamines in chewing tobacco: an international comparison. J Agri Food Chem 33:1178–1181

Colombo APV, Boches SK, Cotton SL, Goodson JM, Kent R, Haffajee AD (2009) Comparisons of subgingival microbial profiles of refractory periodontitis, severe periodontitis, and periodontal health using the human oral microbe identification microarray. J Periodontol 80:1421–1432. https://doi.org/10.1902/jop.2009.090185

Costea DE, Lukandu O, Bui L et al (2010) Adverse effects of Sudanese toombak vs. Swedish snuff on human oral cells. J Oral Pathol Med 39(2):128–140

Djordjevic MV, Fan J, Bush LP, Brunnemann KD, Hoffmann D (1993) Effects of storage conditions on levels of tobacco-specific Nnitrosamines, N-nitrosamines and N-nitrosaminoacids in U.S. moist snuff. J Agri Food Chem 11:1790–1794

Dysvik B, Vasstrand EN, Løvlie R et al (2006) Gene expression profiles of head and neck carcinomas from Sudanese and Norwegian patients reveal common biological pathways regardless of race and lifestyle. Clin Cancer Res 12(4):1109–1120

El-Amin SE-T (2019) School smoking policies and health science students' use of cigarettes, shisha, and dipping Tombak in Sudan. Front Public Health 7:290. https://doi.org/10.3389/fpubh.2019.00290. eCollection 2019

El-Amin A-El, Nwaru BI, Ginawi I, Pisani P, Hakama M (2011) The role of parents, friends and teachers in adolescents' cigarette smoking and tombak dipping in Sudan. Tob Control 20(2):94–99. https://doi.org/10.1136/tc.2010.038091. Epub 2010 Oct 13

Hoare A, Soto C, Rojas-Celis V, Bravo D (2019) Chronic inflammation as a link between periodontitis and carcinogenesis. Rev Mediators Inflamm:1029857 doi: https://doi.org/10.1155/2019/1029857. eCollection 2019

Holt SC, Ebersole JL (2005) Porphyromonas gingivalis, Treponema denticola, and Tannerella forsythia: the "red complex", a prototype polybacterial pathogenic consortium in periodontitis. Periodontol 2000(38):72–122. https://doi.org/10.1111/j.1600-0757.2005.00113.x

Ibrahim SO (1999) *p*53, keratins, human paoilloma virus and proto-oncogenes in oral squamous cell carcinomas from snuff-dippers and non-dippers from The Sudan and Scandinavia. Dr. Odont. thesis. University of Bergen, Bergen, Norway

Ibrahim SO, Lillehaug JR, Dolphine D, Johnson NW, Warnakulasuriya KAAS, Vasstrand EN (2002) Mutations of the cell cycle arrest gene p21WAF1, but not the metastasis-inducing gene S100A4, are frequent in oral squamous cell carcinomas from Sudanese toombak dippers and non-snuff-dippers from The Sudan, Scandinavia, USA and UK. Anticancer Res 22(3):1445–1451

Ibrahim SO, Aarsaether N, Holsve MK et al (2003) Gene expression profile in oral squamous cell carcinomas and matching normal oral mucosal tissues from black Africans and white Caucasians: the case of The Sudan vs. Norway. Oral Oncol 39(1):37–48. https://doi.org/10.1016/s1368-8375(02)00018-0

Idris AM (1992) The etiological association between use of toombak and oral squamous cell carcinoma. Ph.D. thesis. University of Khartoum, Khartoum, Sudan

Idris AM, Nair J, Oshima H, Friesen M, Bronet I, Faustman EM, Bartsch H (1991) Unusually high levels of carcinogenic tobacco-specific nitrosamines in Sudan snuff (toombak). Carcinogenesis 12:1115–1118

Idris AM, Nair J, Friesen M, Oshima H, Bronet I, Faustman EM, Bartsch H (1992) Carcinogenic tobacco-specific nitrosamines are present at unusually high levels in the saliva of oral snuff users in Sudan. Carcinogenesis 13:1001–1005

Idris AM, Ibrahim YE, Warnakulasuriya KA, Cooper DJ, Johnson NW, Nilsen R (1998) Toombak use and cigarette smoking in The Sudan: estimates of prevalence in the Nile State. Children and adolescents (4-17 years). Prev Med 27(4):597–603. https://doi.org/10.1006/pmed.1998.0331

Javed F, Warnakulasuriya S (2016) Is there a relationship between periodontal disease and oral cancer? A systematic review of currently available evidence. Crit Rev Oncol/Hematol 97:197–205. https://doi.org/10.1016/j.critrevonc.2015.08.018

Kallischnigg G, Weitkunat R, Lee PN (2008) Systematic review of the relation between smokeless tobacco and non-neoplastic oral diseases in Europe and the United States. BMC Oral Health:13. https://doi.org/10.1186/1472-6831-8-13

Katarkar A, Saha A, Mukherjee S, Kundu D, Bandyopadhyay P, Chaudhuri K (2015) Telomerase expression in individuals with chronic and aggressive periodontitis. J Periodontol 86:65–65. https://doi.org/10.1902/jop.2015.140540

Kavarthapu A, Gurumoorthy K (2021) Linking chronic periodontitis and oral cancer: a review. Oral Oncol:105375. https://doi.org/10.1016/j.oraloncology.2021.105375. Epub 2021 Jun 1

Kwona TH, Lamsterb IB, Levin L (2021) Current concepts in the management of periodontitis. Concise clinical review. Int Dent J 71(6):462–476

Li T-J, Hao Y-h, Tang Y-l, Liang X-h (2022) Periodontal pathogens: a crucial link between periodontal diseases and oral cancer. Front Microbiol 13:919633. https://doi.org/10.3389/fmicb.2022.919633

Loro LL, Vintermyr OK, Ibrahim SO, Idris AM, Johannessen AC (2000) Apoptosis and expression of Bax and Bcl-2 in snuff- and non-snuff associated oral squamous cell carcinomas. Anticancer Res 20(5A):2855–2860

Moraes RC, Dias FL, Figueredo CM, Fischer RG (2016) Association between chronic periodontitis and oral/oropharyngeal cancer. Brazil Dental J 27:261–266. https://doi.org/10.1590/0103-6440201600754

Nonnenmacher C, Mutters R, De Jacoby LF (2001) Characteristics of subgingival microbiota in adult periodontitis, localized juvenile periodontitis and rapidly progressive periodontitis subjects. Clin Microbiol Infect 7:213–217. https://doi.org/10.1046/j.1469-0691.2001.00210.x

Patil S, Yadalam PK, Hosmani J et al (2023) Modulation of oral cancer and periodontitis using chemotherapeutic agents – a narrative review. Dis Mon 69:101348. https://doi.org/10.1016/j.disamonth.2022.101348

Prokopczyk B, Wu M, Cox JE, Hoffmann D (1992) Bioavailabilty of tobacco-specific nitrosamines to snuff dippers. Carcinogensis 13:863–866

Roman E, Meza-Zepeda LA, Kresse SH, Myklebost O, Vasstrand EN, Ibrahim SO (2008) Chromosomal aberrations in head and neck squamous cell carcinomas in Norwegian and Sudanese populations by array comparative genomic hybridization. Oncol Rep 20(4):825–843

Sami A, Imad Elimairi I, Patangia D, Watkins C, Ryan A, Ross RP, Stanton C (2021) The ultrastructural, metabolomic and metagenomic characterisation of the sudanese smokeless tobacco 'Toombak'. Toxicol Rep 8:1498–1512. https://doi.org/10.1016/j.toxrep.2021.07.008. eCollection 2021

Sapkota D (2011) S100 gene family members in oral squamous cell carcinomas (OSCCs): functional characterization of S100A14 in proliferation and invasion of OSCC derived cells. PhD. Thesis. University of Bergen, Bergen, Norway

Sardi JC, Duque C, Mariano FS, Peixoto IT, Höfling JF, Gonçalves RB (2010) Candida spp. in periodontal disease: a brief review. J Oral Sci 52:177–185. https://doi.org/10.2334/josnusd.52.177

Shi J, Leng W, Zhao L, Deng C, Xu C, Wang J (2018) Tooth loss and cancer risk: a dose–response meta-analysis of prospective cohort studies. Oncotarget 9:15090. https://doi.org/10.18632/oncotarget.23850

Shin Y, Choung H, Lee J, Rhyu I, Kim H (2019) Association of periodontitis with oral cancer: a case-control study. J Dent Res 98:526–533. https://doi.org/10.1177/0022034519827565

Slots J, Slots HJP (2011) Bacterial and viral pathogens in saliva: disease relationship and infectious risk. Periodontol 55:48. https://doi.org/10.1111/j.1600-0757.2010.00361.x

Smyth EM, Kulkarni P, Claye E, Stanfill S, Tyx R, Maddox C, Mongodin EF, Sapkota AR (2017) Smokeless tobacco products harbor diverse bacterial microbiota that differ across products and brands. Appl Microbiol Biotechnol 101(13):5391–5403. https://doi.org/10.1007/s00253-017-8282-9. Epub 2017 Apr 22

Tso TC (1982) Physiology and biochemistry of tobacco plants. Dowden, Hutchinson and Ross, Stroudsburg

Tyx RE, Stanfill SB, Keong LM, Rivera AJ, Satten GA, Watson CH (2016) Characterization of bacterial communities in selected smokeless tobacco products using 16S rDNA analysis. PLoS One 11(1):e0146939. https://doi.org/10.1371/journal.pone.0146939. eCollection 2016

Tyx RE, Rivera AJ, Stanfill SB, Zaatari GS, Watson CH (2022) Shotgun metagenome sequencing of a Sudanese toombak snuff tobacco: genetic attributes of a high tobacco-specific nitrosamine containing smokeless tobacco product. Lett Appl Microbiol 74(3):444–451. https://doi.org/10.1111/lam.13623. Epub 2021 Dec 19

Zhang M, Liu Y, Afzali H, Graves DT (2024) An update on periodontal inflammation and bone loss. Review Front Immunol 15:1385436. https://doi.org/10.3389/fimmu.2024.1385436

Effect of *Mainpuri* on Periodontal and Peri-Implant Health

8

Darshan Devang Divakar and Chitra Jhugroo

Abbreviations

IL Interleukin
MC *Mainpuri* chewers
OHS Oral health status
PA Power analysis
SES Socio-economic status
SSE Sample size estimation
ST Smokeless tobacco

Learning Goals

- Understand the composition and cultural significance of *mainpuri* tobacco, including its regional use and how it is prepared and consumed.
- Identify the oral and periodontal health consequences associated with habitual *mainpuri* use, supported by clinical study data.
- Evaluate the current evidence linking *mainpuri* chewing to periodontal disease, including limitations in existing research.
- Assess the potential pathophysiological mechanisms by which *mainpuri* may negatively affect peri-implant tissues.

D. D. Divakar (✉)
Faculty of Health Sciences, JSS Academy of Higher Education and Research, Vacoas-Phoenix, Mauritius

Nano Dental and Medical Ltd, Solferino, Vacoas, Mauritius

C. Jhugroo
Nano Dental and Medical Ltd, Solferino, Vacoas, Mauritius

F. Javed, S. Warnakulasuriya (eds.), *Smokeless Tobacco and its Effects on Periodontal Health*, https://doi.org/10.1007/978-3-032-16409-4_8

- Recognize the gaps in the current literature, particularly the absence of studies from regions with high *mainpuri* use and the lack of peri-implant health assessments.
- Formulate directions for future research that explore histological and microbiological impacts of *mainpuri* on oral tissues.

8.1 Introduction

Mainpuri is a city located in the northern state of Uttar Pradesh, India; and serves as the administrative headquarters of the Mainpuri district (Fig. 8.1). According to the 2011 Census of India, Mainpuri city had a population of approximately 1.4 million, with a literacy rate of around 85%. The district has a sex ratio of 876 females per 1000 males, reflecting the broader demographic trends of the region. Besides its cultural and historical heritage, Mainpuri City is famous to produce smokeless tobacco (ST), "*Mainpuri* tobacco", which is widely consumed both locally and in surrounding regions. *Mainpuri* is typically hand-prepared, reflecting its deep cultural and social integration in rural and semi-urban communities.

Mainpuri use is not restricted to India and has several users in other countries including Pakistan, Nepal and Bangladesh (Akhtar et al. 2017; Channa and Khan 2014; Zhao et al. 2021). This product is a mixture of sun-dried crushed tobacco, slaked-lime (aqueous calcium hydroxide), areca nut (AN) (also known as betel nut), and finely powdered *catechu* (an extract of the acacia tree) (Figs. 8.2, 8.3, 8.4, and 8.5).

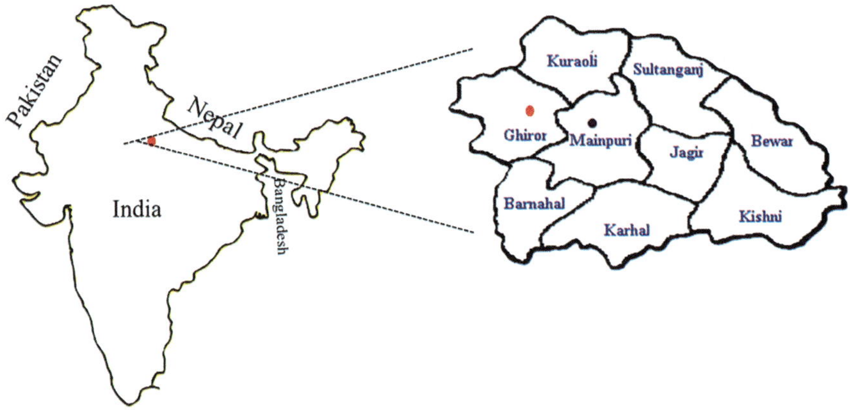

Fig. 8.1 Mainpuri city, located in the state of Uttar Pradesh, India. (The location of Mainpuri depicted is approximate and intended for general reference purposes only)

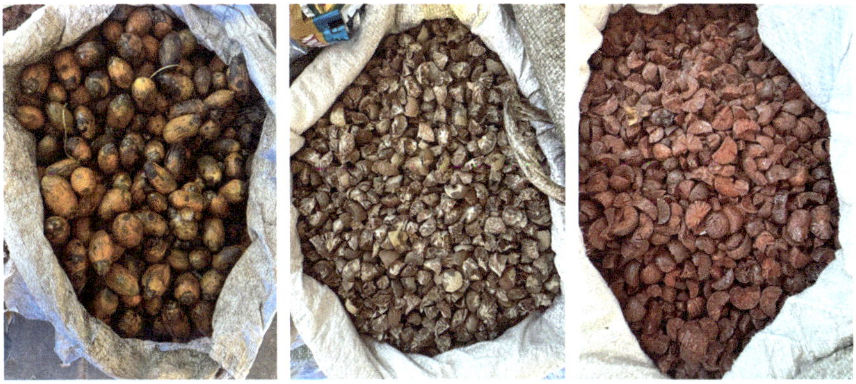

Fig. 8.2 *Mainpuri* (Ingredients) Different quality and size cut betel nuts

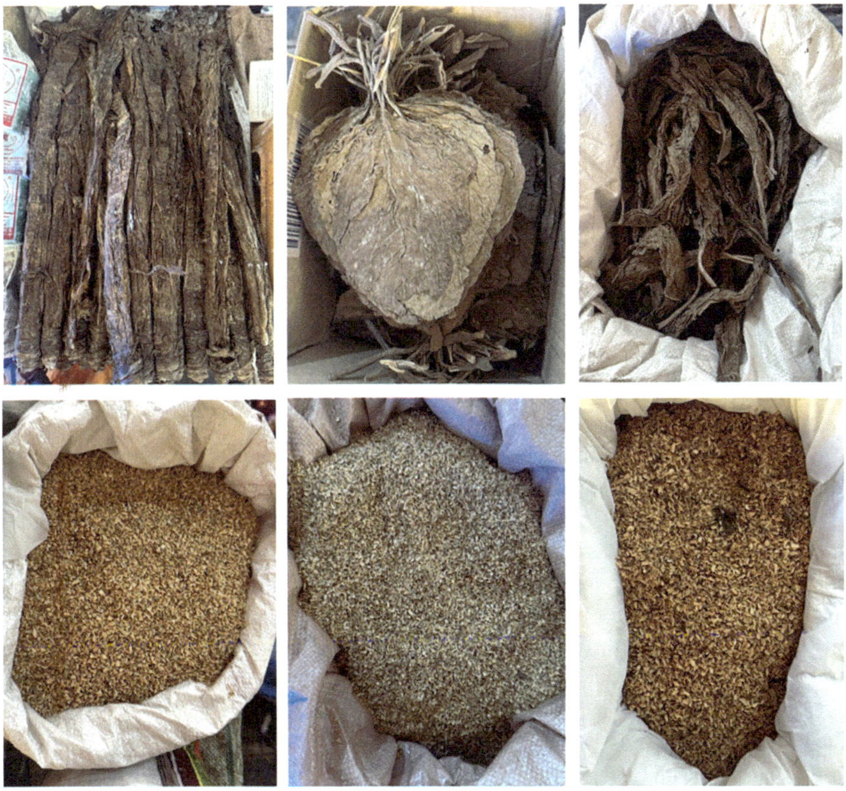

Fig. 8.3 *Mainpuri* (Ingredients) Different quality rolled and pieces of tobacco leaves

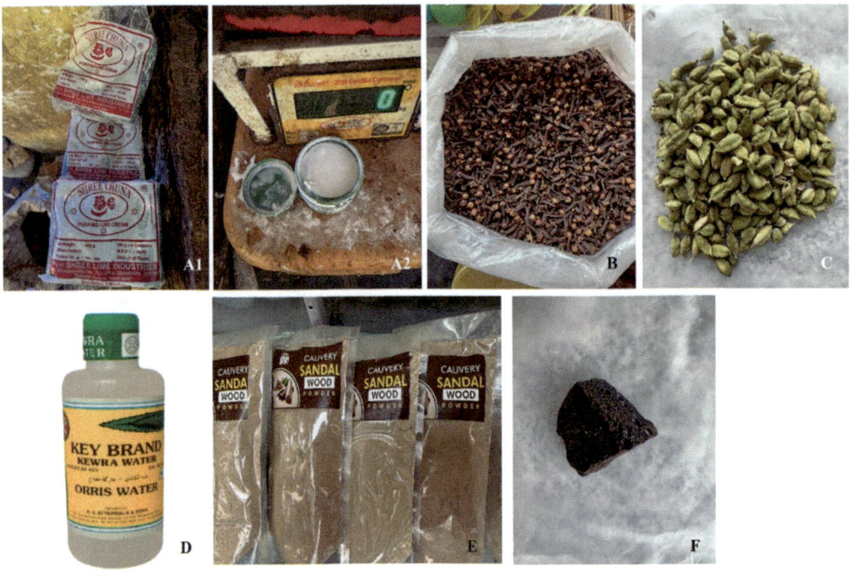

Fig. 8.4 *Mainpuri* (Ingredients) (**a**1, **a**2) Slaked Lime. (**b**) Cloves. (**c**) Cardamom. (**d**) Kewara Water (Extracted from the fragrant flower of *Pandanus Odoratissimus*). (**e**) Sandalwood Powder. (**f**) Catechu

Occasionally, other aromatic additives such as cinnamon, clove, and camphor (a terpenoid and a cyclic ketone) are included to enhance its flavour and appeal (Channa and Khan 2014). *Mainpuri* is typically sold in non-branded plastic pouches lacking any health warning (Fig. 8.1). The precise prevalence of *mainpuri* usage in the Indian subcontinent and around the world remains unknown; however, it has been reported that in the Mainpuri district in India, every second male and every third female uses this ST product (Channa and Khan 2014).

Users take a small pinch of *Mainpuri* between their fingers and place it under the lip, along the gum line, or in the cheek pouch. The placement allows for prolonged contact with the oral mucosa. Once placed, users may occasionally chew or manipulate the mixture with their tongue to release the flavours and active compounds, including nicotine and arecoline. Chewing also facilitates the absorption of these substances through the oral mucosa. The active compounds are absorbed directly into the bloodstream through the mucous membranes in the mouth, providing a rapid psychoactive effect without the need for smoking. After the desired effects have been achieved, the residue is typically spat out. However, some users may swallow small amounts, which can exacerbate health risks due to systemic absorption of harmful substances.

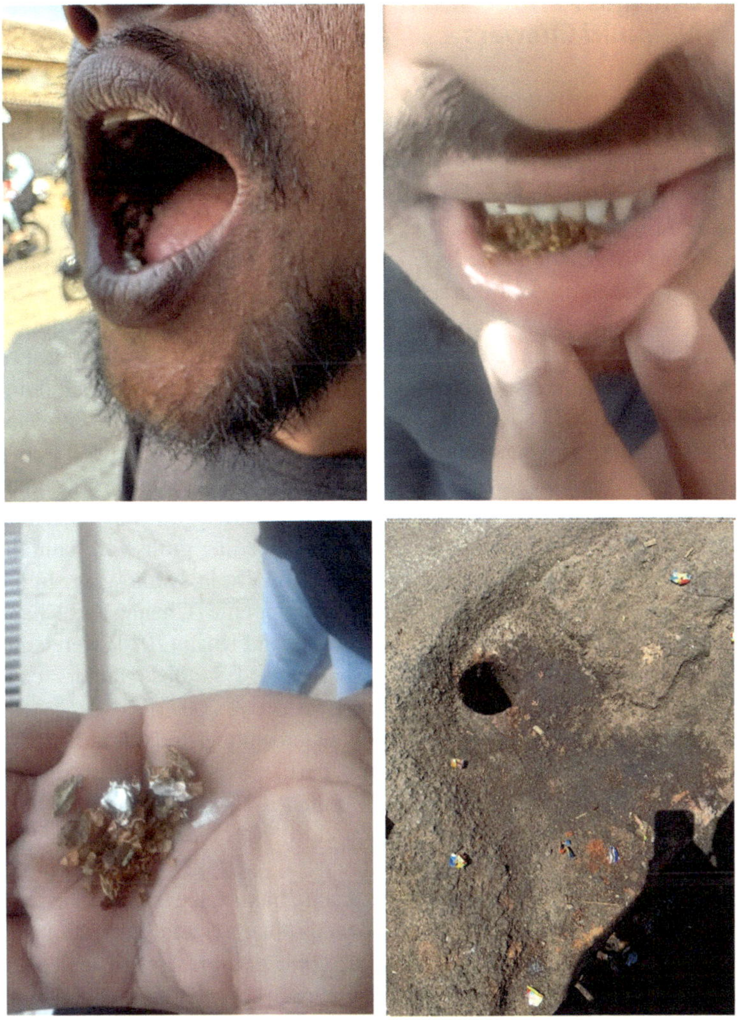

Fig. 8.5 *Mainpuri* kept in buccal and labial mucosa, held at hand and spitting zone

Key Points

- *Mainpuri* is a city in Uttar Pradesh, India, with a population of around 1.4 million, as of the 2011 census.
- *Mainpuri* tobacco is a hand-prepared ST product that is culturally and socially ingrained in rural and semi-urban communities in *Mainpuri* and surrounding regions.
- *Mainpuri* typically contains sun-dried tobacco, slaked lime, areca nut, and catechu, with optional aromatic additives like cinnamon and camphor.
- *Mainpuri* is sold in non-branded plastic pouches that lack health warnings.

8.2 Oral and Periodontal Health Status Among *Mainpuri* Chewers

A limited number of original clinical studies have assessed the oral health status (OHS) among *mainpuri* chewers (MC) and non-chewers (controls). Nearly a decade ago, Channa and Khan (2014) performed an observational cross-sectional study in the city of Hyderabad, Pakistan, to compare the OHS among MC and controls. In this study, 114 MC and 119 controls with ages ranging between 15 and 45 years were included. A questionnaire based on 75 items was administered to all participants. Besides gathering data on age, gender, and socio-economic status (SES) of the participants, the study reported in general terms information regarding "mouth condition" and "different complications" was collected using a questionnaire. However, these parameters were not explicitly detailed in the study's methodology (Channa and Khan 2014). All self-reported MC were young males with ages ranging between 15 and 30 years (mean age was not reported). Moreover, poor education ($P < 0.001$) and a deprived SES ($P < 0.001$) were significantly associated with *mainpuri* chewing habit. Regarding self-rated OHS, the following symptoms were more often manifested in MC than controls: (a) bleeding gums; (b) pain on chewing; (c) difficulty in mouth opening; and (d) difficulty in swallowing. In addition, most of the MC were underweight due to loss of appetite (Channa and Khan 2014). Although the participants in the study by Channa and Khan (2014) were educationally deprived and possessed an underprivileged SES, these factors cannot be regarded as definitive indicators of ST use (Imam et al. 2007).

Results from a cross-sectional study conducted among students at a medical university showed that nearly 22% of the study participants had at least tried chewing ST products and 6.4% were lifetime ST product users including *mainpuri* (Imam et al. 2007). However, in this study (Imam et al. 2007), the precise prevalence of *mainpuri* use population was not reported.

A cross-sectional study conducted in Karachi, Pakistan, evaluated the patterns of periodontal diseases among 377 users of ST products, including *mainpuri* (Nasir et al. 2023). Participants were 15–45 years old, and most were males (61.3%). Eighteen percent ($n = 68$) of the study population were self-reported habitual *mainpuri* chewers. Although the results of this study (Nasir et al. 2023) were not exclusively based on *mainpuri* usage, nearly 55% of the participants were chewing ST products for at least 5 years and were keeping it in the mouth for at least 5 min. This study did not compare the periodontal status among ST product users and non-users; but rather reported the frequency of periodontal inflammatory parameters in this cohort (Fig. 8.3). In summary, periodontal health status of ST users (including MC) showed significant deterioration. Community Periodontal Index (CPI) scores of 3 and 4 were observed in approximately 69% of MC, indicating moderate to severe periodontitis. Additionally, nearly 66% of ST users presented with class II to IV gingival recession, approximately 96% had no or mild furcation involvement. Tooth mobility was noted in approximately 14% of ST users, and 21% had missing teeth. These findings suggest that habitual *mainpuri* use is associated with significant periodontal deterioration, necessitating further research and public health interventions (Fig. 8.3). Based on the results, it seems that all ST products including *mainpuri* compromised periodontal health. Therefore, it is demanding to assess the extent of periodontal inflammation induced exclusively by *mainpuri*. Nevertheless, nearly 22% of the ST product users reported that they never brushed their teeth, which by itself is a common risk factor for periodontal disease (Fig. 8.6).

Whether *mainpuri* users who diligently adhere to daily oral hygiene maintenance practices, such as toothbrushing and flossing, exhibit superior periodontal health compared to those who do not consistently follow such protocols warrants further studies. A split-mouth, cross-sectional in vivo study conducted in India compared the periodontal status among ST chewers in relation to unilateral ST-related keratosis (Nimbal et al. 2023). The contralateral site served as control in this study (Nimbal et al. 2023). In this study, 6% male ST chewers self-reported that they were MC. The individuals were using ST products since approximately a decade and were nearly 30 years old (Nimbal et al. 2023). Furthermore nearly 50% of the study population reported that they brushed teeth once daily and nearly 11% of these individuals reported to have never visited a dentist. Approximately 64% of the study participants were placing the ST product in the right buccal vestibule for over 5 min. The results showed that gingival bleeding, probing depth, and clinical attachment loss were significantly higher in sites associated with ST-induced keratosis than the contralateral side (Nimbal et al. 2023). Since *mainpuri* contains areca nut as a chief ingredient, it is possible that chewing and prolonged placement of this form of ST product in the buccal vestibule causes keratosis as well as periodontal inflammation. Table 8.1 provides an overview of studies that assessed the periodontal health status among *mainpuri* chewers and non-chewers. However, to date, there are no studies that have histologically compared the buccal mucosal tissues from the chewing and contra-lateral side among MC.

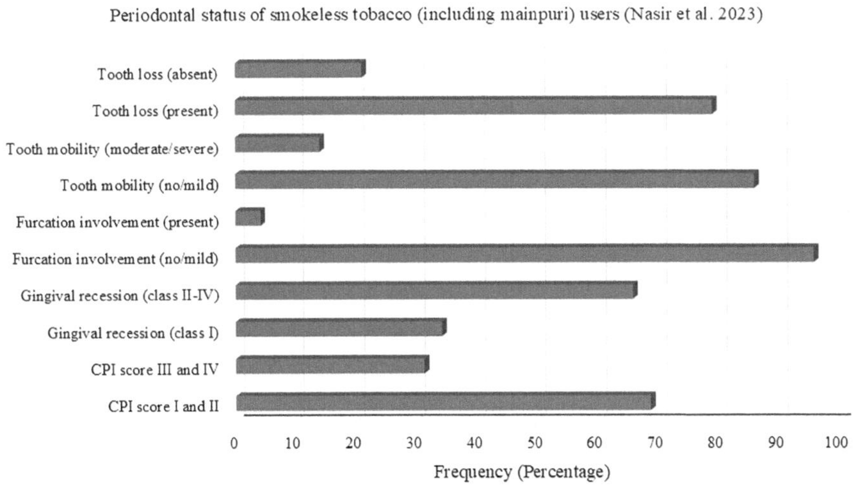

Fig. 8.6 Periodontal status of smokeless tobacco (including *mainpuri* chewers) users. (Modified from the study by Nasir et al. (2023))

Table 8.1 Overview of studies that assessed the periodontal health status among *mainpuri* chewers and non-chewers

Authors et al. (year)	Location	Age of participants	Study groups (*n*)	Results	Power analysis?
Channa and Khan (2014)	Pakistan	15–45 years	MC: 114 Controls: 119	Bleeding gums and pain on chewing were more common in MC than in controls	No
Nasir et al. (2023)	Pakistan	15–45 years	MC: 68 Controls: none	68.7% of MC had CPI scores between 3 and 4. 65.8% of MC had GR between class II and IV. 95.8% of MC had no or mild furcation involvement. 14.1% of MC had moderate to severe tooth mobility. 21% of MC had missing teeth	No
Nimbal et al. (2023)	India	18–35 years	96 ST product users 6% were MC	Increased gingival bleeding on the side of ST-induced keratosis[a]. Increased probing depth on the side of ST-induced keratosis[a]. Increased attachment loss on the side of ST-induced keratosis[a]	No

MC Mainpuri chewers, *ST* smokeless tobacco, *Controls* Individuals not using nicotinic products
[a]Compared to contralateral side

Key Points

- *Mainpuri* users are typically young males with low education and deprived socio-economic backgrounds.
- *Mainpuri* chewers frequently report bleeding gums, pain while chewing, difficulty opening the mouth, and trouble swallowing, indicating compromised oral health status compared to non-chewers.
- Habitual use of *mainpuri* is linked to moderate to severe periodontitis, gingival recession, tooth mobility, and tooth loss.
- A substantial proportion of ST users, including *mainpuri* users, reported inadequate oral hygiene practices, such as never brushing their teeth.
- Most studies do not isolate the effects of *mainpuri* from other ST products, making it difficult to assess its specific impact on periodontal health.

From a statistical point of view, it is worth mentioning that none of the studies referenced above were power-adjusted (Channa and Khan 2014; Nasir et al. 2023; Nimbal et al. 2023). Further well-designed and power adjusted studies are needed to assess the effect of *mainpuri* on periodontal health.

8.2.1 Peri-Implant Health Status in *Mainpuri* Chewers

A vigilant review of indexed scientific literature showed that to date, there are no studies that have assessed the impact of *mainpuri* chewing on peri-implant soft and osseous tissues. Nevertheless, the authors of the present chapter perceive that *mainpuri* jeopardizes peri-implant tissues through several potential pathophysiological mechanisms:

- Compromised vascularity: Chewing ST leads to prolonged exposure of peri-implant tissues to nicotine, which induces vasoconstriction by activating the sympathetic nervous system, reducing local blood flow to the peri-implant tissues (Clarke and Shephard 1984; Rifai et al. 2020). Reduced vascularity compromises oxygen and nutrient delivery essential for osseointegration and soft tissue healing, leading to delayed or incomplete healing after implant placement.
- Inflammatory dysregulation: The ST contains carcinogens, such as nitrosamines, and pro-inflammatory compounds that stimulate chronic inflammation. This heightened inflammatory response potentially increases levels of destructive inflammatory cytokines like interleukin (IL)-6, IL-1 beta and matrix metalloproteinases in the saliva, and peri-implant tissues and sulci (Javed et al. 2015; Sgambato et al. 2018).
- Persistent inflammation degrades the peri-implant soft tissue and bone, predisposing the site to peri-implant mucositis and peri-implantitis.
- Disruption in osseous remodelling: Nicotine impairs osteoblast function and enhances osteoclast activity tipping the balance of bone remodelling towards resorption (Gruber et al. 2023; Martinez et al. 2022). This imbalance weakens the osseointegration process, jeopardizing the primary stability and most likely compromising the likelihood of long-term survival of dental implants.
- Mechanical trauma: *Mainpuri* contains AN as a chief ingredient. It is therefore likely that chronic placement of *mainpuri* in the oral vestibule adjacent to the implant site/s exposes peri-implant tissues to mechanical trauma as well as chemical irritation. It is hypothesized that repeated *mainpuri* exposure weakens the epithelial barrier and makes tissues more susceptible to microbial invasion, inflammation, and eventual crestal bone loss.

Further clinical and experimental studies are needed to evaluate the impact of *mainpuri* on peri-implant tissues.

Key Points

- No studies to date have specifically evaluated the effects of *mainpuri* chewing on peri-implant soft and osseous tissues, highlighting a gap in the literature.
- *Mainpuri* contains carcinogens and pro-inflammatory agents that may elevate inflammatory cytokines (e.g., IL-6, IL-1β, MMPs), increasing the risk of peri-implant mucositis and peri-implantitis.

- Chronic *mainpuri* placement in the vestibule can cause direct mechanical trauma and chemical irritation, weakening the epithelial barrier and facilitating microbial invasion and tissue breakdown.
- There is a strong need for clinical and experimental studies to validate the hypothesized pathophysiological mechanisms of *mainpuri's* impact on peri-implant health.

8.3 Limitations of This Chapter and Recommendations

A major limitation of this chapter is the limited number of studies that have assessed the impact of *mainpuri* on periodontal and peri-implant health. While existing research suggests a potential link between *mainpuri* use and adverse oral health outcomes, the findings are often confounded by other forms of ST mixed with *mainpuri* or poor oral hygiene practices. Notably, no studies have been reported from Mainpuri district where this habit is most prevalent. Additionally, no studies have investigated the specific effects of *mainpuri* on peri-implant tissues, making it difficult to draw definitive conclusions about its role in peri-implant inflammation and bone loss. The lack of power-adjusted studies further weakens the reliability of current findings, necessitating caution when interpreting the available data. To address these gaps, future studies should focus on well-designed, prospective clinical studies that specifically evaluate the periodontal and peri-implant clinical (including plaque and gingival indices, probing depths, gingival recessions, and loss of attachment) and radiographic parameters (marginal and crestal bone levels) of habitual *mainpuri* users. In addition, future studies should include control groups comprising of individuals who do not use any form of tobacco product/s to establish clearly defined comparative groups. Furthermore, it is recommended that future studies should be based on power-adjusted data to enhance the statistical validity of the findings. Investigations utilizing histological and microbiological analyses of peri-implant tissues in MC are also warranted to elucidate potential pathophysiological mechanisms.

Key Points

- There is a scarcity of studies examining the impact of *mainpuri* use on periodontal and peri-implant health
- The absence of power-adjusted studies reduces the statistical reliability of current findings.

8.4 Conclusion

Habitual *mainpuri* use is a risk-factor of periodontal as well as peri-implant diseases. Further well-designed and power-adjusted studies are needed to assess the effect of *mainpuri* on periodontal and peri-implant tissues. Furthermore, it is imperative to educate patients about the detrimental effects of ST products on oral, periodontal, peri-implant, and overall health. Routine anti-tobacco public health awareness programmes in the Mainpuri district in India can play a significant role in this context.

References

Akhtar A, Afridi HI, Kazi TG, Talpur FN, Arain SS, Baig JA, Khan N et al (2017) Chromium exposure in the adult population, consuming different types of smokeless tobacco products in Pakistan. Biol Trace Elem Res 175:312–321

Channa NA, Khan A (2014) Hazards of Mainpuri chewing in Hyderabad and adjoining areas, Pakistan. Rawal Med J 39:216–219

Clarke NG, Shephard BC (1984) The effects of epinephrine and nicotine on gingival blood flow in the rabbit. Arch Oral Biol 29:789–793

Gruber MD, Gibbs D, Vignolles-Jeong J, Viljoen S, Grossbach AJ, Xu D (2023) The effects of nicotine- and cigarette-related products on osteogenesis, bone formation, and bone mineralization: a systematic review. Neurosurgery 93:247–256

Imam SZ, Nawaz H, Sepah YJ, Pabaney AH, Ilyas M, Ghaffar S (2007) Use of smokeless tobacco among groups of Pakistani medical students – a cross sectional study. BMC Public Health 7:231

Javed F, Al-Kheraif AA, Al Amri MD, Mikami T, Vohra F, Warnakulasuriya S, Romanos GE (2015) Periodontal parameters and whole salivary cytokine profiles among habitual gutka chewers and non-chewers. J Periodontol 86:689–695

Martinez IKC, Sparks NRL, Madrid JV, Talbot P, Zur Nieden NI (2022) Exposure to cigarette smoke impedes human osteoblast differentiation independently of nicotine. Nicotine Tob Res 24:1921–1926

Nasir SM, Sultana T, Hashmi S, Ahmed M (2023) Patterns and predictors of periodontal disease and tooth loss among users of smokeless tobacco. BMC Oral Health 23:428

Nimbal AV, Kharkar SP, Vishwakarma AP, Patil AA, Patil SS, Patil RA (2023) Comparative analysis of dentition and periodontal status in patients with unilateral smokeless tobacco pouch keratosis. Cureus 15:e48923

Rifai M, Aoun G, Majzoub Z (2020) Evaluation of the papillary gingival vasculature in smokers and nonsmokers with chronic periodontitis: a clinical in vivo study. J Int Soc Prev Community Dent 10:368–375

Sgambato JA, Jones BA, Caraway JW, Prasad GL (2018) Inflammatory profile analysis reveals differences in cytokine expression between smokers, moist snuff users, and dual users compared to non-tobacco consumers. Cytokine 107:43–51

Zhao L, Mbulo L, Twentyman E, Palipudi K, King BA (2021) Disparities in smokeless tobacco use in Bangladesh, India, and Pakistan: findings from the Global Adult Tobacco Survey, 2014–2017. PLoS One 16:e0250144

Effect of Khat (*Catha edulis*) on Periodontal and Peri-Implant Health

9

Sukumaran Anil, Saravanan Sampoornam Pape Reddy, Delfin Lovelina Francis, and Vishnupriya K. Sweety

Abbreviations

CAL	Clinical attachment loss
CI	Calculus index
CPITN	Community Periodontal Index of Treatment Needs
GCF	Gingival crevicular fluid
GI	Gingival index
GR	Gingival recession
IL-1β	Interleukin 1-beta
IL-6	Interleukin-6
MMPs	Matrix metalloproteinases
MMP-8	Matrix metalloproteinase-8
MMP-9	Matrix metalloproteinase-9
OPG	Osteoprotegerin
PI	Plaque index
RANKL	Receptor Activator of Nuclear Factor Kappa-B Ligand
ROS	Reactive oxygen species
TNF-α	Tumour necrosis factor-alpha

S. Anil (✉)
Department of Dentistry, Hamad Medical Corporation, Oral Health Institute, Qatar University, Doha, Qatar
e-mail: asukumaran1@hamad.qa

S. S. P. Reddy
Department of Periodontology, Army Dental Centre (Research & Referral), New Delhi, India

D. L. Francis
Saveetha Dental College & Hospitals, Saveetha University, Saveetha Institute of Medical and Technical Sciences (SIMATS), Chennai, India

V. K. Sweety
Pushpagiri Institute of Medical Sciences, Thiruvalla, Kerala, India

F. Javed, S. Warnakulasuriya (eds.), *Smokeless Tobacco and its Effects on Periodontal Health*, https://doi.org/10.1007/978-3-032-16409-4_9

Learning Goals

- *Understand the botany and chemical composition of khat (Catha edulis)* and identify its primary psychoactive constituents, including cathinone and cathine.
- *Describe the traditional usage patterns and cultural significance* of khat chewing in East African and Arabian Peninsula societies, and how these impact oral health behaviours.
- *Explain the pharmacological mechanisms* by which khat affects oral and periodontal tissues, focusing on vasoconstriction, oxidative stress, and inflammatory cytokine release.
- *Evaluate the pathophysiological mechanisms* through which khat contributes to gingival recession, clinical attachment loss, and alveolar bone destruction.
- *Analyse the impact of chronic khat use on salivary flow and xerostomia,* and its implications for periodontal disease progression.
- *Recognize the characteristic oral manifestations* associated with khat chewing, including tooth wear, pigmentation changes, mucosal lesions, and halitosis.
- *Assess the effects of khat use on peri-implant tissues,* particularly its influence on osseointegration, bone metabolism, and peri-implant soft tissue healing.
- *Interpret and critically appraise epidemiological data* from clinical studies assessing the relationship between khat use and periodontal or peri-implant outcomes.
- *Develop culturally sensitive strategies for patient management* in populations that habitually use khat, integrating evidence-based periodontal and implant care principles.
- *Identify current knowledge gaps and research needs* regarding the long-term effects of khat on periodontal and peri-implant health, and propose potential future research directions.

9.1 Introduction

Chewing khat (*Catha edulis*) is one of the most significant psychostimulant habits in Eastern Africa and the Arabian Peninsula, with deep historical roots extending back thousands of years. This evergreen plant, native to the Horn of Africa, has evolved from a localized cultural phenomenon to a global public health consideration, particularly regarding its impacts on periodontal and peri-implant health (Abdelwahab et al. 2015). The systematic examination of khat's effects on periodontal tissues has gained increasing importance as dental practitioners encounter patients from khat-using populations or regions where its use is prevalent (Kalakonda et al. 2017).

The historical narrative of khat consumption traces back to the highlands of Ethiopia, where archaeological evidence suggests cultivation and use as early as the first century CE, with documented regular use by the thirteenth century. From these origins, the practice spread throughout the Horn of Africa, becoming deeply embedded in the cultural fabric of countries including Ethiopia, Somalia, and Djibouti, before establishing a significant presence in Yemeni society (Gebissa 2010). Contemporary usage patterns reflect both traditional consumption and modern globalization, with prevalence rates reaching 90% among adult males in Yemen, 75–80% in Somalia, and 30–50% among adults in Ethiopia.

The socio-cultural dimensions of khat use extend beyond its pharmacological effects, embodying deep-rooted traditional practices and social customs. In many communities, particularly in Yemen and East Africa, khat ceremonies are vital social institutions that facilitate cultural exchange, business discussions, and community decision-making (Al Shubbar 2024). However, the periodontal health implications of this widespread practice have become increasingly evident through clinical observations and research studies.

Despite growing research interest, several critical knowledge gaps persist in understanding the full impact of khat on periodontal health. These include the need for comprehensive longitudinal studies examining long-term periodontal health outcomes and peri-implant tissue responses, and detailed investigations of biological mechanisms, including molecular pathways of periodontal tissue damage (Algutaini et al. 2024). This chapter aims to address these gaps by providing a comprehensive examination of khat's effects on periodontal and peri-implant health, offering a detailed analysis of impacts on periodontal tissues, clinical implications for treatment planning, and evidence-based recommendations for patient care.

Key Points

- Khat (*Catha edulis*), also known as qat or miraa is a historically entrenched psychostimulant habit in Eastern Africa and the Arabian Peninsula, with use dating back to the first century CE.
- While initially a regional practice, khat use has evolved into a global public health concern.
- Khat chewing serves important social functions in many communities.
- Despite the growing body of evidence, significant gaps remain regarding the long-term effects of khat on oral tissues.

9.2 Botany and Chemistry of Khat (*Catha edulis*)

Catha edulis, known as khat, qat, or miraa, belongs to the Celastraceae family. This evergreen shrub or tree typically grows to 1–20 metres under optimal conditions (Fig. 9.1). However, cultivated plants are usually maintained at smaller heights through regular pruning to facilitate harvest and maximize young shoot production. The leaves, which constitute the primary consumable portion, display serrated margins and a distinct pattern of venation (Wabe 2011).

The chemical composition of khat reveals a complex array of bioactive compounds, with phenylalkylamines representing the primary psychoactive constituents. The most significant psychoactive compounds include cathinone (α-aminopropiophenone), cathine (norpseudoephedrine), and norephedrine, which are structurally related to amphetamine (Table 9.1). Cathinone, considered the most potent of these compounds, is predominantly found in fresh leaves, with concentrations highest in newly emerged shoots (Gashawa and Getachew 2014).

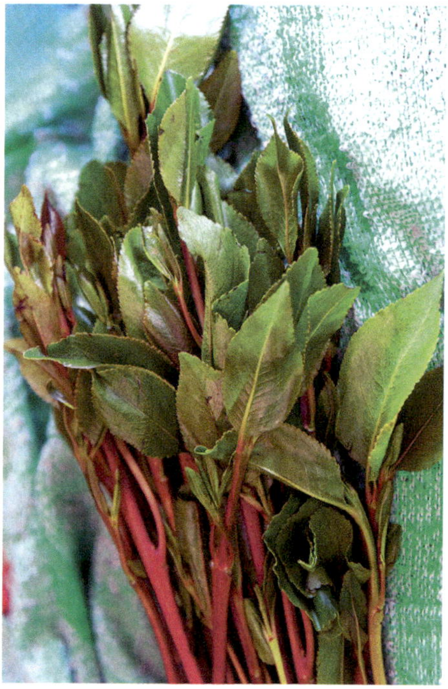

Fig. 9.1 Khat plant (*Catha edulis*)

Table 9.1 Chemical constituents of khat and their effects on oral/periodontal structures

Constituent	Concentration (range)	Primary effects	Periodontal health impact	Mechanism of action
Cathinone	0.1–2.0% (fresh leaves)	CNS stimulant, vasoconstriction	Gingival ischaemia, delayed periodontal healing, reduced blood flow	α-adrenergic receptor activation
Cathine	0.1–0.8%	Mild stimulant, sympathomimetic	Xerostomia, increased expression of pro-inflammatory markers such as IL-1β, TNF-α, and MMPs in the GCF	β-adrenergic receptor stimulation
Norephedrine	0.05–0.3%	Vasoconstriction	Compromised gingival perfusion	Noradrenergic pathway activation
Tannins	7–14% by weight	Astringent, chromogenic	Gingival irritation, tissue inflammation	Direct tissue contact irritation
Flavonoids	1–3%	Antioxidant	Potential anti-inflammatory effects	Free radical scavenging (beneficial effect)
Silica bodies	Variable	Abrasive	Mechanical trauma to periodontal tissues	Physical abrasion during chewing
Cellulose fibres	15–25%	Structural	Plaque retention, trauma to tissues	Mechanical entrapment

GCF Gingival crevicular fluid, *IL-1β* Interleukin 1-beta, *TNF-α* Tumour necrosis factor-alpha, *MMPs* Matrix metalloproteinases

Key Points

- *Catha edulis* is an evergreen shrub or tree from the Celastraceae family typically growing 1–20 metres tall.
- The young leaves and shoots, which contain the highest concentrations of psychoactive compounds, are the primary parts consumed.
- Khat contains a variety of bioactive substances, with phenylalkylamines being the main psychoactive components responsible for its stimulant effects.
- The principal psychoactive constituents, cathinone, cathine, and norephedrine, are structurally similar to amphetamines, with cathinone being the most potent and most concentrated in fresh, young leaves.

9.3 Traditional Processing and Usage

The traditional processing and consumption of khat represent a culturally rich practice. The preparation begins with careful harvesting practices, with young shoots and tender leaves preferentially selected as they contain the highest concentrations of active compounds (Gebissa 2010; Pendl et al. 2021).

Consumption patterns exhibit significant regional variations while retaining commonalities (Al-Mugahed 2008). In Yemen, khat sessions typically begin in the early afternoon and last several hours, with users gradually accumulating a bolus of masticated leaves in their cheeks. This prolonged unilateral chewing pattern creates asymmetric mechanical stress on periodontal tissues. The method of consumption follows relatively consistent patterns: users begin by removing leaves from stems, then place them in the mouth, and slowly chew until a substantial portion collects in one cheek, typically on the preferred side (Santos et al. 2024). Sessions usually last 4–8 h, during which continuous mechanical stress is applied to periodontal structures on the chewing side. This extended exposure and chemical irritation from khat constituents create conditions conducive to periodontal tissue breakdown (Al-Maweri et al. 2018).

Key Points

- Cathinone, cathine, and norephedrine are the main psychoactive compounds found in khat.
- These compounds share structural similarities with amphetamines, contributing to their stimulant effects on the central nervous system.
- Cathinone is the most potent alkaloid, exerting the strongest psychoactive effects.
- The highest concentration of cathinone is present in fresh khat leaves, making them the preferred part for consumption.

9.4 Pharmacology and Mechanisms of Action

9.4.1 Pharmacokinetics

Khat alkaloids show extensive tissue distribution, with oral tissues experiencing significantly higher concentrations due to direct contact during mastication (Atlabachew et al. 2016). Metabolism primarily occurs in the liver, where cathinone undergoes reduction to norephedrine and cathine, with elimination primarily through renal excretion (Al-Duais and Al-Awthan 2021). Khat affects oral tissues through multiple mechanisms, including alterations in cellular proliferation, differentiation, and survival pathways (Al-Duais and Al-Awthan 2021). The vasoconstrictive properties of khat alkaloids compromise tissue perfusion and oxygen delivery, creating zones of relative ischaemia in areas contacted by the khat bolus

(Al-Maweri et al. 2018). Chronic exposure leads to adaptive changes in epithelial tissues, including increased keratinization and altered cell turnover rates, manifesting as white lesions and hyperkeratotic areas. These changes extend to cell signalling pathways and inflammatory mediator production, affecting tissue homeostasis and repair (Abou-Elhamd et al. 2021).

Key Points

- Khat alkaloids accumulate in oral tissues at significantly higher levels due to prolonged direct contact during chewing.
- Cathinone, the primary active alkaloid in khat, is metabolized in the liver into norephedrine and cathine, and is primarily eliminated through the kidneys.
- Khat interferes with oral tissue homeostasis by altering cellular proliferation, differentiation, and survival.
- The vasoconstrictive action of khat alkaloids reduces blood flow, causing ischaemic zones, and chronic exposure induces hyperkeratosis, epithelial thickening, and inflammatory dysregulation.

9.4.2 Pathophysiological Mechanisms Affecting Periodontal Health

The pharmacokinetics of khat's active compounds significantly influence periodontal health through both local and systemic pathways. During chewing, compounds are released into the oral cavity, with the buccal and sublingual mucosa serving as primary sites of absorption. Cathinone exhibits rapid absorption, with detectable plasma levels within 15–30 min, but more importantly, periodontal tissues experience direct, prolonged exposure to these compounds (Toennes et al. 2003). The distribution pattern shows particularly high concentrations in periodontal tissues due to direct contact during mastication. This localized exposure creates zones of chemical irritation and altered cellular metabolism in the gingival and periodontal ligament tissues. The vasoconstrictive properties compromise tissue perfusion, creating relative ischaemia in areas contacted by the khat bolus (Al-Maweri et al. 2018).

The inflammatory mediator profile in khat-affected periodontal tissues demonstrates significant alterations, with elevated levels of pro-inflammatory cytokines including interleukin-1β (IL-1β), tumour necrosis factor-alpha (TNF-α), and interleukin-6 (IL-6). These elevated cytokine levels create a persistent inflammatory state within periodontal tissues, contributing to progressive tissue destruction (Chepukosi et al. 2021). Oxidative stress emerges as a significant component of khat-induced periodontal damage. Khat constituents increase reactive oxygen species (ROS) production while compromising cellular antioxidant defences. This enhanced oxidative burden leads to lipid peroxidation and protein oxidation within periodontal tissues, contributing to accelerated tissue breakdown (Hassan et al. 2020).

Matrix metalloproteinase (MMP) expression undergoes significant modification, with enhanced expression of MMP-2, MMP-8, and MMP-9 in khat-affected periodontal tissues. This increased MMP activity leads to accelerated degradation of periodontal ligament collagen and other extracellular matrix components. The balance between MMPs and their inhibitors (TIMPs) becomes disrupted, favouring tissue destruction (Luchian et al. 2022). Bone metabolism alterations represent critical mechanisms affecting periodontal health. Khat compounds influence osteoblast and osteoclast activity, affecting the Receptor Activator of Nuclear Factor Kappa-B Ligand/osteoprotegerin ratio and enhancing bone resorption. These changes compromise alveolar bone support for teeth and may affect osseointegration in implant cases (Silva et al. 2022).

Key Points

- Khat's active constituents, especially cathinone, are rapidly absorbed through the oral mucosa during chewing, resulting in high localized concentrations in periodontal tissues.
- The vasoconstrictive properties of khat compromise gingival and periodontal perfusion, creating ischaemic zones that impair nutrient delivery and healing capacity.
- Khat-affected periodontal tissues exhibit increased levels of pro-inflammatory cytokines such as IL-1β, TNF-α, and IL-6, which promote chronic inflammation and drive progressive periodontal destruction.
- Khat increases ROS production while weakening the antioxidant defence system, leading to oxidative damage such as lipid peroxidation and protein degradation in periodontal structures.
- There is a marked upregulation of MMP-2, MMP-8, and MMP-9 in khat chewers, causing excessive degradation of periodontal ligament collagen and extracellular matrix.
- Khat compounds affect bone metabolism by altering osteoblast and osteoclast function and disturbing the RANKL/OPG ratio, enhancing bone resorption and undermining alveolar bone support and osseointegration.

9.5 Khat Chewing and Its Effects on Periodontal Health

9.5.1 Gingival Changes and Recession in Khat Users

Habitual khat chewing is strongly associated with detrimental gingival alterations, most notably increased gingival inflammation, bleeding, and clinically significant gingival recession (Table 9.2). A cross-sectional study of 730 Yemeni participants (336 chewers, 394 non-chewers) found significantly higher gingival bleeding in khat chewers (Al-Kholani 2010). Histopathological examinations reveal severe

Table 9.2 Effects of khat chewing on periodontal health: summary of clinical studies

Study (year)	Participants (*n*)	Key periodontal findings
Dhaifullah et al. (2015)	122 Khat chewers 238 Non-chewers	Khat chewers had significantly more sextants with bleeding and pockets than non-chewers
Al-Maweri et al. (2014)	235 Khat chewers 174 Non-chewers	Khat chewers had significantly higher PI, CAL, and GR than non-chewers; the chewing side had more prominent gingival recession
Al-Sharabi et al. (2013)	400 Khat chewers 100 Non-chewers	CPI and attachment loss are significantly associated with khat chewing; higher parameters on chewing sides
Al-Hajri et al. (2013)	25 Khat chewers 30 Non-chewers	Chewing khat has negative effects on periodontal tissues
Al-Sharabi (2011)	490 Khat chewers 160 Non-chewers	Khat chewing caused GR at chewing sites, especially in the buccal area
Al-Bayaty et al. (2011)	1216 Males[a] 1290 Females[a]	Both male and female khat chewers had significantly more tooth loss, especially in mandibular teeth
Al-Kholani (2010)	336 Khat chewers 394 Non-chewers	51% GR vs. 26% in controls; associated oral hygiene changes
Yarom et al. (2010)	47 Khat chewers 55 Non-chewers	GR is significantly higher among chewers; lower GI and pocket depth on the chewing side; associated with CAL
Sultan et al. (2008)	66 Khat chewers 66 Non-chewers	Gingival recession on the chewing side
Ali (2007)	1528 Khat chewers 972 Non-chewers	Khat chewers had more periodontal pocketing (31.8% pocketing vs. 12% in non-chewers), higher GI, and increased GR; there was a significant association with frequency and duration
Mengel et al. (1996)	359 Khat chewers 642 Non-chewers	Khat chewers had significantly higher CPITN, CI, and CAL than non-chewers; higher CAL scores on the chewing side

[a]An exact number of khat chewers was not reported. *CAL* Clinical Attachment Loss, *CI* Calculus Index, *CPI* Community Periodontal Index, *CPITN* Community Periodontal Index of Treatment Needs, *GI* Gingival Index, *GR* Gingival Recession, *n* Number of participants, *I* Plaque Index, *vs*. versus

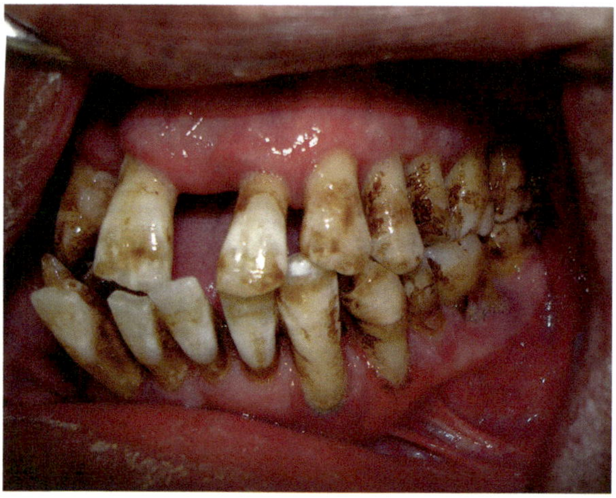

Fig. 9.2 Periodontal effects of chronic khat chewing. An intraoral photograph shows teeth with marked gingival recession, exposed root surfaces with characteristic brown staining, and inflamed gingival tissues consistent with long-term khat use. Note the dark discolouration and tissue damage typical of mechanical trauma from habitual khat chewing

inflammation characterized by dense plasma cell infiltration, termed plasma cell gingivitis, suggesting an immunological response to khat components.

Gingival recession represents the most consistently reported consequence of khat chewing. Halboub et al. (2009) reported gingival recession in khat chewers (Fig. 9.2). Al-Hajj et al. (2020) noted increased gingival recession specifically on the chewing side. A systematic review by Kalakonda et al. (2017) confirmed that khat chewing significantly increases the odds of gum recession. The mechanisms underlying khat-induced gingival recession are likely multifactorial. The direct mechanical irritation from the fibrous khat bolus being held against the gingiva for prolonged periods is a significant contributing factor. This chronic friction can lead to physical trauma and gradual displacement of the gingival margin. Additionally, the chemical constituents of khat, including alkaloids and tannins, may exert irritant or cytotoxic effects on the gingival tissues, further promoting inflammation and tissue breakdown. The vasoconstrictive properties of cathinone, a primary active compound in khat, could reduce blood flow to the gingival tissues, impairing their health and repair capacity. However, this specific link to recession requires more direct research. Furthermore, poorer oral hygiene practices are often observed among khat chewers, which can exacerbate gingival inflammation and contribute to recession. Khat-induced xerostomia further impairs natural cleansing mechanisms, potentially increasing plaque accumulation and gingival inflammation. A dose–response relationship exists, with long-term regular users presenting more pronounced gingival recession than occasional users (Astatkie et al. 2015).

Key Points

- Habitual khat chewing is significantly associated with increased gingival inflammation and bleeding.
- Gingival recession is the most consistent and prevalent periodontal manifestation among khat chewers, especially pronounced on the habitual chewing side.
- Histopathological findings show plasma cell gingivitis in khat chewers, indicating a potential immunological response to khat's chemical components.
- The multifactorial aetiology of gingival recession includes chronic mechanical trauma from the fibrous khat bolus and the cytotoxic effects of khat constituents such as cathinone and tannins.
- Vasoconstrictive effects of cathinone may reduce gingival perfusion and impair healing, contributing to tissue breakdown, though this link warrants further research.
- Poor oral hygiene habits and khat-induced xerostomia in habitual chewers exacerbate gingival inflammation and recession, with more severe outcomes observed in long-term chewers.

9.5.2 Periodontal Attachment Loss and Alveolar Bone Changes

Clinical attachment loss (CAL) is significantly more pronounced in khat users compared to non-users. In their meta-analysis, Al-Akhali and Al-Moraissi (2017) concluded that khat users had higher odds of periodontal pocketing, directly correlating with attachment loss. Al-Sharabi et al. (2013) found that 78.3% of individuals with periodontitis were khat chewers compared to 21.7% non-chewers in 730 Yemeni adults.

Al-Maweri et al. (2018) observed that attachment loss was particularly pronounced on the chewing side, creating asymmetric periodontal damage. Mengel et al. (1996) found that CAL was positively correlated with both duration and frequency of khat use. Al-Kholani (2010) documented a dose–response relationship between khat use duration and periodontal parameters. The mechanisms involve mechanical trauma from prolonged chewing sessions, which directly damage periodontal ligament fibres, while chemical constituents (cathinone, tannins) contribute to chronic inflammation. This activates host immune responses, releasing pro-inflammatory cytokines and matrix metalloproteinases (MMPs) that degrade periodontal tissues.

Alveolar bone resorption is a hallmark of periodontitis, and chronic khat use has been associated with significant bone loss due to several mechanisms. Prolonged khat chewing induces chronic inflammation in periodontal tissues, leading to the release of pro-inflammatory cytokines such as interleukin-1β (IL-1β) and tumour necrosis factor-alpha (TNF-α). These cytokines stimulate osteoclast activity, resulting in alveolar bone loss (Al-Kholani 2010). Moreover, the sympathomimetic compounds in khat (cathinone and cathine) cause vasoconstriction, reducing blood flow to periodontal tissues, thereby impairing tissue repair and accelerating bone resorption (Abebe 2018). A comparative study by Al-Akhali and Al-Moraissi (2017) examined radiographic bone levels in khat chewers and non-chewers, revealing significantly greater alveolar bone loss in khat users. The study attributed this to both mechanical and pharmacological effects of khat.

Key Points

- Khat users exhibit significantly greater CAL compared to non-users.
- Mechanical trauma from unilateral habitual khat chewing contributes to localized periodontal destruction.
- The severity of CAL is positively correlated with both the duration and frequency of khat use.
- Khat constituents, such as cathinone and tannins, induce chronic inflammation and immune responses that elevate pro-inflammatory cytokines (such as IL-1β, TNF-α) and MMPs leading to degradation of periodontal structures.
- Chronic khat use contributes to significant alveolar bone resorption through increased osteoclast activity stimulated by inflammatory mediators and impaired blood flow due to vasoconstriction.
- Khat users experience markedly greater alveolar bone loss than non-users, attributable to both mechanical irritation and the pharmacological effects of khat.

9.5.3 Xerostomia and Reduced Salivary Flow

Khat use causes xerostomia through sympathomimetic effects of cathinone and cathine on adrenergic receptors, affecting salivary gland function (Ali Quadri and Mohan 2022). Research indicates oral dryness occurs within 30 min of khat chewing, with long-term reduction in salivary quantity and quality (Badulla and Ben Yahiya 2019). Clinical manifestations include difficulty speaking, dysphagia, increased thirst, and altered oral comfort (Astatkie et al. 2015). Reduced salivary flow compromises protective functions, including lubrication, acid buffering, and antimicrobial activity, creating conditions conducive to periodontal disease progression. Changes in oral pH from diminished buffering capacity, often exacerbated by concurrent sugary beverage consumption, may favour acidogenic bacteria growth (Badulla and Ben Yahiya 2019).

Key Points

- Khat causes xerostomia through sympathomimetic effects of cathinone and cathine on adrenergic receptors.
- Oral dryness occurs within 30 min of khat chewing.
- Clinical manifestations of khat-induced xerostomia include difficulty in speech, dysphagia, increased thirst, and altered oral comfort.
- Khat-induced xerostomia compromises salivary buffering capacity and antimicrobial activity, creating conditions conducive to periodontal disease progression.
- Khat-induced xerostomia facilitates the growth of acidogenic bacteria.

9.5.4 Tooth Wear Patterns in Khat Users

Tooth wear patterns in chronic khat users present clinically significant challenges directly impacting periodontal health. Research demonstrates that mechanical forces during khat chewing can exceed normal masticatory pressures, with studies indicating sustained forces of up to 100–150 Newtons on the preferred chewing side during sessions lasting 4–8 h (Sayed et al. 2017). The wear process involves complex interactions between attrition (tooth-to-tooth contact), abrasion (from silica bodies in khat leaves), and erosion (from acidic compounds). This creates altered occlusal relationships that can affect periodontal health through modified force distribution and potential development of trauma from occlusion (Mohamed Abdoul-Latif et al. 2024). Clinical manifestations include flattening of cuspal inclines and development of wear facets, predominantly affecting the chewing side. Advanced cases may present with compromised vertical dimension of occlusion, leading to compensatory dental eruption and potential temporomandibular joint complications that further affect periodontal health (Al Moaleem et al. 2020).

Key Points

- Chronic khat users exert unusually high mechanical chewing forces, ranging from 100–150 Newtons.
- Tooth wear in khat users results from a combination of attrition (tooth-to-tooth contact), abrasion (due to silica bodies in khat leaves), and erosion (from acidic plant compounds).
- The chewing side shows more significant clinical manifestations such as flattened cuspal inclines and prominent wear facets, leading to occlusal imbalance.
- Extensive tooth wear compromises the vertical dimension of occlusion, prompting compensatory tooth eruption that can further destabilize occlusion.
- Long-term occlusal alterations may result in TMJ complications, such as joint pain and functional limitations.

9.5.5 Tooth Loss in Khat Users

Chronic khat use significantly increases the risk of tooth loss, representing the end-stage of periodontal disease progression. Al-Sharabi et al. (2013) documented 1.6 times greater odds of multiple tooth loss among khat users in 730 Yemeni adults, while Astatkie et al. (2015) reported a 2.3-fold increased risk of premature tooth loss in users with >10 years of use compared to non-users. The pathophysiology involves chronic periodontal inflammation from khat's chemical constituents (cathinone, tannins), mechanical trauma from prolonged chewing sessions, and compromised periodontal healing responses. The characteristic asymmetric pattern predominantly affects the chewing side, leading to posterior tooth loss and functional challenges, with complex prosthetic requirements. Concurrent tobacco use increases risk by 1.8–2.4 times, while users >15 years show markedly higher loss rates (Al-Maweri et al. 2018; Erawati and Fitriana 2024).

Key Points

- The risk of tooth loss is 1.6–2.3 times higher in khat chewers than non-chewers.
- Tooth loss in khat users is primarily driven by chronic periodontal inflammation, mechanical trauma from prolonged chewing, and impaired healing.
- The risk of tooth loss is further amplified by concurrent tobacco use and longer durations of khat chewing, with users exceeding 15 years exhibiting the most severe outcomes.

9.5.6 Other Oral Manifestations

While this chapter focuses primarily on periodontal and peri-implant health, khat use is associated with several other oral manifestations that provide important clinical context. White keratotic lesions represent the most prevalent manifestations, typically presenting as frictional keratosis, hyperkeratosis, and leukoedema on the buccal mucosa corresponding to the preferred chewing side, with prevalence rates of 33.3% in khat users versus 7.7% in non-users (Schmidt-Westhausen et al. 2014). Histopathological examination reveals characteristic acanthosis, hyperkeratosis, and inflammatory cell infiltration (Lukandu et al. 2015). Distinctive brown-to-greenish tooth staining occurs in up to 85% of regular users within the first year due to tannin deposition, with chromogenic compounds penetrating up to 150 micrometres into the enamel surface, creating permanent aesthetic concerns that resist conventional cleaning methods (Al-Akhali et al. 2023; Al-Bayaty et al. 2011). Pigmentation changes manifest as brown discolouration affecting teeth, gingiva, and oral mucosa, primarily due to increased melanin production in the basal epithelial layer (Al-Maweri et al. 2014, 2018). The relationship with dental caries presents complex patterns, with risk factors including frequent consumption of sugary beverages during chewing sessions and khat-induced xerostomia. However, some studies suggest khat's antimicrobial properties may provide protective effects (Al-Alimi et al. 2018). Additional manifestations include temporomandibular joint disorders from prolonged unilateral chewing, presenting as joint pain, clicking sounds, and limited mouth opening, with radiographic evidence of condylar flattening in long-term users (Al-Maweri et al. 2018; Mohamed Abdoul-Latif et al. 2024), as well as halitosis resulting from mechanical retention of khat particles and decreased salivary flow (Al Moaleem et al. 2020). Regarding oral cancer risk, the evidence remains inconclusive due to significant confounding factors, particularly concurrent tobacco use among many khat users, making direct causality difficult to establish (Al-Maweri et al. 2018). While these conditions are clinically relevant, they occur alongside more pronounced periodontal manifestations, which represent the primary oral health concern requiring clinical intervention in khat users.

Key Points

- White keratotic lesions such as frictional keratosis, hyperkeratosis, and leukoedema are significantly more prevalent among khat users than non-users.
- White keratotic lesions are more often manifested on the buccal mucosa of the preferred chewing side, with histopathological features including acanthosis and inflammatory infiltration.
- Oral pigmentation changes in khat users manifest as brown discoloration of teeth, gingiva, and oral mucosa, primarily due to increased melanin synthesis in the basal epithelial layers.
- Dental caries risk in khat users is influenced by reduced salivary flow and frequent intake of sugary beverages during chewing sessions, although khat's potential antimicrobial effects may offer some protective influence.
- Temporomandibular joint disorders may develop in long-term khat users due to prolonged unilateral chewing, leading to joint pain, clicking, limited mouth opening, and radiographic evidence of condylar changes.

9.6 Khat Use and Dental Implant Treatment

9.6.1 Effects on Osseointegration

Khat consumption significantly influences osseointegration outcomes through multiple mechanisms that compromise implant success. The vasoconstrictive properties of cathinone and cathine sustain vasoconstriction in periosteal and endosseous blood vessels, resulting in reduced oxygen tension and compromised delivery of essential nutrients for bone formation (Al-Motarreb and Broadley 2003). Khat alkaloids directly affect osteoblast function during the critical osseointegration phase, altering their proliferation and differentiation. Research demonstrates modified expression patterns of key osteogenic markers, including alkaline phosphatase and osteocalcin. The disruption of bone morphogenetic protein (BMP) signalling cascades leads to suboptimal bone formation around implant surfaces (Silva et al. 2022). Long-term implant stability remains challenging due to altered bone metabolism. The prolonged duration of khat chewing sessions exposes implants to extended periods of mechanical loading, which, combined with altered bone metabolism, may exceed the physiological adaptive capacity of peri-implant tissues (Sayed et al. 2017).

Key Points

- Khat's active compounds, cathinone, and cathine, induce vasoconstriction in periosteal and endosseous vessels, reducing oxygen and nutrient delivery critical for bone healing and osseointegration.
- The alkaloids in khat interfere with osteoblast proliferation and differentiation, leading to altered expression of osteogenic markers (such as alkaline phosphatase and osteocalcin) and disrupted BMP signalling, which compromises bone formation around implants.
- Chronic khat chewing imposes prolonged mechanical loading on implants and alters bone metabolism, potentially exceeding the adaptive capacity of peri-implant tissues and threatening long-term implant success.

9.6.2 Peri-Implant Soft Tissue Response

Peri-implant soft tissues in khat users exhibit significant architectural changes and modifications in inflammatory status. The most notable change is pronounced epithelial keratinization at sites directly contacted by the khat bolus. While this hyperkeratotic response may offer protection against mechanical trauma, it interferes with normal peri-implant soft tissue architecture (Lukandu et al. 2015). Inflammatory changes present a complex pattern of acute and chronic responses. Studies demonstrate elevated levels of pro-inflammatory cytokines (IL-1β, TNF-α, IL-6) in peri-implant crevicular fluid of khat users. The vascular response shows significant modifications, with reduced capillary density and altered vascular architecture affecting tissue oxygenation and nutrient delivery (Al-Maqtari et al. 2024; Ali et al. 2015). The normal wound healing cascade exhibits alterations characterized by modified fibroblast activity and collagen synthesis patterns. This may lead to accelerated tissue breakdown and compromised healing following therapeutic interventions, affecting long-term peri-implant health (Alhazmi et al. 2022).

Key Points

- Hyperkeratinization of peri-implant tissues is a common response in khat users.
- Inflammatory mediator levels, including IL 1β, TNF-α, and IL-6, are elevated in the peri-implant crevicular fluid of khat chewers than non-users.
- Vascular and fibroblast dysfunction, characterized by reduced capillary density, impaired nutrient delivery, and altered collagen synthesis leads to delayed wound healing and increased risk of peri-implant tissue breakdown in khat chewers than non-users.

9.7 Summary

This comprehensive examination of the effects of khat (*Catha edulis*) reveals significant impacts on periodontal and peri-implant health beyond simple mechanical trauma. The complex interplay between khat's chemical constituents, particularly cathinone, cathine, and tannins, and prolonged mechanical stress creates a unique pathophysiological environment that significantly compromises periodontal health. Key findings demonstrate that khat chewers face substantially elevated risks for gingival recession, periodontal attachment loss, and alveolar bone loss compared to non-users. These effects show clear dose–response relationships, with longer duration of use correlating with more severe periodontal destruction. The characteristic asymmetric pattern of tissue damage, predominantly affecting the habitual chewing side, creates unique clinical challenges for diagnosis and treatment.

For dental implant therapy, khat use presents significant concerns through compromised osseointegration, altered bone metabolism, and modified peri-implant soft tissue responses. The vasoconstrictive properties of khat alkaloids and mechanical trauma from prolonged chewing sessions may compromise initial implant stability and long-term success rates. The evidence necessitates modified clinical approaches for khat-using populations, including enhanced assessment protocols, adjusted treatment timelines, and intensive maintenance programs. While cessation remains the optimal intervention, the deep cultural significance of khat use requires culturally sensitive approaches that balance oral health objectives with patient autonomy and cultural respect.

Key Points

- Khat chewing significantly compromises periodontal health, with chemical constituents like cathinone and tannins, combined with mechanical trauma, leading to gingival recession, attachment loss, and alveolar bone destruction—often in a dose-dependent and asymmetric manner.
- Khat use adversely affects dental implant outcomes by impairing osseointegration, altering bone metabolism, and modifying peri-implant soft tissue healing, thereby increasing the risk of implant failure.
- Effective management of khat-using patients requires tailored clinical protocols that account for cultural sensitivity, including enhanced diagnostics, modified treatment planning, and rigorous maintenance strategies to mitigate the risks associated with khat consumption.

References

Abdelwahab SI, Alsanosy RM, Rahim BE, Mohan S, Taha S, Mohamed Elhassan M, El-Setouhy M (2015) Khat (Catha edulis Forsk) dependence potential and pattern of use in Saudi Arabia. Biomed Res Int 2015:604526. https://doi.org/10.1155/2015/604526

Abebe W (2018) Khat and synthetic cathinones: emerging drugs of abuse with dental implications. Oral Surg Oral Med Oral Pathol Oral Radiol 125(2):140–146. https://doi.org/10.1016/j.oooo.2017.11.015

Abou-Elhamd AS, Kalamegam G, Ahmed F, Assidi M, Alrefaei AF, Pushparaj PN, Abu-Elmagd M (2021) Unraveling the Catha edulis extract effects on the cellular and molecular signaling in SKOV3 cells [original research]. Front Pharmacol 12:666885. https://doi.org/10.3389/fphar.2021.666885

Al Moaleem MM, Porwal A, Al Ahmari NM, Shariff M, Homeida H, Khalid A (2020) Khat chewing induces a floral shift in dental material-associated microbiota: a preliminary study. Med Sci Monit 26:e918219. https://doi.org/10.12659/MSM.918219

Al Shubbar MD (2024) Understanding Khat: its sociocultural and health implications in Saudi Arabia. Cureus 16(3):e56657. https://doi.org/10.7759/cureus.56657

Al-Akhali MS, Al-Moraissi EA (2017) Khat chewing habit produces a significant adverse effect on periodontal, oral health: a systematic review and meta-analysis. J Periodontal Res 52(6):937–945. https://doi.org/10.1111/jre.12468

Al-Akhali AAM, Al-Hamzi M, Al-Shami IZ, Al-Kholani AI, Madfa AA (2023) Effect of khat extract on color stability of digitally and manually fabricated provisional restorations: an in vitro comparative study. BMC Oral Health 23(1):700. https://doi.org/10.1186/s12903-023-03425-w

Al-Alimi KR, Razak AAA, Saub R (2018) Is Khat chewing habit a risk factor for occlusal caries progression? Afr Health Sci 18(4):1036–1045. https://doi.org/10.4314/ahs.v18i4.25

Al-Bayaty FH, Ali N, Bulgiba AM, Masood M, Hussain SF, Abdulla MA (2011) Tooth mortality in khat and non khat chewer in Sana'a Yemen. Sci Res Essays 6:1039–1045

Al-Duais MA, Al-Awthan YS (2021) Khat chewing and lipid profile in human and experimental animals. Biomed Res Int 2021(1):6001885. https://doi.org/10.1155/2021/6001885

Algutaini SA, Al-Ameri A, Abdo BAM (2024) The impact of Qat chewing on health and social life: a cross-sectional study among Yemeni adults. J Med Health Res Psychiatry 01:1–11

Al-Hajj W, Hwaiti H, Shamala A, Al-Azazi H, Alwesabi M (2020) Association of Khat chewing, smoking, age and sex with periodontal status among Yemeni adults. Braz Dent Sci 23(1):8

Al-Hajri M, El Refaey M, Fathalla G, El-Firt E (2013) Apoptosis due to Khat chewing analyzed by p53 expression in gingival tissue. Egypt Dent J 59:1–9

Alhazmi HA, Bakri MA, Mohzari YA, Alshigaify YG, Al Bratty M, Javed SA, Najmi A, Rehman Z, Ahsan W, Taha MME (2022) Study of influence of Catha edulis (Khat) chewing on oral pharmacokinetics of irbesartan in rats using a newly developed HPLC-UV method. Saudi Pharm J 30(3):237–244. https://doi.org/10.1016/j.jsps.2022.01.002

Ali AA (2007) Qat habit in Yemen society: a causative factor for oral periodontal diseases. Int J Environ Res Public Health 4(3):243–247. https://doi.org/10.3390/ijerph2007030008

Ali Quadri MF, Mohan S (2022) Khat (Catha edulis) and oral health. In: Patel VB, Preedy VR (eds) Handbook of substance misuse and addictions. Springer International Publishing, pp 1751–1766. https://doi.org/10.1007/978-3-030-92392-1_90

Ali EH, Hegazy HG, Mosaad RM (2015) Interaction between pro-inflammatory cytokines and brain oxidative stress biomarkers of khat, cathinone and pseudoephedrine hydrochloride intoxication in male mice. Afr J Pharm Pharmacol 9(23):585–594

Al-Kholani AI (2010) Influence of Khat chewing on periodontal tissues and oral hygiene status among Yemenis. Dent Res J (Isfahan) 7(1):1–6. https://www.ncbi.nlm.nih.gov/pubmed/21448439

Al-Maqtari MA, Al-Tahami MA, Hameed DA, Ali RS (2024) Impact of Khat (Catha edulis) chewing on inflammatory markers and advanced glycation end products among Yemeni women. Sana'a Univ J Appl Sci Technol 2(1):96–102

Al-Maweri SA, Alaizari NA, Al-Sufyani GA (2014) Oral mucosal lesions and their association with tobacco use and qat chewing among Yemeni dental patients. J Clin Exp Dent 6(5):e460–e466. https://doi.org/10.4317/jced.51706

Al-Maweri SA, Warnakulasuriya S, Samran A (2018) Khat (Catha edulis) and its oral health effects: an updated review. J Investig Clin Dent 9(1). https://doi.org/10.1111/jicd.12288

Al-Motarreb AL, Broadley KJ (2003) Coronary and aortic vasoconstriction by cathinone, the active constituent of khat. Auton Autacoid Pharmacol 23(5–6):319–326. https://doi.org/10.1111/j.1474-8673.2004.00303.x

Al-Mugahed L (2008) Khat chewing in Yemen: turning over a new leaf. Bull World Health Organ 86(10):741–742. https://doi.org/10.2471/blt.08.011008

Al-Sharabi AK (2011) Conditions of Oral Mucosa due to Takhzeen al-Qat. Yemeni J Med Sci 5(1):1–6. https://doi.org/10.20428/yjms.v5i1.256

Al-Sharabi AK, Shuga-Aldin H, Ghandour I, Al-Hebshi NN (2013) Qat chewing as an independent risk factor for periodontitis: a cross-sectional study. Int J Dent 2013:317640. https://doi.org/10.1155/2013/317640

Astatkie A, Demissie M, Berhane Y, Worku A (2015) Oral symptoms significantly higher among long-term khat (Catha edulis) users in Ethiopia. Epidemiol Health 37:e2015009. https://doi.org/10.4178/epih/e2015009

Atlabachew M, Combrinck S, Viljoen AM, Hamman JH, Gouws C (2016) Isolation and in vitro permeation of phenylpropylamino alkaloids from Khat (Catha edulis) across oral and intestinal mucosal tissues. J Ethnopharmacol 194:307–315. https://doi.org/10.1016/j.jep.2016.09.012

Badulla WFS, Ben Yahiya AR (2019) Effect of Khat chewing on the salivary pH before and after using mouthwashes. Addict Health 11(3):148–155. https://doi.org/10.22122/ahj.v11i3.237

Chepukosi KW, Nyariki JN, Jillani NE, Okanya PW, Isaac AO (2021) Manganese exacerbated chronic khat-induced neurological deficits, inflammation and organ toxicity in a mouse model. Toxicol Environ Heal Sci 13(4):337–350. https://doi.org/10.1007/s13530-021-00091-9

Dhaifullah E, Al-Maweri SA, Al-Motareb F, Halboub E, Elkhatat E, Baroudi K, Tarakji B (2015) Periodontal health condition and associated factors among university students, Yemen. J Clin Diagn Res 9(12):Zc30–Zc33. https://doi.org/10.7860/jcdr/2015/16435.6964

Erawati S, Fitriana D (2024) The effect of one-sided chewing habits on the occurrence of caries, calculus, and oral status hygiene in students of SMP Islam Terpadu Nurul Fadhilah, Percut Sei Tuan District, Deli Serdang Regency, Indonesia. Community Med Educ J 5(1):433–437

Gashawa A, Getachew T (2014) The chemistry of khat and adverse effect of khat chewing. Am Sci Res J Eng Technol Sci 9(1):35–46

Gebissa E (2010) Khat in the Horn of Africa: historical perspectives and current trends. J Ethnopharmacol 132(3):607–614. https://doi.org/10.1016/j.jep.2010.01.063
Halboub E, Dhaifullah E, Abdulhuq M (2009) Khat chewing and smoking effect on oral mucosa: a clinical study. Acta Medica (Hradec Kralove, Czech Republic) 52(4):155–158. https://doi.org/10.14712/18059694.2016.122
Hassan AA, Hobani YH, Mosbah N, Abdalla SE, Zaino M, Mohan S, El-Setouhy M (2020) Chronic khat (Catha edulis) chewing and genotoxicity: the role of antioxidant defense system and oxidative damage of DNA. Pharmacogn Mag 16(68):168
Kalakonda B, Al-Maweri SA, Al-Shamiri HM, Ijaz A, Gamal S, Dhaifullah E (2017) Is Khat (Catha edulis) chewing a risk factor for periodontal diseases? A systematic review. J Clin Exp Dent 9(10):e1264–e1270. https://doi.org/10.4317/jced.54163
Luchian I, Goriuc A, Sandu D, Covasa M (2022) The role of matrix metalloproteinases (MMP-8, MMP-9, MMP-13) in periodontal and peri-implant pathological processes. Int J Mol Sci 23(3):1806. https://doi.org/10.3390/ijms23031806
Lukandu OM, Koech LS, Kiarie PN (2015) Oral lesions induced by chronic Khat use consist essentially of thickened Hyperkeratinized epithelium. Int J Dent 2015(1):104812. https://doi.org/10.1155/2015/104812
Mengel R, Eigenbrodt M, Schunemann T, Flores-de-Jacoby L (1996) Periodontal status of a subject sample of Yemen. J Clin Periodontol 23(5):437–443. https://doi.org/10.1111/j.1600-051x.1996.tb00571.x
Mohamed Abdoul-Latif F, Ainane A, Merito A, Houmed Aboubaker I, Mohamed H, Cherroud S, Ainane T (2024) The effects of Khat chewing among Djiboutians: dental chemical studies, gingival histopathological analyses and bioinformatics approaches. Bioengineering (Basel) 11(7). https://doi.org/10.3390/bioengineering11070716
Pendl E, Pauritsch U, Kollroser M, Schmid MG (2021) Determination of cathinone and cathine in Khat plant material by LC-MS/MS: fresh vs. dried leaves. Forensic Sci Int 319:110658. https://doi.org/10.1016/j.forsciint.2020.110658
Santos IC, Maia D, Dinis-Oliveira RJ, Barbosa DJ (2024) New psychoactive substances: health and legal challenges. Psychoactives 3(2):285–302. https://www.mdpi.com/2813-1851/3/2/18
Sayed ME, Hamdi AD, Hakami BM, Mugri MH, Bhandi SH (2017) Tooth wear patterns among Khat and Shammah users in Jazan City, Kingdom of Saudi Arabia: a cross-sectional survey. J Contemp Dent Pract 18(6):429–436. https://doi.org/10.5005/jp-journals-10024-2060
Schmidt-Westhausen AM, Al Sanabani J, Al-Sharabi AK (2014) Prevalence of oral white lesions due to qat chewing among women in Yemen. Oral Dis 20(7):675–681. https://doi.org/10.1111/odi.12188
Silva B, Soares J, Rocha-Pereira C, Mladenka P, Remiao F, On Behalf of the Oemonom, R (2022) Khat, a cultural chewing drug: a toxicokinetic and toxicodynamic summary. Toxins (Basel) 14(2). https://doi.org/10.3390/toxins14020071
Sultan M, Alhadad KA, Alsanaban F (2008) Tooth lost and gingival recession as a risk factor of khat chewing in Yemen. Cairo Dent J 2:171–176
Toennes SW, Harder S, Schramm M, Niess C, Kauert GF (2003) Pharmacokinetics of cathinone, cathine and norephedrine after the chewing of khat leaves. Br J Clin Pharmacol 56(1):125–130. https://doi.org/10.1046/j.1365-2125.2003.01834.x
Wabe NT (2011) Chemistry, pharmacology, and toxicology of khat (catha edulis forsk): a review. Addict Health 3(3–4):137–149. https://www.ncbi.nlm.nih.gov/pubmed/24494129
Yarom N, Epstein J, Levi H, Porat D, Kaufman E, Gorsky M (2010) Oral manifestations of habitual khat chewing: a case-control study. Oral Surg Oral Med Oral Pathol Oral Radiol Endod 109(6):e60–e66. https://doi.org/10.1016/j.tripleo.2010.02.022

10 The Effects of Snuff and Snus on Periodontal and Peri-Implant Health

Harriet Rumgay, Delfin Lovelina Francis,
and Saravanan Sampoornam Pape Reddy

10.1 Overview of Snuff and Snus

Snuff and snus are smokeless tobacco products that are used in different forms across the world. Although snuff and snus are both derived from tobacco, they differ in their geographical presence, preparation, chemical composition including nitrosamine content, and modes of consumption (International Agency for Research on Cancer 2007). The use of these products has been associated with various health risks, including oral and systemic diseases.

While various snuff products exist globally, this chapter provides a detailed overview of moist snuff and Swedish snus, as commonly used in North America and Europe, the patterns of their use and regulatory landscape, and implications for periodontal and peri-implant health.

10.1.1 Historical Context and Consumption Patterns of Snuff and Snus

Snuff was first used by indigenous populations in Central and South America (International Agency for Research on Cancer 2007). After the arrival of European settlers in the Americas in the fifteenth century, the use of snuff spread to parts of Europe, particularly France, England, and the Netherlands where it became

H. Rumgay (✉)
International Agency for Research on Cancer, World Health Organization, Lyon, France
e-mail: rumgayh@iarc.who.int

D. L. Francis
Saveetha Dental College & Hospitals, Saveetha Institute of Medical and Technical Sciences (SIMATS), Saveetha University, Chennai, India

S. S. P. Reddy
Department of Periodontology, Army Dental Centre (Research & Referral), New Delhi, India

F. Javed, S. Warnakulasuriya (eds.), *Smokeless Tobacco and its Effects on Periodontal Health*, https://doi.org/10.1007/978-3-032-16409-4_10

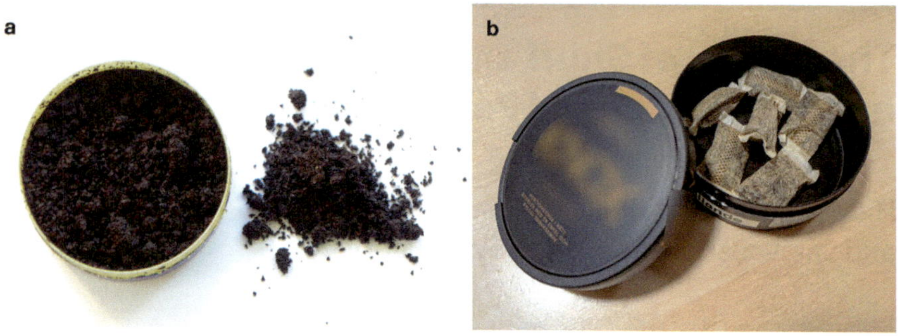

Fig. 10.1 (**a**) Loose moist snuff. (**b**) Pouches of portioned snus. (Credits: Uffe Johansson)

common among the upper social classes (International Agency for Research on Cancer 2007). Snuff, as used in earlier centuries, was typically dry and inhaled through the nose or placed in the mouth. Over time, the use of snuff or "dip" became popular in other parts of the world including the United States (US), Japan, and China (International Agency for Research on Cancer 2007). In the nineteenth and twentieth centuries, however, the use of snuff began to decline, primarily due to the rising popularity of cigarettes (International Agency for Research on Cancer 2007). Despite this, snuff is still consumed particularly in the USA, where it is primarily used as a "dip" placed in the mouth (Fig. 10.1a) (International Agency for Research on Cancer 2007). Use of moist snuff is most common among rural populations in the Midwest states of the USA, with 5.2 million adults (2.1% of the US population) reporting daily use of smokeless tobacco, including chewing tobacco, snuff, dip, and snus in 2021 (Cornelius et al. 2023).

Swedish-type moist snuff (snus) is a type of ground tobacco product that is commonly sold as loose or portioned snus in small pouches in Sweden and across Scandinavia (Fig. 10.1b) (International Agency for Research on Cancer 2007). To use snus, the user places the pouch under the upper lip and absorbs the tobacco without inhaling or chewing. Similar to snuff, the origins of snus date back to the early eighteenth century when it was introduced to Sweden from Europe. Since the introduction of cigarettes in the 1940s, snus has been marketed as a safer alternative to smoking, particularly in Sweden where it is promoted as a less harmful tobacco product than cigarettes (International Agency for Research on Cancer 2007). The prevalence of using snus has increased in Sweden since 2014 and in 2024, 22% of men and 4% of women reported daily use of snus, while snus has gained popularity in Norway and Finland (Raitasalo et al. 2022).

10.1.2 Composition of Snuff and Snus Products

Moist snuff is made from finely ground tobacco leaves that have been air- or fire-cured, with added salt, flavourings, and sometimes sweeteners (Table 10.1) (Gupta et al. 2022). Depending on the kind of tobacco and preparation, its nicotine content

Table 10.1 Types of snuff and snus products, ingredients, mode of consumption, and chemical features

Type of snuff product	Alternative name(s) and geographic location (National Cancer Institute and Centers for Disease Control Prevention 2014)	Main ingredients (National Cancer Institute and Centers for Disease Control Prevention 2014)	Mode of consumption (National Cancer Institute and Centers for Disease Control Prevention 2014)	pH (National Cancer Institute and Centers for Disease Control Prevention 2014)	Nicotine concentration (mg/g) (Gupta et al. 2022)	TSNA concentration (µg/g) (Gupta et al. 2022)
Dry snuff	Scotch snuff, snuff (USA, Canada, Germany, South Africa, Nigeria)	Tobacco (air- or fire-cured, fermented), flavourings	Held in the mouth or inhaled through the nose	5.41–7.96	1.2–17.2	1.7–20.5
Moist snuff	Dip, spit tobacco (USA, Canada, Mexico, South Africa)	Tobacco (air- or fire-cured, fermented), flavourings, inorganic salts, humectants	Held in the mouth	5.49–8.62	3.9–40.1	0.3–76.5
Swedish snus	Sweden, Norway, Iceland, Finland, Denmark, USA, Canada, Brazil, South Africa	Tobacco (air-cured, pasteurized), moisturizers, sodium carbonate, salt, sweeteners, flavourings	Held in the mouth	6.48–7.70	7.8–15.2	0.6–0.7

TSNA Tobacco-specific nitrosamine

ranges from 3.9 to 40.1 mg per gram of tobacco (Gupta et al. 2022). The primary ingredients in snus are tobacco, moisturisers, salt, and other flavouring agents (Gupta et al. 2022). In the production of snus, the tobacco is generally pasteurized which results in lower concentrations of tobacco-specific nitrosamines (TSNAs) often produced by fermentation in other smokeless tobacco and combustible tobacco products (Gupta et al. 2022). The concentration of nicotine in snus differs by brand and the type of tobacco and usually ranges from 7.8 to 15.2 mg per gram of tobacco (Gupta et al. 2022).

10.1.3 Health Risks of Snuff and Snus

The most reported health risks associated with using snuff or snus are their links to oral diseases such as gingivitis, gingival recession, periodontitis, tooth loss, oral leukoplakia or snus-induced lesions, and oral cancer (Bhandari and Bhatta 2021). The nicotine contained in snuff and snus products can also lead to addiction and might increase the risk of cardiovascular diseases, including hypertension, stroke, and coronary heart disease (Titova et al. 2021). Furthermore, the use of snus during pregnancy is associated with an increased risk of preterm birth, low birth weight, and other adverse pregnancy outcomes (Brinchmann et al. 2023).

10.1.4 Regulatory Landscape of Snuff and Snus

The production, sale, and consumption of snuff and snus are regulated in different ways when comparing one country to another. For example, in the USA, snuff is regulated by the Food and Drug Administration (FDA) as per the Family Smoking Prevention and Tobacco Control Act (Deyton 2011). It is important to note that while the FDA has the authority to regulate the manufacture, labelling, and advertising of all commercial products of snuff, the agency has not yet fully addressed the potential health risks for the use of snuff (Deyton 2011).

As for snus, its sale has been authorised in the USA since 2019 when it was approved by the government as a "Modified Risk Tobacco Product" compared to traditional cigarettes. In Sweden, snus is available with no restrictions and has been promoted as a less harmful alternative to smoking (International Agency for Research on Cancer 2007). The European Union, however, has prohibited the sale of snus in the majority of its member states, with concerns over the high addiction rates and wider health risks (International Agency for Research on Cancer 2007). In addition, the sales and marketing of smokeless tobacco products including snuff and snus are strictly regulated in other countries such as Canada and Australia (Chugh et al. 2023).

10.2 Epidemiology of Periodontal and Peri-Implant Health in Users of Snuff and Snus

There is evidence that snuff and snus cause local periodontal destruction and may predispose users to peri-implant disease at the sites where these products are placed. While individual effects depend on the user and product, the burden of periodontal and peri-implant conditions in the population is a function of regional consumption patterns, product composition, and behaviours among users of snuff and snus.

10.2.1 Prevalence of Poor Periodontal Health in Users of Snuff and Snus

Oral snuff and snus are associated with negative periodontal and peri-implant outcomes; however, their severity and presentation depend on the product composition and user behaviour (Richter et al. 2008). Mild to moderate periodontitis is the most common presentation, but outcomes may be as severe as advanced periodontal breakdown in long-term, high-frequency users, especially those with poor oral hygiene, diabetes, or genetic predispositions (Richter et al. 2008).

Epidemiological studies have shown a consistently greater level of periodontal inflammation, attachment loss, and bone resorption among snuff users in comparison to non-users. A cross-sectional study based on the US National Health and Nutrition Examination Survey (NHANES III) analysed 295 current users of smokeless tobacco, mainly moist snuff, and found that odds of having severe active periodontal disease, defined as at least one tooth with 6 mm or more attachment loss and bleeding on the same tooth, was double the odds among never users (odds ratio 2.1, $p < 0.05$) (Fisher et al. 2005). Another study of 33 moist snuff users in Sweden found that 42% of users had gingival recession versus 17% among controls ($p = 0.006$) and the mean clinical attachment loss was 0.2 and 0.1 mm in snuff-users and controls, respectively ($p > 0.05$) (Montén et al. 2006). Finally, one study of 1094 professional baseball players and staff examined in 1988 found that sites adjacent to smokeless tobacco-induced mucosal lesions in current users of snuff or chewing tobacco showed significantly greater prevalence of gingival recession (30% of mandibular sites with smokeless tobacco-induced lesions, $p < 0.05$) and attachment loss compared to non-users (17% of sites) or sites not adjacent to smokeless tobacco-induced lesions in current users (17%) (Robertson et al. 1990).

10.2.2 Peri-Implant Health in Users of Snuff and Snus

The influence of snuff and snus on peri-implant health could be significant, as this area has a specific biological and microbiome habitat compared to the structure around natural teeth. Unlike natural teeth, dental implants do not have a periodontal ligament, which can withhold peri-implant-based tissues from being sterile and mechanically traumatized (Jia et al. 2024).

10.2.3 Population Groups at Increased Susceptibility of Poor Periodontal or Peri-Implant Health When Using Snuff or Snus

Factors like genotypic susceptibility or patterns of oral hygiene and tobacco exposure can influence the risk of poor periodontal health in those who use snuff or snus, either amplifying or alleviating it. People who carry a genetic polymorphism in matrix metalloproteinase-3 may also have a more aggressive periodontal breakdown via the interleukin-1 beta (IL-1β) or receptor activator of nuclear factor kappa-B ligand (RANKL) pathways when they are additionally exposed to snuff or snus (Hu et al. 2024a).

One of the greatest concerns is a possible synergistic action of snuff or snus in populations with pre-existing systemic disorders such as diabetes mellitus. Chronic hyperglycaemia affects neutrophil function and collagen metabolism, which makes individuals with diabetes mellitus prone to rapid periodontal disease progression (Saotome et al. 2025). For these patients, use of snus or snuff may represent an additional risk factor, causing accelerated tissue destruction and diminished responsiveness to periodontal therapy (Chung et al. 2024).

10.3 Effects of Snuff and Snus on Periodontal Health

10.3.1 Biological Mechanisms of Effects of Snuff and Snus on Periodontal Health

The mechanisms through which snuff and snus impact periodontal health are mediated through a complex, dynamic interplay of biochemical, microbiological, and inflammatory pathways. Snuff and snus adversely affect periodontal health through vascular, inflammatory, immune-modulatory, and microbial mechanisms.

Nicotine-induced vasoconstriction is one of the most studied biological effects of smokeless tobacco use, including snuff and snus. Nicotine is significantly attracted to nicotinic acetylcholine receptors (nAChRs) that are abundant in endothelial cells (Duerrschmidt et al. 2012). After nicotine binds, it prompts the release of catecholamines such as epinephrine and norepinephrine, which has been shown to cause continued vasoconstriction of gingival blood vessels in animal models (Duerrschmidt et al. 2012). Reduced blood perfusion and oxygenation hinders the transport of biological nutrients and immune cells thus delaying healing and predisposing the host to periodontal destruction similar to nicotine-induced changes in smoking (Ng et al. 2015). Adequate blood flow is required to maintain collagen synthesis and fibroblast proliferation, as well as to promote tissue regeneration during periodontal disease; therefore, chronic exposure to nicotine can hinder the antioxidant response of the periodontium and limit its ability to self-repair after mechanical or bacterial insults following use of snuff or snus.

Immune modulation and inflammation dysregulation are also common mechanisms driven by snuff or snus to further compound periodontal health. Individuals who use snuff or snus show increased pro-inflammatory cytokines in the gingival crevicular fluid, such as IL-1β, tumour necrosis factor-alpha (TNF-α), and prostaglandin E2 (PGE2) (Pandey et al. 2015). These cytokines are key mediators of tissue destruction in periodontitis, promoting connective tissue breakdown and alveolar bone resorption (Hugoson and Rolandsson 2011). TNF-α, also triggers osteoclastogenic pathways through RANKL, and thus promotes bone loss in patients with periodontitis. In snuff and snus users, higher activity of matrix metalloproteinase (MMP), especially MMP-8 and MMP-9, is also reported, which causes collagen breakdown and loss of attachment between the periodontal ligament and the cementum surrounding the root surfaces of the teeth (Ando et al. 2024).

In addition to vascular and inflammatory mechanisms, the use of snuff and snus could lead to dysbiosis of the oral microbiome, enhancing the proliferation of periodontal pathogens. Studies have demonstrated that tobacco users have an increased prevalence of anaerobic bacteria including the "red complex" bacteria, which comprises of *Porphyromonas gingivalis*, *Tannerella forsythia*, and *Treponema denticola*, and which are highly correlated with aggressive forms of periodontitis (Al Kawas et al. 2021). Snuff or snus products with a highly alkaline pH might worsen this pathway by increasing bacterial adherence and virulence. Due to the nicotine content of snuff and snus, their use could also be associated with increased colonization of *Candida* fungi that may exacerbate mucosal dysbiosis and inflammation of periodontal tissues (Negi et al. 2019).

Moreover, smokeless tobacco products also contain TSNAs such as N-nitrosonornicotine (NNN) and 4-(methylnitrosamino)-1-(3-pyridyl)-1-butanone (NNK), that are strong carcinogens and play an important role in periodontal tissue destruction (Hecht et al. 2016). TSNAs cause oxidative stress and induce DNA damage leading to an inflammatory microenvironment that accelerates periodontal destruction by disrupting the balance between microbial homeostasis and host immune defence (Hecht et al. 2016).

The regular placement of snuff and snus, which come into direct contact with the gingival tissues, can be a source of mechanical irritation which, together with chemical assault from snuff and snus, appears to increase the risk of chronic inflammation, gingival recession, and periodontal disease.

10.3.2 Clinical Presentation of Changes in Periodontal Health in Users of Snuff or Snus

In clinical settings, users of snuff and snus have been reported to show localized gingival recession, plaque accumulation, and attachment loss. In regular users, periodontal pockets can occur, especially since nicotine is highly addictive and could lead to prolonged exposure, alongside increased likelihood of poor oral hygiene in users (Rahim et al. 2022). Compared with non-users, the risk of gingivitis and periodontitis is significantly higher among consumers of snuff and snus.

Gingival recession is the most commonly reported clinical presentation of poor periodontal health in snuff and snus users, specifically in sites where the product is regularly placed (Fig. 10.2) (Chu et al. 2010). A study from Pakistan reported that 65.8% of daily smokeless tobacco users have localized gingival recession adjacent to the site of placement (Nasir et al. 2023). This gingival recession is typically due to chronic mechanical irritation enhanced by nicotine-induced vasoconstriction that decreases blood supply to the gingiva. Such recession may also be commonly associated with more plaque formation which potentiates inflammatory disease and loss of periodontal tissue.

In addition to gingival recession, the pocket probing depth and clinical attachment loss of snuff and snus users can also be higher than non-users (Fig. 10.3), although the evidence is mixed (Montén et al. 2006). Many clinical studies have documented higher bleeding on probing scores in snus users, indicating a defective host immune response to microbial biofilms, where as there may be limited presence of alveolar bone loss (>2 mm) (Abrahamsson et al. 2006). This is different from what is seen in smokers, where bleeding on probing is usually suppressed due to chronic vasoconstriction, suggesting that the vascular reactivity is not completely compromised in snus or snuff users, so that periodontal inflammation can still be detected in its early forms (Prakash et al. 2014).

Hyperkeratosis and leukoplakic lesions in the mucosa around the placement site are further distinguishing features of consumers of snuff and snus (Figs. 10.4 and 10.5) (Kopperud et al. 2023). Though lesions such as these demonstrate no direct link to periodontal disease, they can cause soft tissue aberrations and secondary bacterial colonization that indirectly worsen periodontal inflammation (Tebbutt et al. 2020).

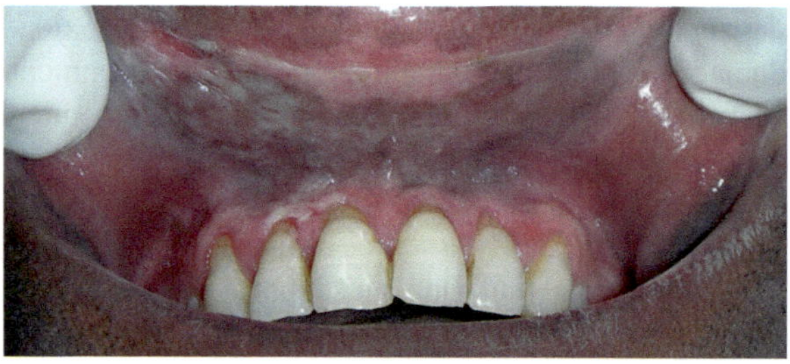

Fig. 10.2 Clinical presentation of a consumer of snus with localized gingival recession (tooth number #6 to #10)

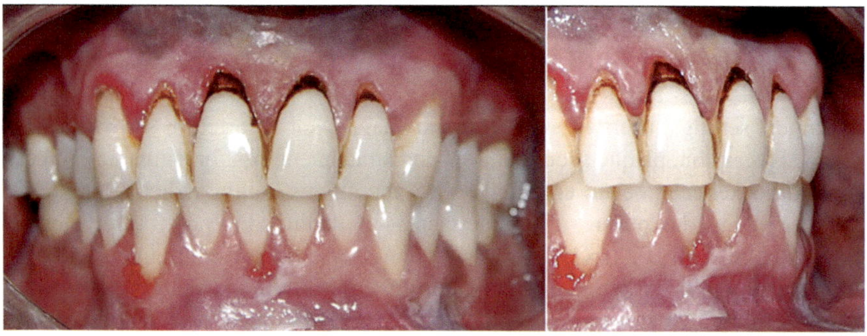

Fig. 10.3 Clinical presentation of a consumer of snus with multiple gingival recessions and white lesions in the oral cavity. Presentation demonstrated increased tendency of bleeding on probing

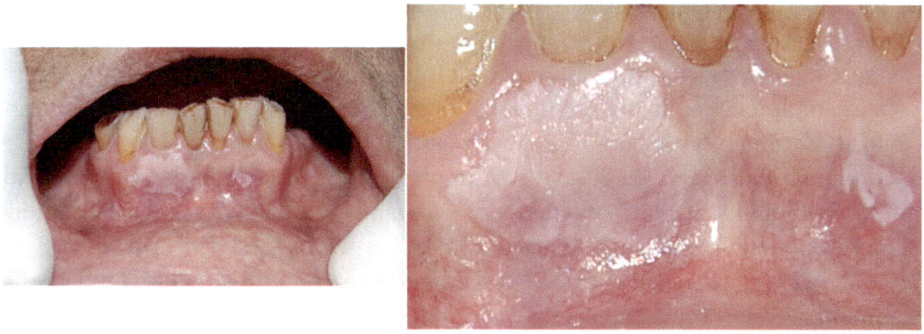

Fig. 10.4 Clinical appearance of a snus-associated white lesion with hyperkeratosis after chronic snus use

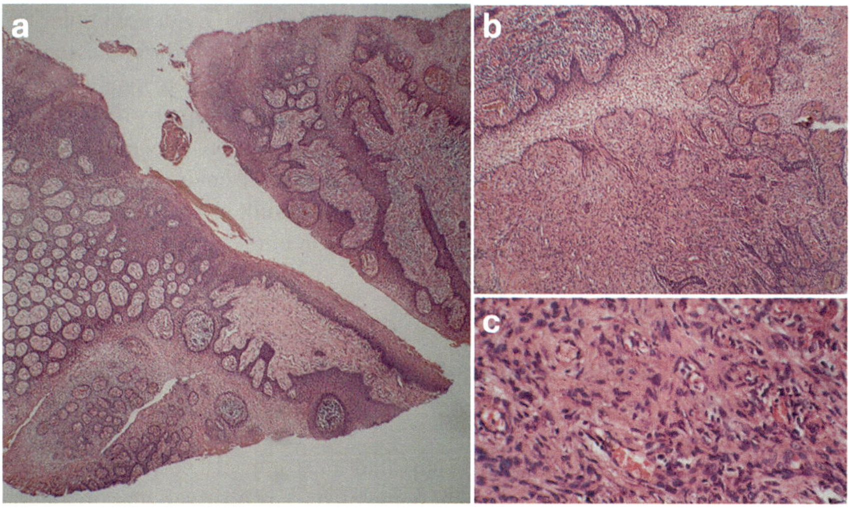

Fig. 10.5 Histopathological features of a snus-associated white lesion in (**a**) low power (10X) exhibiting hyperparakeratosis, (**b**) subepithelial band of inflammatory cell infiltration and (**c**) at high power (40X) showing plasma cell infiltration

10.4 Effects of Snuff and Snus on Peri-Implant Health

10.4.1 Comparison of Effects of Snuff and Snus on Peri-Implant Health with Effects on Periodontal Health

Less is known about peri-implant health in users of snuff and snus compared with periodontal health. The available evidence indicates that using these products might be pro-inflammatory and impair peri-implant tissue integration in an environment which is already susceptible to inflammatory insults, microbial dysbiosis, and host-mediated tissue destruction. An initial inflammatory condition of the soft tissue surrounding the implant, known as peri-implant mucositis, may occur at a higher rate in users of snuff or snus compared with non-users (Hu et al. 2024b). Without treatment, peri-implant mucositis can develop into peri-implantitis which is a more serious condition that involves inflammation and bone loss around the implant, subsequently leading to implant failure (Vámos et al. 2024).

Although both periodontal and peri-implant tissues can become inflamed with microbial biofilms, the lack of a periodontal ligament in implants provides a unique pathophysiologic pathway of tobacco-induced tissue damage. In periodontitis, the periodontal ligament can alleviate mechanical stress and inflammatory responses, supplying vessels for immune defence and healing. In peri-implant tissues, the absence of capability for fibroblastic repair indicates that inflamed peri-implant tissues heal less well than inflamed tissues surrounding a natural tooth (Zhang et al. 2022).

In addition, gingival fibroblasts in periodontal tissue also have stronger regenerative ability than peri-implant soft tissues (Huang et al. 2024). Evidence implicating snuff and snus on the host response suggests that nicotine exposure is associated with decreased fibroblast proliferation, compromised collagen synthesis, and increased apoptosis, all of which lead to delayed wound healing and reduced peri-implant tissue stability (Javed et al. 2019; Şahin 2024). As peri-implant soft tissues are unable to recreate the same depth sensation or reparative environment characteristic of natural gingiva, an inflammatory or microbial insult in the presence of snuff or snus could result in a more accelerated destruction of the peri-implant apparatus (Vámos et al. 2024).

10.4.2 Biological Mechanisms of Effects of Snuff and Snus on Peri-Implant Health

Similar to periodontal health, using snuff and snus impacts peri-implant health through biological mechanisms that are complex and involve vascular, inflammatory, and microbial features.

The reduction in oxygen delivery to healing peri-implant tissues is one of the most significant effects of nicotine due to its capacity to induce vasoconstriction (Hu et al. 2024b). The ischaemic surroundings hinder normal peri-implant connective tissue to sufficiently respond to immune-mediated reactions which increases the risk for early acute peri-implant mucositis and impaired osseointegration (D'Ambrosio et al. 2022).

The nicotine in snuff and snus has also been proven to have a stimulating effect on osteoclastic activity and an inhibitory effect on osteoblastic function, disrupting the necessary balance between bone resorption and formation which is essential for the stability of implants (Nilawati et al. 2023). Multiple in vitro studies have shown that nicotine decreases the activity of alkaline phosphatase, an enzyme important for bone mineralization and represses the expression of bone morphogenetic proteins which are necessary for bone formation (Gruber et al. 2023). These findings imply that implant osseointegration in chronic snuff and snus users could be impaired, thereby increasing the risk of early implant failure.

Compared with non-users, the immune response towards the biofilms surrounding dental implants could also differ in snuff and snus users (Jia et al. 2024). Neutrophil dysfunction induced by chronic nicotine exposure is characterized by impaired chemotaxis, reduced phagocytosis, and increased oxidative stress (Brembach et al. 2023). These immunological defects result in an excessive inflammatory response with increased levels of IL-1β, TNF-α, and MMPs (Al-Shibani et al. 2011). Specifically, increased MMP activity correlates with abnormal degradation of the extracellular matrix which leads to increased risk of peri-implant soft tissue deficiency and exposure of the implant surface leading to additional bacterial colonization.

Microbial dysbiosis is another crucial factor affecting peri-implant health among snuff and snus users. Habitual placement of snuff or snus could be associated with colonization of periodontopathogenic bacteria such as *P. gingivalis*, *Fusobacterium nucleatum*, and *T. forsythia*. These species are important facilitators of peri-implant inflammation, leading to the progression of peri-implant mucositis to peri-implantitis (Di Spirito et al. 2024). In addition, the alkaline pH of snuff and snus could increase the pathogenicity of these bacteria.

10.4.3 Clinical Presentation of Changes in Peri-Implant Health in Users of Snuff and Snus

Few observational studies have reported the clinical presentation of peri-implant outcomes in users of snuff and snus. This might be because cessation of snuff or snus use, similar to smoking cessation, is often a prerequisite to installation of implant and thus the pool of current snuff or snus users would be limited. Nevertheless, snuff and snus users could have a significantly altered soft tissue response to implants in addition to impaired stability such as that seen in smokers, although data among continuing users are not available (Alghamdi et al.). Existing research among smokers has shown that continuing use can lead to increased frequency of peri-implant attachment loss, which results in decreased stability of the peri-implant tissues (Alghamdi et al. 2020). Such instability of the soft tissues could lead snuff and snus consumers to be at risk for early peri-implant disease and higher maintenance needs over the long term, as seen in smokers (Vámos et al. 2024).

In addition, experimental studies also showed that nicotine exposure decreases the biomechanical stability of implants. In animal models, the bone implant contact ratios were lower with implants inserted into nicotine-exposed bone, as well as bone density and thickness of the peri-implant connective tissue layer, indicating that nicotine undermines the integrity of bone–implant interface.

10.5 Comparing the Effects of Snuff and Snus on Periodontal Health with Smoking and Other Nicotine-Delivery Devices

10.5.1 Comparison with Smoking

Compared with people who smoke, the risk of severe periodontitis is lower in those who use snuff or snus (smoking OR 6.50, $p = 0.001$; snus OR 0.82, $p > 0.05$ relative to non-users), according to the latest follow-up (2003) of a pooled analysis of cross-sectional studies in Sweden (Hugoson and Rolandsson 2011). Smoking was associated with a higher frequency of pocket probing depth ≥4 mm ($p = 0.001$), and lower bone level index ($p = 0.001$) than using snus, whereas the frequency of gingivitis was similar between both behaviours (Hugoson and Rolandsson 2011). Localized tissue damage in periodontal tissue and gingival recession in users of snuff or snus indicates that the underlying pathogenesis is primarily represented by both mechanical trauma and chemical irritations, in contrast to the systemic effects due to inhaled toxins in smoking-related periodontitis (Hugoson and Rolandsson 2011).

While smokers have increased frequency of severe periodontal disease, snus users do not appear to have similar global attachment loss or pocket formation; however, they do show signs of localized clinical attachment loss and are generally found to have higher levels inflammatory biomarkers in the gingival crevicular fluid (Hugoson and Rolandsson 2011).

10.5.2 Comparison with Oral Nicotine Pouches and Other Nicotine-Delivery Devices

Oral nicotine pouches have been available in several markets since 2022 (Fig. 10.6). These products are visually similar to Swedish snus and are also consumed by holding between the lip and gum, but do not contain tobacco (Jackson et al. 2023). Due to the similar method of using oral nicotine pouches, gingival recession due to mechanical irritation is the most likely effect expected on periodontal health compared to snuff and snus pouches (Jackson et al. 2023). Their high flavouring content has also been associated with microbial dysbiosis and inflammation at the site of regular contact (Ye and Rahman 2023). The concentration of nicotine in these products is comparable to snuff and snus (up to 11 mg per pouch) (Jackson et al. 2023), and would likely result in similar vasoconstriction, although the novelty of these products means there is little evidence comparing their effects on periodontal and peri-implant health with other nicotine-delivery devices (Ye and Rahman 2023).

Comparisons between the effects of e-cigarettes or vaping on periodontal health versus those from snuff or snus are not readily available. There is evidence that e-cigarette use could lead to inflammation which could be relevant for periodontal health (Ye and Rahman 2023). Using e-cigarettes has been associated with a higher prevalence of gingivitis than non-use ($p = 0.012$), (Garcia et al. 2024) but

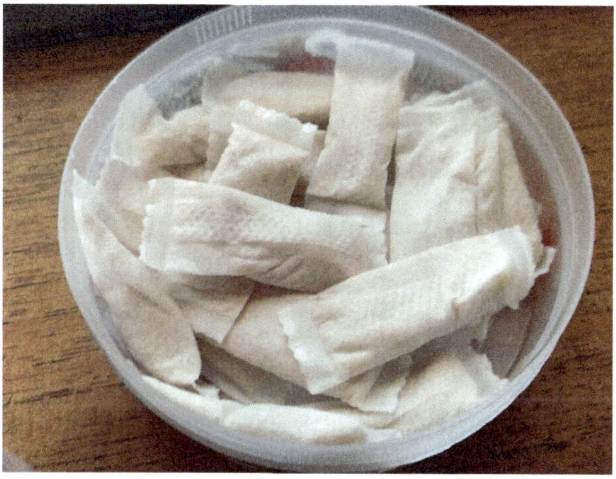

Fig. 10.6 Oral nicotine pouches. (Credits: L.V. Olavi Rantala)

comparisons with snuff or snus are not available. Dysbiosis of the oral microbiome is also more present in e-cigarette users than non-users, possibly favouring colonization of disease-associated pathogens and periodontal disease (Scherer et al. 2024; Pushalkar et al. 2020).

Nicotine replacement therapy is available in several forms such as patches, lozenges, gum, mouth or nasal spray, and have limited side effects compared with continuing tobacco use, especially with regard to periodontal and peri-implant health (Alayadi 2024). Considering the topical application of nicotine patches, their periodontal effects are limited. However, some short-term effects have been reported due to the vasoconstrictive effects of nicotine on blood vessels which can impair gingival healing and decrease the effectiveness of the immune response to oral bacteria, along with the resulting reduction of saliva production leading to dry mouth (Jackson et al. 2023; Alayadi 2024). While nicotine gum and oral sprays might enhance vasoconstriction and changes in the oral mucosa and disrupt the oral microbiome in the short term, the long-term effects are not significant (Wallström et al. 1999).

10.6 Implications for Clinical Practice

Clinicians should be aware that use of snuff and snus is a substantial, yet preventable, risk factor for poor periodontal and peri-implant health. Although these products may seem safer than smoking in terms of health in general, their localized vasoconstrictive and inflammatory effects represent a challenge for the durability of implants and oral health as a whole.

Early detection and individualized maintenance protocols to address snuff and snus use are the cornerstone of not just good management, but good clinical practice. Normalizing appropriate screening of snuff and snus use, including smoking history, smokeless tobacco history, and increasing awareness among patients about potential risks through education, may positively change the long-term treatment outcomes (Fu and Wang 2020). Considering the risks involved, early intervention, tobacco use cessation, extensive peri-implant monitoring, and patient education is critical in clinical management.

10.6.1 Risk Assessment of Patients Who Use Snuff or Snus

In patients who use snuff or snus, risk assessment, patient education, and tailored periodontal maintenance strategies are necessary for their management. The rising use of snuff and snus in young adolescents represents a new challenge for dental practitioners, especially in relation to the diagnosis, treatment, and maintenance of periodontal and peri-implant health (Németh et al. 2024). These products are commonly promoted as safer alternatives to smoking; however, an increasing body of evidence indicates that these products compromise the integrity of periodontium and peri-implant tissues, and a specific approach to risk assessment, patient education, and treatment planning is necessary (Parihar et al. 2024). Clinical management of snuff and snus users must take an integrative approach that considers both the biological effects of nicotine and tobacco-specific nitrosamines, and also behavioural and patient monitoring concerns that may alter oral health outcomes.

Adequate risk assessment is the basis of successful treatment of periodontal and peri-implant disease in users of snuff and snus. Clinicians should take a detailed tobacco history, assessing how often and how long snuff and snus is being used including pack-years, frequency, duration, and placement site in the oral cavity. Patients who use snuff or snus have an increased risk of localized gingival recession, peri-implant soft tissue inflammation, or further complications. Routine dental check-ups are excellent opportunities to implement tobacco-specific risk assessment tools such the Fagerstrom Test for Nicotine Dependence with the aim of identifying patients who could be referred to tobacco cessation programmes (Salhi et al. 2021; Benjamin et al. 2024).

The assessment of soft tissue and peri-implant structures via clinical examination by regular periodontal probing, to evaluate clinical attachment loss and bleeding on probing, must be done to diagnose the early inflammatory changes of periodontitis before irreversible damage occurs. On probing the depths of peri-implant sites, when depths are ≥4 mm and bleeding or suppuration occurs, immediate intervention is warranted (Ramseier 2024). These are early signs of peri-implant mucositis or peri-implantitis which need professional management.

Furthermore, peri-implant failure is especially severe in patients with other risk factors such as diabetes mellitus, poor plaque control, or a history of periodontitis (Linghu et al. 2025). A full assessment of other existing conditions is thus necessary for efficient and informative risk assessment before deciding whether treatment with implant therapy is appropriate.

10.6.2 Recommendations for Management and Maintenance of Periodontal Health in Users of Snuff or Snus

For patients with periodontal disease who use snuff or snus, treatment strategies should adhere to recommended protocols. Models of periodic periodontal maintenance (once every 3–4 months) to verify disease progression are of paramount importance. Emphasis on oral hygiene, including interproximal cleaning and antimicrobial mouth rinses, hydrogen peroxide gels, or photodynamic therapy, is recommended to minimize further complications by microbial insults (Roosaar et al. 2006).

Non-surgical periodontal therapy in snuff or snus users should mostly involve scaling and root planing and focus on management of microbial biofilms (Ramanauskaite et al. 2020). In cases with residual inflammation, adjunctive therapies such as local delivery of antimicrobial agents may be helpful. Considering the site-specific periodontal destruction associated with snuff and snus consumption, clinicians should focus on site-specific augmentation procedures such as soft tissue grafting to treat gingival recession (Kharazmi et al. 2014; Hoge and Kirkham 1983).

The effect of snuff and snus on periodontal treatment outcomes, such as healing after scaling and root planing or periodontal surgery, will probably be slower, which may be attributed to the diminished vascular supply and inhibition of fibroblast proliferation. The literature contains reports of sub-optimal regenerative responses among smokeless tobacco users treated with guided tissue regeneration or bone grafting, which are likely due to impaired angiogenesis and increased inflammation.

Advances in personalized medicine and precision medicine approaches could be adopted in future clinical research with snuff and snus users to improve the efficacy of treatment and management of periodontal problems. These could include integration of genetic risk profiling and microbiome analysis in addition to advanced regenerative therapies.

10.6.3 Recommendations for Management and Maintenance of Peri-Implant Health in Users of Snuff or Snus

Due to the increased risk of peri-implant disease progression among users of snuff or snus, clinicians should implement preventive and therapeutic strategies to counteract these effects. Thus, snuff and snus consumers should be subjected to a comprehensive peri-implant risk characterization prior to dental implant placement (Ciurescu et al. 2025). Smoking and smokeless tobacco cessation counselling should be strongly encouraged as cessation of smokeless tobacco before implant surgery may enhance wound healing and implant osseointegration (Natto et al. 2019).

Close monitoring of peri-implant soft tissues for early signs of inflammation and increased probing depths is warranted in current and former users of snuff or snus. This should be accompanied by regular peri-implant maintenance visits (every 3–4 months) for early detection of peri-implant mucositis (Satpathy et al. 2024). Adjunctive microbiological therapies such as chlorhexidine rinses, local antibiotic delivery, and laser decontamination may contribute to managing microbial load, particularly in high-risk patients (Kim et al. 2024). Non-surgical and, if necessary, surgical approaches should also be carried out, including implantoplasty or regenerative peri-implant treatments in patients with peri-implantitis. Providing advice on oral hygiene is also necessary and could incorporate promoting the use of interdental brushes, soft-tissue stimulators, and implant-compatible dental flossing methods.

If diagnosed early, peri-implant mucositis can be reversed with mechanical debridement combined with localized antibiotic therapy and behavioural changes regarding risk factors. Patients with signs of early-stage peri-implantitis, such as increased pocket depth, suppuration, or bone loss ≥2 mm, should receive timely treatment with non-surgical periodontal therapy, including laser decontamination, subgingival irrigation, and systemic antibiotics (metronidazole and amoxicillin). In the advanced stages of peri-implantitis, surgical procedures such as guided bone regeneration and implantoplasty may be required to prevent peri-implant bone loss (Levine et al. 2025). In aesthetically sensitive sites, soft tissue grafting is recommended in cases of considerable gingival recession resulting from the use of snuff and snus.

For implant patients, soft tissue augmentation has been established to enhance peri-implant keratinized tissue width and mitigate additional peri-implant soft tissue deficiency (Zucchelli et al. 2020). When restoring implants, attention should be paid to creating smooth prosthetic contours and ideal crown emergence profiles to reduce plaque accumulation. Higher biofilm formation has been reported when rough-surfaced zirconia abutments are utilized which is of relevance for snuff and snus users (Selamet et al. 2025). Because of this, highly polished titanium abutments may be preferable to rough surfaced zirconia abutments to minimize bacterial proliferation (Sun et al. 2024). However, studies have shown that platelet concentrates and enamel matrix derivatives may improve the healing process of soft tissues in peri-implant sites compromised due to smokeless tobacco usage (Liu et al. 2025; Cardaropoli et al. 2024). Previous research has reported that low level laser therapy decreases peri-implant inflammation and enhanced wound healing in high-risk patients (Zou et al. 2024).

10.6.4 Patient Education and Intervention for Cessation of Snuff and Snus

Many users of snuff and snus falsely believe that these products are harmless or consider them to be less dangerous than smoking. Clinicians should deliver evidence-based counselling that underscores their localized and systemic effects (Chahar et al. 2023). Evidence suggests that cessation of snuff and snus is likely to improve periodontal treatment outcomes and avoid peri-implant complications, which can contribute to implant failure and aesthetic problems. Patients using snuff or snus should therefore be counselled regarding the impact that delayed wound healing and microbial dysbiosis may have on the success of regenerative periodontal procedures or peri-implant therapies.

Though complete cessation of tobacco use in all forms is the best outcome, many patients are not willing or able to stop right away. Clinicians should use motivational interviewing strategies to suggest gradual reduction of snuff and snus, focusing on the oral health benefits of reduced exposure (Holliday et al. 2021). Nicotine replacement therapy, behavioural counselling, and digital cessation tools such as mobile apps or online support groups could improve quit rates among users (Holliday et al. 2021). A reasonable time for referral to cessation is at least 4–6 weeks in the perioperative period for the patients requiring the periodontal or implant therapy considering the positive effect on osseointegration and peri-implant tissue healing, and could also be considered for cessation of snuff and snus.

10.7 Gaps in the Evidence and Future Directions for Research

Future studies investigating the effects of snuff and snus use on periodontal and peri-implant health are needed, particularly focusing on the long-term impacts and in comparison to other nicotine-delivery products. This evidence will ultimately guide best clinical practices, inform health policies, and encourage healthier behaviours. Continued research in these domains could address the detrimental effects of snuff and snus in terms of oral health and provide strategies for mitigating or reversing the progression of periodontal and peri-implant disease in users of snuff or snus.

A relevant focus is the initiation of large, longitudinal studies and multicenter clinical trials that follow snus users over an extended period of time to assess periodontal disease trajectory. Such studies should investigate the relationship between periodontal disease and snus users, compared with both non-users and smokers, to help determine whether use of snus carries unique risks, or whether the effects of use are similar to those noted in smoking. Such studies could also determine whether snus use was associated with the stage of periodontitis, tooth loss, and other complications.

It is necessary to elucidate the molecular mechanisms that underlie the adverse consequences of snus on periodontal tissues. More research must be targeted at the mechanism of how nicotine, tobacco-specific nitrosamines, and other detrimental substances in snuff and snus play a role in inducing periodontal disease. By investigating the immune response, oxidative stress, and inflammatory mediators that are triggered and perpetuated in snuff or snus users, it could be possible to uncover mechanisms that promote degenerative processes in the periodontium and impair tissue repair.

It would also be of value to compare studies on snus with other tobacco or nicotine-delivery products, including smoking, e-cigarettes, and other novel products as they become available. This would allow further evaluation to clarify the effects of snuff or snus use on periodontal health and disease progression when compared to other tobacco use patterns and to corroborate the benefits of recommended nicotine replacement therapy. Assessment of any additive or synergistic effects of smoking and snuff or snus use on periodontal and peri-implant health could also be examined in relation to duration and frequency of use, although dual use is currently less common among smoking populations and could prove difficult to represent in large studies.

Genetic studies may help explain why some snus users develop periodontal disease while others do not. Determining genetic factors that render certain individuals more susceptible to periodontal problems from snus use may aid in implementing personalized prevention measures and specialized interventions.

Another crucial area of research is to develop preventive and therapeutic strategies that are specific to snus users. This should be coupled with a considerable effort in education around public health, making sure the public is aware that snus is harmful for periodontal and peri-implant health. As large populations use snus in many countries, campaigns raising awareness regarding the potential periodontal risk of snus use will help reduce usage and eventually promote awareness towards healthier lifestyles.

Disclaimer Where authors are identified as personnel of the International Agency for Research on Cancer/World Health Organization, the authors alone are responsible for the views expressed in this chapter and they do not necessarily represent the decisions, policy, or views of the International Agency for Research on Cancer/World Health Organization.

Conflict of Interest Statement The authors declare no conflicts of interest.

References

Abrahamsson KH, Koch G, Norderyd O, Romao C, Wennström JL (2006) Periodontal conditions in a Swedish city population of adolescents: a cross-sectional study. Swed Dent J 30(1):25–34

Al Kawas S, Al-Marzooq F, Rahman B, Shearston JA, Saad H, Benzina D, Weitzman M (2021) The impact of smoking different tobacco types on the subgingival microbiome and periodontal health: a pilot study. Sci Rep 11(1):1113. https://doi.org/10.1038/s41598-020-80937-3

Alayadi H (2024) The impact of nicotine patches on gingival and oral health: a narrative review. Cureus 16(9):e70571. https://doi.org/10.7759/cureus.70571

Alghamdi O, Alrabiah MA-O, Al-Hamoudi N, AlKindi M, Vohra FA-O, Abduljabbar TA-O (2020) Peri-implant soft tissue status and crestal bone loss around immediately-loaded narrow-diameter implants placed in cigarette-smokers: 6-year follow-up results. Clin Implant Dent Relat Res 22(2):220–225. (1708–8208 (Electronic))

Al-Shibani NK, Labban NY, Kowolik MJ, Ruby JD, Windsor LJ (2011) Responses of human neutrophils to nicotine and/or Porphyromonas gingivalis. J Periodontol 82(10):1504–1508. https://doi.org/10.1902/jop.2011.100757

Ando Y, Tsukasaki M, Huynh NC-N, Zang S, Yan M, Muro R, Nakamura K, Komagamine M, Komatsu N, Okamoto K, Nakano K, Okamura T, Yamaguchi A, Ishihara K, Takayanagi H (2024) The neutrophil–osteogenic cell axis promotes bone destruction in periodontitis. Int J Oral Sci 16(1):18. https://doi.org/10.1038/s41368-023-00275-8

Benjamin N, Choubey V, Bhasin M, Sushma B, Choudhary A, Thomas PA (2024) Analysis of tobacco cessation programs in dental settings. J Pharm Bioallied Sci 16(Suppl 4):S3290–s3292. https://doi.org/10.4103/jpbs.jpbs_710_24

Bhandari A, Bhatta N (2021) Tobacco and its relationship with oral health. JNMA J Nepal Med Assoc 59(243):1204–1206. https://doi.org/10.31729/jnma.6605

Brembach TC, Sabat R, Witte K, Schwerdtle T, Wolk K (2023) Molecular and functional changes in neutrophilic granulocytes induced by nicotine: a systematic review and critical evaluation. Front Immunol 14:1281685. https://doi.org/10.3389/fimmu.2023.1281685

Brinchmann BC, Vist GE, Becher R, Grimsrud TK, Elvsaas I, Underland V, Holme JA, Carlsen KCL, Kreyberg I, Nordhagen LS, Bains KES, Carlsen KH, Alexander J, Valen H (2023) Use of Swedish smokeless tobacco during pregnancy: a systematic review of pregnancy and early life health risk. Addiction 118(5):789–803. https://doi.org/10.1111/add.16114

Cardaropoli D, Tamagnone L, Roffredo A, Costanzo L (2024) The use of enamel matrix derivative to modulate wound healing of peri-implant soft tissues. Int J Periodontics Restorative Dent 44(4):408–421. https://doi.org/10.11607/prd.6573

Chahar P, Mohanty VR, Y BA, Rijhwani K (2023) Correlates of nicotine dependence among patients visiting a tobacco cessation centre in India: a retrospective analysis. Natl Med J India 36(5):301–304. https://doi.org/10.25259/nmji_677_21

Chu YH, Tatakis DN, Wee AG (2010) Smokeless tobacco use and periodontal health in a rural male population. J Periodontol 81(6):848–854. https://doi.org/10.1902/jop.2010.090310

Chugh A, Arora M, Jain N, Vidyasagaran A, Readshaw A, Sheikh A, Eckhardt J, Siddiqi K, Chopra M, Mishu MP, Kanaan M, Rahman MA, Mehrotra R, Huque R, Forberger S, Dahanayake S, Khan Z, Boeckmann M, Dogar O (2023) The global impact of tobacco control policies on smokeless tobacco use: a systematic review. Lancet Glob Health 11(6):e953–e968. https://doi.org/10.1016/S2214-109X(23)00205-X

Chung YL, Lee JJ, Chien HH, Chang MC, Jeng JH (2024) Interplay between diabetes mellitus and periodontal/pulpal-periapical diseases. J Dent Sci 19(3):1338–1347. https://doi.org/10.1016/j.jds.2024.03.021

Ciurescu CE, Dima L, Gheorghiu A, Ciurescu VA, Festila DG, Moga MA, Vesa S, Cosgarea R (2025) Prevalence of peri-implant diseases in a private practice and potential risk indicators. Oral Health Prev Dent 23:43–49. https://doi.org/10.3290/j.ohpd.c_1805

Cornelius ME, Loretan CG, Jamal A, Davis Lynn BC, Mayer M, Alcantara IC, Neff L (2023) Tobacco product use among adults - United States, 2021. MMWR Morb Mortal Wkly Rep 72(18):475–483. https://doi.org/10.15585/mmwr.mm7218a1

D'Ambrosio F, Pisano M, Amato A, Iandolo A, Caggiano M, Martina S (2022) Periodontal and peri-implant health status in traditional vs. heat-not-burn tobacco and electronic cigarettes smokers: a systematic review. Dent J (Basel) 10(6):103

Deyton LR (2011) FDA tobacco product regulations: a powerful tool for tobacco control. Public Health Rep 126(2):167–169. https://doi.org/10.1177/003335491112600206

Di Spirito F, Giordano F, Di Palo MP, D'Ambrosio F, Scognamiglio B, Sangiovanni G, Caggiano M, Gasparro R (2024) Microbiota of peri-implant healthy tissues, peri-implant mucositis, and peri-implantitis: a comprehensive review. Microorganisms 12(6):1137

Duerrschmidt N, Hagen A, Gaertner C, Wermke A, Nowicki M, Spanel-Borowski K, Stepan H, Mohr FW, Dhein S (2012) Nicotine effects on human endothelial intercellular communication via α4β2 and α3β2 nicotinic acetylcholine receptor subtypes. Naunyn Schmiedeberg's Arch Pharmacol 385(6):621–632. https://doi.org/10.1007/s00210-012-0738-y

Fisher MA, Taylor GW, Tilashalski KR (2005) Smokeless tobacco and severe active periodontal disease, NHANES III. J Dent Res 84(8):705–710. https://doi.org/10.1177/154405910508400804

Fu JH, Wang HL (2020) Breaking the wave of peri-implantitis. Periodontol 2000 84(1):145–160. https://doi.org/10.1111/prd.12335

Garcia BFS, Nascimento BB, Marques EF, Jesus CBD, Santana Neto IC, Rocha LST, Oliveira GMS, Bazaglia da Silva MI, Kasai MLHI, Takahama Junior A (2024) The use of electronic cigarettes and other tobacco products among university students and their potential relationship with oral health: a cross-sectional study. J Am Dent Assoc 155(8):647–656. https://doi.org/10.1016/j.adaj.2024.04.012

Gruber MD, Gibbs D, Vignolles-Jeong J, Viljoen S, Grossbach AJ, Xu D (2023) The effects of nicotine- and cigarette-related products on osteogenesis, bone formation, and bone mineralization: a systematic review. Neurosurgery 93(2):247–256. https://doi.org/10.1227/neu.0000000000002412

Gupta AK, Kanaan M, Siddiqi K, Sinha DN, Mehrotra R (2022) Oral cancer risk assessment for different types of smokeless tobacco products sold worldwide: a review of reviews and meta-analyses. Cancer Prev Res 15(11):733–746. https://doi.org/10.1158/1940-6207.Capr-21-0567

Hecht SS, Stepanov I, Carmella SG (2016) Exposure and metabolic activation biomarkers of carcinogenic tobacco-specific nitrosamines. Acc Chem Res 49(1):106–114. https://doi.org/10.1021/acs.accounts.5b00472

Hoge HW, Kirkham DB (1983) Clinical management and soft tissue reconstruction of periodontal damage resulting from habitual use of snuff. J Am Dent Assoc 107(5):744–745. https://doi.org/10.14219/jada.archive.1983.0327

Holliday R, Hong B, McColl E, Livingstone-Banks J, Preshaw PM (2021) Interventions for tobacco cessation delivered by dental professionals. Cochrane Database Syst Rev 2(2):Cd005084. https://doi.org/10.1002/14651858.CD005084.pub4

Hu A, Wang X, Ai L, Liu K, Kong L (2024a) Association between matrix metalloproteinase-3 gene polymorphism and susceptibility to chronic periodontitis: a systematic review and meta-analysis. J Med Biochem 43(5):655–663. https://doi.org/10.5937/jomb0-49044

Hu R, Qian H, Wang X, Peng B, Huang D (2024b) Nicotine promotes pathogenic bacterial growth and biofilm formation in peri-implant. J Med Microbiol 73(10). https://doi.org/10.1099/jmm.0.001897

Huang Y, Tang Y, Zhang R, Wu X, Yan L, Chen X, Wu Q, Chen Y, Lv Y, Su Y (2024) Role of periodontal ligament fibroblasts in periodontitis: pathological mechanisms and therapeutic potential. J Transl Med 22(1):1136. https://doi.org/10.1186/s12967-024-05944-8

Hugoson A, Rolandsson M (2011) Periodontal disease in relation to smoking and the use of Swedish snus: epidemiological studies covering 20 years (1983–2003). J Clin Periodontol 38(9):809–816. https://doi.org/10.1111/j.1600-051X.2011.01749.x

International Agency for Research on Cancer (2007) IARC Monographs on the Evaluation of Carcinogenic Risks to Humans Volume 89. Smokeless Tobacco and Some Tobacco-specific N-Nitrosamines. World Health Organization. https://publications.iarc.who.int/Book-And-Report-Series/Iarc-Monographs-On-The-Identification-Of-Carcinogenic-Hazards-To-Humans/Smokeless-Tobacco-And-Some-Tobacco-specific-Em-N-Em--Nitrosamines-2007

Jackson JM, Weke A, Holliday R (2023) Nicotine pouches: a review for the dental team. Br Dent J 235(8):643–646. https://doi.org/10.1038/s41415-023-6383-7

Javed F, Rahman I, Romanos GE (2019) Tobacco-product usage as a risk factor for dental implants. Periodontol 2000 81(1):48–56. https://doi.org/10.1111/prd.12282

Jia P, Guo X, Ye J, Lu H, Yang J, Hou J (2024) Microbiome of diseased and healthy implants-a comprehensive microbial data analysis. Front Cell Infect Microbiol 14:1445751. https://doi.org/10.3389/fcimb.2024.1445751

Kharazmi M, Carlsson AP, Hallberg P, Modig M, Björnstad L, Hirsch JM (2014) Surgical approach to snus-induced injury of the oral mucosa. J Oral Sci 56(1):91–94. https://doi.org/10.2334/josnusd.56.91

Kim YJ, Song YW, Park SY, Cha JK, Lee HJ, Yang SM, Park JB, Koo KT (2024) Current understanding of the etiology, diagnosis, treatment, and management of peri-implant diseases: a narrative review for the consensus report of the Korean Academy of Periodontology. J Periodontal Implant Sci 54(6):377–392. https://doi.org/10.5051/jpis.2403920196

Kopperud SE, Vibeke A, Ibrahimu M, Rune B, Valen H (2023) Oral lesions associated with daily use of snus, a moist smokeless tobacco product. A cross-sectional study among Norwegian adolescents. Acta Odontol Scand 81(6):473–478. https://doi.org/10.1080/00016357.2023.2178502

Levine RA, Monje A, Saleh MHA, Dias DR, Kalani K, Pinsky HM, Ganeles J, Renouard F, Araújo MG (2025) Eight keys for the reconstructive therapy of peri-implantitis-related intrabony defects. Compend Contin Educ Dent 46(3):120–127

Linghu D, Zhang D, Liu M (2025) Predictors of implant failure: a comprehensive analysis of risk factors in oral implant restoration for patients with partial defects of dentition. Biomol Biomed. https://doi.org/10.17305/bb.2024.11668

Liu R, Chen S, Wang P, Bi R (2025) Using platelet concentrates to treat maxillofacial tissue lesions. Front Bioeng Biotechnol 12. https://doi.org/10.3389/fbioe.2024.1523225

Montén U, Wennström JL, Ramberg P (2006) Periodontal conditions in male adolescents using smokeless tobacco (moist snuff). J Clin Periodontol 33(12):863–868. https://doi.org/10.1111/j.1600-051X.2006.01005.x

Nasir SM, Sultana T, Hashmi S, Ahmed M (2023) Patterns and predictors of periodontal disease and tooth loss among users of smokeless tobacco. BMC Oral Health 23(1):428. https://doi.org/10.1186/s12903-023-03087-8

National Cancer Institute, Centers for Disease Control Prevention (2014) Smokeless tobacco and public health: a global perspective. U.S. Department of Health and Human Services, Centers for Disease Control and Prevention and National Institutes of Health, National Cancer Institute, Bethesda

Natto ZS, Almeganni N, Alnakeeb E, Bukhari Z, Jan R, Iacono VJ (2019) Peri-implantitis and peri-implant mucositis case definitions in dental research: a systematic assessment. J Oral Implantol 45(2):127–131. https://doi.org/10.1563/aaid-joi-D-18-00097

Negi M, Sepolia N, Panwar SS, Kumar M, Singla J, Aggarwal RK (2019) Prevalence of oral parameters in smokeless tobacco-associated precancer. J Family Med Prim Care 8(12):3956–3961. https://doi.org/10.4103/jfmpc.jfmpc_667_19

Németh O, Sipos L, Mátrai P, Szathmári-Mészáros N, Iványi D, Simon F, Kivovics M, Pénzes D, Mijiritsky E (2024) Snus use in adolescents: a threat to oral health. J Clin Med 13(14). https://doi.org/10.3390/jcm13144235

Ng TK, Huang L, Cao D, Yip YW-Y, Tsang WM, Yam GH-F, Pang CP, Cheung HS (2015) Cigarette smoking hinders human periodontal ligament-derived stem cell proliferation, migration and differentiation potentials. Sci Rep 5(1):7828. https://doi.org/10.1038/srep07828

Nilawati N, Widyastuti W, Rizka Y, Kurniawan H (2023) Dental implant osseointegration inhibition by nicotine through increasing nAChR, NFATc1 expression, osteoclast numbers, and decreasing osteoblast numbers. Eur J Dent 17(4):1189–1193. https://doi.org/10.1055/s-0042-1758794

Pandey V, Salam SA, Moda A, Agarwal P, Nath S, Pulikkotil SJ (2015) Effect of the use of snuff on the levels of interleukin-1 β and interleukin-8 in the gingival crevicular fluid of periodontitis patients. Dent Res J (Isfahan) 12(5):461–468. https://doi.org/10.4103/1735-3327.166222

Parihar AS, Shinkre R, Boddun M, Das A, Gupta G, Chandgothia N, Laddha R (2024) Innovations in screening and diagnosis of periodontal disease in tobacco users: a review. J Pharm Bioallied Sci 16(Suppl 3):S1962–s1964. https://doi.org/10.4103/jpbs.jpbs_172_24

Prakash P, Rath S, Mukherjee M, Malik A, Boruah D, Sahoo NK, Dutta V (2014) Comparative evaluation of the marginal gingival epithelium in smokers and nonsmokers: a histomorphometric and immunohistochemical study. Int J Periodontics Restorative Dent 34(6):781–786. https://doi.org/10.11607/prd.1823

Pushalkar S, Paul B, Li Q, Yang J, Vasconcelos R, Makwana S, González JM, Shah S, Xie C, Janal MN, Queiroz E, Bederoff M, Leinwand J, Solarewicz J, Xu F, Aboseria E, Guo Y, Aguallo D, Gomez C, Kamer A, Shelley D, Aphinyanaphongs Y, Barber C, Gordon T, Corby P, Li X, Saxena D (2020) Electronic cigarette aerosol modulates the oral microbiome and increases risk of infection. iScience 23(3):100884. https://doi.org/10.1016/j.isci.2020.100884

Rahim A, Syed K, Ahad B, Farooq A, Ayub Z, Batool SM (2022) Comparison of severity of periodontal clinical parameters among naswar/snuff users: cross sectional study. PLoS One 17(9):e0273288. https://doi.org/10.1371/journal.pone.0273288

Raitasalo K, Bye EK, Pisinger C, Scheffels J, Tokle R, Kinnunen JM, Ollila H, Rimpelä A (2022) Single, dual, and triple use of cigarettes, e-cigarettes, and snus among adolescents in the Nordic countries. Int J Environ Res Public Health 19(2):683

Ramanauskaite E, Sakalauskaite UM, Machiulskiene V (2020) The efficacy of adjunctive aids in periodontal maintenance therapy: a systematic literature review and meta-analysis. Oral Health Prev Dent 18(4):889–910. https://doi.org/10.3290/j.ohpd.a45406

Ramseier CA (2024) Diagnostic measures for monitoring and follow-up in periodontology and implant dentistry. Periodontol 2000 95(1):129–155. https://doi.org/10.1111/prd.12588

Richter P, Hodge K, Stanfill S, Zhang L, Watson C (2008) Surveillance of moist snuff: total nicotine, moisture, pH, un-ionized nicotine, and tobacco-specific nitrosamines. Nicotine Tob Res 10(11):1645–1652. https://doi.org/10.1080/14622200802412937

Robertson PB, Walsh M, Greene J, Ernster V, Grady D, Hauck W (1990) Periodontal effects associated with the use of smokeless tobacco. J Periodontol 61(7):438–443. https://doi.org/10.1902/jop.1990.61.7.438

Roosaar A, Johansson ALV, Sandborgh-Englund G, Nyrén O, Axéll T (2006) A long-term follow-up study on the natural course of snus-induced lesions among Swedish snus users. Int J Cancer 119(2):392–397. https://doi.org/10.1002/ijc.21841

Şahin T (2024) Investigation of the relationships between peri-implant diseases, periodontal diseases, and conditions: a cross-sectional study. PeerJ 12:e18663. https://doi.org/10.7717/peerj.18663

Salhi L, Seidel L, Albert A, Lambert F (2021) Fagerström test for nicotine dependence as an indicator in tobacco-related studies in periodontology. J Periodontol 92(2):298–305. https://doi.org/10.1002/jper.20-0019

Saotome M, Kuraji R, Numabe Y (2025) Hyperglycemia exacerbates periodontal destruction via systemic suppression of regulatory T cell number and function. J Periodontal Res 60(6):590–603. https://doi.org/10.1111/jre.13366

Satpathy A, Grover V, Kumar A, Jain A, Gopalakrishnan D, Grover HS, Kolte A, Melath A, Khatri M, Dani N, Thakur R, Tiwari V, Yadav VS, Thomas B, Chahal GS, Bhasin MT, Pandit N, Lawande SA, Manjunath RGS, Sachdeva S, Bhardwaj A, Pradeep AR, Nichani AS, Singh B, Ganesh PR, Deshpande NC, Reddy SSP, Raj SC (2024) Indian society of periodontology good clinical practice recommendations for peri-implant care. J Indian Soc Periodontol 28(1):6–31. https://doi.org/10.4103/jisp.jisp_124_24

Scherer G, Pluym N, Scherer M (2024) Oral health risks in adults who use electronic nicotine delivery systems and oral nicotine pouches: a critical review of the literature and qualitative synthesis of the available evidence. Harm Reduct J 21(1):229. https://doi.org/10.1186/s12954-024-01147-y

Selamet SM, Kumbuloglu O, Sahiner A, Ozdemir G (2025) Assessment of surface roughness and microbiological retention on custom abutments produced by different techniques and materials. Eur J Oral Sci 133(1):e13038. https://doi.org/10.1111/eos.13038

Sun J, Ding Q, Chen Y, Li J, Wang Z, Wei Z, Ge X, Zhang L (2024) Effects and underlying mechanism of micro-nano-structured zirconia surfaces on biological behaviors of human gingival fibroblasts under inflammatory conditions. Acta Biomater 183:356–370. https://doi.org/10.1016/j.actbio.2024.05.031

Tebbutt J, Khan Z, Ariyaratnam R (2020) A case report of oral nicotine-associated keratosis and a review of oral mucosal changes in tobacco and similar products. Br Dent J 228(10):757–760. https://doi.org/10.1038/s41415-020-1530-x

Titova OE, Baron JA, Michaëlsson K, Larsson SC (2021) Swedish snuff (snus) and risk of cardiovascular disease and mortality: prospective cohort study of middle-aged and older individuals. BMC Med 19(1):111. https://doi.org/10.1186/s12916-021-01979-6

Vámos O, Komora P, Gede N, Hegyi P, Kelemen K, Varga G, Mikulás K, Kerémi B, Kispélyi B (2024) The effect of nicotine-containing products on peri-implant tissues: a systematic review and network meta-analysis. Nicotine Tob Res 26(10):1276–1285. https://doi.org/10.1093/ntr/ntae085

Wallström M, Sand L, Nilsson F, Hirsch JM (1999) The long-term effect of nicotine on the oral mucosa. Addiction 94(3):417–423. https://doi.org/10.1046/j.1360-0443.1999.94341711.x

Ye D, Rahman I (2023) Emerging oral nicotine products and periodontal diseases. Int J Dent 2023(1):9437475. https://doi.org/10.1155/2023/9437475

Zhang Y, Niazi SA, Yang Y, Wang Y, Cao X, Liu Y, Li Y, Zhou Q (2022) Smoking by altering the peri-implant microbial community structure compromises the responsiveness to treatment. Front Cell Infect Microbiol 12:1040765. https://doi.org/10.3389/fcimb.2022.1040765

Zou Q, Zhang S, Jiang C, Xiao S, Wang Y, Wen B (2024) Low-level laser therapy on soft tissue healing after implantation: a randomized controlled trial. BMC Oral Health 24(1):1477. https://doi.org/10.1186/s12903-024-05258-7

Zucchelli G, Tavelli L, McGuire MK, Rasperini G, Feinberg SE, Wang HL, Giannobile WV (2020) Autogenous soft tissue grafting for periodontal and peri-implant plastic surgical reconstruction. J Periodontol 91(1):9–16. https://doi.org/10.1002/jper.19-0350

Impact of Smokeless Tobacco Product Usage on Systemic Health

11

Fawad Javed, Khalid Almas, and Saman Warnakulasuriya

Abbreviations

ALT	Alanine aminotransferase
AST	Aspartate aminotransferase
BP	Blood pressure
BUN	Blood urea nitrogen
CKD	Chronic kidney disease
CPS	Cancer prevention study
CVD	Cardiovascular disease
DBP	Diastolic blood pressure
DM	Diabetes mellitus
FEV1	Forced expiratory volume in 1 s
FVC	Forced vital capacity
GIT	Gastrointestinal tract
H. Pylori	*Helicobacter pylori*
HIF	Hypoxia inducible factor
HR	Heart rate
IARC	International Agency for Research on Cancer
MI	Myocardial infarction

F. Javed (✉)
Department of Orthodontics and Dentofacial Orthopedics, Eastman Institute for Oral Health, University of Rochester, Rochester, NY, USA
e-mail: fawad_javed@urmc.rochester.edu

K. Almas
Preventive Dental Sciences Department, Division of Periodontics, Imam Abdulrahman Bin Faisal University, College of Dentistry, Dammam, Saudi Arabia

S. Warnakulasuriya
Faculty of Dentistry, Oral & Craniofacial Sciences, King's College London, London, UK

F. Javed, S. Warnakulasuriya (eds.), *Smokeless Tobacco and its Effects on Periodontal Health*, https://doi.org/10.1007/978-3-032-16409-4_11

MS	Metabolic syndrome
OR	Odds ratios
SBP	Systolic blood pressure
ST	Smokeless tobacco
TSNA	Tobacco-specific nitrosamines

Learning Goals

- Understand the composition of smokeless tobacco (ST) products.
- Assess the association between ST use and cardiovascular diseases such as hypertension, myocardial infarction, and stroke.
- Evaluate the role of ST use in the development of metabolic syndrome and type-2 diabetes, with emphasis on nicotine-induced insulin resistance and systemic inflammation.
- Explain the adverse effects of ST on male and female reproductive systems, including menstrual irregularities, placental damage, stillbirth risks, and reduced sperm quality.
- Analyse the limited evidence linking ST use with compromised pulmonary function and respiratory symptoms.
- Summarize the evidence for ST-related damage to the gastrointestinal tract, including mucosal lesions, increased *Helicobacter pylori* infections, and elevated cancer risks.
- Identify how ST products contribute to liver and kidney damage.
- Evaluate the epidemiological and experimental evidence linking ST use to various cancers, particularly pancreatic, oral, oesophageal, and stomach cancers.
- Discuss the importance of education, policy, and regulation in mitigating ST-related health risks and promoting cessation through community and clinical interventions.

11.1 Background

The global burden of tobacco use remains a significant public health challenge with smokeless tobacco (ST) emerging as a crucial contributor to morbidity and mortality. The ST products contain a complex mixture of carcinogens, nitrosamines, heavy metals, and other bioactive compounds (Li and Hecht 2022). Notably, nicotine and tobacco-specific nitrosamines (TSNA) play pivotal roles in mediating systemic toxicity. Nicotine is rapidly absorbed through oral mucosa, leading to cardiovascular stimulation, insulin resistance, and neurophysiological effects. Moreover, TSNA, such as N-nitrosonornicotine and 4-(methylnitrosamino)-1-(3-pyridyl)-1-butanone, are potent carcinogens implicated in various malignancies (Li and Hecht 2022;

Peterson et al. 2024; Stanfill et al. 2023). Furthermore, exposure to reactive oxygen species and inflammatory mediators perpetuates oxidative stress, endothelial dysfunction, and systemic inflammation, forming the foundation for multiple disease processes (Bagchi et al. 1996; Stich and Anders 1989; Zhao et al. 2021).

It is well-known that habitual use of ST products is a significant risk factor for periodontal diseases such as periodontitis (Al-Askar et al. 2017; Javed et al. 2010, 2013, 2015; Nasir et al. 2023). Moreover, habitual use of ST increases the risk of oral malignant diseases such as oral squamous cell carcinoma and periodontal and peri-implant diseases (Muthukrishnan and Warnakulasuriya 2018; Vámos et al. 2024; Warnakulasuriya and Kerr 2016; Warnakulasuriya et al. 2021). However, the detrimental effects of ST use extend beyond the oral cavity posing significant threats to systemic health. For instance, data from the National Family Health Survey conducted in India reported that ST is an independent risk factor for hypertension (Vidya et al. 2022). Similarly, results from an experimental study in Wistar rats showed that ST damages the biochemical and histological profiles of liver and kidney in a dose-dependent manner (Al-Mukhaini et al. 2017). This chapter aims to review the systemic health consequences of ST use addressing the global burden of this often-overlooked public health issue.

Key Points

- Smokeless tobacco (ST) is a major public health concern, significantly contributing to global morbidity and mortality.
- ST products contain toxic substances, including nicotine, tobacco-specific nitrosamines (TSNAs), heavy metals, and carcinogens, which are responsible for systemic toxicity, oxidative stress, and inflammation.
- Nicotine and TSNAs are central to ST's harmful effects, leading to cardiovascular stimulation, insulin resistance, neurophysiological changes, and increased cancer risk.
- ST use is strongly linked to oral and periodontal diseases, such as periodontitis, oral squamous cell carcinoma, and peri-implant diseases.
- The systemic effects of ST use include elevated risks of hypertension and organ damage, with studies showing dose-dependent liver and kidney toxicity in experimental models.

11.2 Effect of Smokeless Tobacco Products on Systemic Health

11.2.1 Cardiovascular System

The American Heart Association published a comprehensive overview of cardiovascular implications associated with ST use (Piano et al. 2010). The statement highlights that ST use is associated with an increased risk of fatal myocardial infarction (MI) and stroke (Piano et al. 2010). Notably, in individuals with pre-existing coronary artery disease, nicotine and other constituents in ST can decrease coronary blood flow, potentially exacerbating ischaemic conditions (Asplund 2003). Additionally, ST use has been linked to elevated blood pressure (BP) and heart rate (HR), contributing to the overall cardiovascular risk profile (Table 11.1). Nicotine, a primary and addictive component of ST can stimulate the sympatho-adrenal system (Benowitz 1997a; Benowitz and Gourlay 1997). Moreover, the relatively high sodium content and occasional presence of liquorice in ST may impact BP (Benowitz 1988; Benowitz 1997b). Table 11.1 summarizes the outcomes of studies that have investigated the acute effects of ST on BP levels (Bolinder and de Faire 1998; Bolinder et al. 1997; Simon and Iglauer 1960; Vidya et al. 2022). In the study by Bolinder and de Faire (1998), a statistically significant correlation between 24-h systolic and diastolic blood pressures (SBP and DBP, respectively) and blood cotinine levels was observed among ST users (SBP: $r = 0.48$, $P < 001$; DBP: $r = 0.41$, $P < 0.01$) compared with non-chewers (SBP: $r = -0.12$, $P = 0.47$; DBP, $r = -0.03$; $P = 0.84$). Similar results were reported by Vidya et al. (2022). In this study (Bolinder and de Faire 1998), 32% of the total patient population reported a family history of hypertension; however, this relationship was only among smokers. It is worth mentioning that hypertension is a significant predictor of future cardiovascular events including MI and stroke. Thus, determination of the impact of ST product use on the development of hypertension is critical. The INTERHEART study was a case-control study involving 15,152 individuals experiencing their first MI, conducted across 52 countries in Asia, Europe, Africa, the Middle East, Australia, and America (Teo et al. 2006). Participants used various forms of smokeless tobacco (ST), including chewing tobacco, snuff, and betel-quid. A sub-analysis assessed the risk of MI based on the type of ST product used (Teo et al. 2006). The results of this study showed that individuals who exclusively chewed ST had a significantly higher likelihood of experiencing a first MI, with an odds ratio (OR) of 2.23 (95% CI: 1.41–3.52) compared to those who had never used tobacco (Teo et al. 2006). Nevertheless, controversial results have also been reported. A study from India estimated the risk of hypertension among ST-chewers and non-chewers. The results showed no significant association between ST-chewing and hypertension (OR: 1.24 CI: 0.98–1.58; *P*-value 0.656) (Anand and Sk 2017).

Stroke is a major cause of disability in adults (Lawes et al. 2004). Studies (Accortt et al. 2002; Bolinder et al. 1994; Haglund et al. 2007; Henley et al. 2005; Hergens et al. 2008) with conflicting results have explored the link between ST use and the risk of fatal and non-fatal strokes (Table 11.2). In the US-based Cancer Prevention Study (CPS)-I and CPS-II, male ST-chewers (snuff or chewing tobacco) were monitored for 12 and 18 years, respectively (Henley et al. 2005). After adjusting the data for confounders including race, education level, alcohol consumption, physical activity, aspirin use, body mass index (BMI), and dietary fat intake, the results showed that ST use in CPS-I and CPS-II was associated with a higher hazard ratio for mortality from cerebrovascular disease (Henley et al. 2005). The CPS-II study assessed the frequency and duration of ST use; however, a clear dose–response

Table 11.1 An overview of studies that assessed the impact of smokeless tobacco on diastolic and systolic blood pressure

Authors et al. (Year)	Type of ST	Average age (range)	Gender (n)	Study groups	Average amount of ST chewed/day	Results
Simon and Iglauer (1960)	Snuff	51.1 years (34–71 years)	Male	ST-chewers (24) and placebo gum chewers (NR)	10 grams/day	Increase in pulse rate among ST-chewers, range of increase (1–24 beats/min) SBP increased by 17.9 mmHg (range: 10–45 mmHg) in 16 ST-chewers DBP increased by 11.8 mmHg (range: 5–20 mmHg) in 15 ST-chewers No change in BP among gum-chewers
Anand and SK MK (2017)	NR	NR (10–≥70 years)	Male and female	2327 ST-chewers	10 grams/day	No association between ST chewing and hypertension (OR 1.24 [0.98–1.58] P value 0.656)
Bolinder et al. (1997)	Snuff	45 ± 6 years (35–60 years)	Male	ST-chewers (50) and non-chewers (68)	27 ± 15 grams/day	No significant difference in BP among ST-chewers and non-chewers
Bolinder and de Faire (1998)	Snuff	NR (35–60 years)	Male	ST-chewers (47) and non-chewers (59)	27 ± 15 grams/day	Heart rate was significantly higher in ST-users (69 ± 14 beats/min) than non-chewers (63 ± 12 beats/min) SBP was significantly higher in ST-chewers (131 ± 10 mmHg) than non-chewers (126 ± 8 mmHg) No difference in DBP in both groups
Vidya et al. (2022)	Gutka, BQ, Khaini, snuff	30.9 ± 10 years	13.8% males 86.2% females	National Family Health Survey	NR	ST use was a risk factor for hypertension for females OR-1.1 (1.08–1.13) and males OR-1.07 (1.03–1.1)

BP Blood pressure, *BQ* Betel-quid, *DBP* Diastolic blood pressure, *NR* Not reported, *OR* Odds ratios, *SBP* Systolic blood pressure, *ST* Smokeless tobacco

Table 11.2 An overview of studies assessing the association between smokeless tobacco chewing and stroke

Authors et al. (Year)	Country/design/ population	Sample-size and cases of events	Results
Bolinder et al. (1994)	Cohort study 12-years follow-up Swedish construction workers	Non-users (*n* = 13,784, stroke mortality cases = 16) Current ST users: 35–54 years old (*n* = 1672, stroke mortality cases = 4) Current ST users: 55–65 years old (*n* = 1734, stroke mortality cases = 26)	No significant increase in RR for stroke mortality among 35–54-year olds (RR 1.9; 95% CI: 0.6–5.7) or among 55–65-year olds (RR 1.2; 95% CI: 0.7–1.8)
Accortt et al. (2002)	Cohort study Epidemiological survey at 10, 15, and 20 years of follow-up	Exclusive ST users (*n* = 414) (mean age, 64.9 years) Non-chewers (*n* = 5192) (mean age, 54 years) Total stroke cases were not reported	No significant increase in death due to stroke among ST chewers than non-chewers
Henley et al. (2005)	Cohort study Cancer prevention study-I, 12 years follow-up Cancer prevention study-II, 18 years follow-up	CPS-I: *n* = 69,662, cerebrovascular-related mortality cases = 1451 CPS-II: *n* = 111,482, cerebrovascular-related mortality cases = 1451	CPS-I: ST use was associated with a significantly greater CVD-related mortality (HR 1.46; 95% CI: 1.31–1.64) CPS-II: ST use was associated with a significantly greater CVD-related mortality (HR 1.40; 95% CI: 1.10–1.79)
Haglund et al. (2007)	Cohort study 14–16 years of follow-up Swedish national survey	Non-chewers: *n* = 2579; non-fatal stroke cases = 126 ST-chewers: *n* = 721; non-fatal stroke cases = 19	No increase in stroke incidence (IRR 1.07; 95% CI: 0.65–1.77) in ST-chewers
Hergens et al. (2008)	Cohort study. 18 years of follow-up Swedish national survey	Non-chewers: *n* = 84,110; cases of all types of stroke = 2805. ST-chewers *n* = 34,354, cases for all types of stroke = 412	Among current ST-chewers, no increase in RR for non-fatal stroke was found (RR 1.02; 95% CI: 0.91–1.14) There was an increase in RR for fatal stroke (RR 1.38; 95% CI: 0.99–1.91)

CI Confidence interval, *CPS* Cancer prevention study, *CVD* Cardiovascular disease, *HR* Hazard ratio, *IRR* Incidence ratio risk, *RR* Relative risk, *ST* Smokeless tobacco

relationship between cardiovascular disease (CVD) and ST use was not established (Henley et al. 2005). The authors of this chapter suggest that this result should be cautiously interpreted as the number of stroke cases in both the frequency and duration groups was limited (e.g., only seven stroke cases in the ST duration category of

1–10 years) (Henley et al. 2005). In contrast, another study, which used data from the US National Health and Nutrition Examination Survey follow-up study reported no association between ST use and death due to stroke among ST-chewers after adjustment for multiple confounders, including age, sex, race, alcohol consumption, BMI, BP, serum cholesterol. and family history of cancer (Accortt et al. 2002). Likewise, results by Haglund et al. (2007) reported no increase in the incidence of stroke or mortality among Swedish snuff users in the Swedish Survey of Living Conditions; however, the number of mortality cases was low ($n = 4$). Similar results were reported by Bolinder et al. (1994). In a prospective study on Swedish construction workers, the age-adjusted relative risk (RR) for non-fatal stroke showed no significant increase among individuals who had ever used or were current users of ST (snuff) (Hergens et al. 2008). However, the RR for fatal stroke was elevated in both groups (Hergens et al. 2008). Overall, while some evidence points to a potential link between ST use and fatal stroke, inconsistencies across studies highlight the need for further well-controlled, large-scale prospective studies to clarify the impact of ST on cerebrovascular health. Public health policies and clinical recommendations should consider these uncertainties when advising individuals on the risks associated with ST consumption.

Key Points

- ST use is associated with an increased risk of fatal myocardial infarction and stroke, especially in individuals with existing coronary artery disease.
- Nicotine and sodium content in ST products stimulate the sympathoadrenal system and may raise blood pressure and heart rate.
- According to a case-control study, ST users have significantly higher odds of deaths from first-time myocardial infarction than non-users.
- Long-term studies have linked ST use to higher cerebrovascular mortality, but others did not find significant associations with stroke incidence or mortality.
- More robust, well-controlled, and large-scale research is needed to conclusively determine the cardiovascular and cerebrovascular risks of ST use.

11.2.2 Metabolic Syndrome and Diabetes Mellitus

Nicotine, the key addictive substance in ST, plays a significant role in altering glucose metabolism and insulin responsiveness (Carlsson et al. 2017; Vu et al. 2014). By activating the sympathoadrenal system, nicotine triggers the release of catecholamines, which subsequently elevate blood glucose levels while impairing insulin sensitivity (Vu et al. 2014). Moreover, chronic nicotine exposure has been shown to cause pancreatic beta-cell dysfunction, impairing insulin secretion (Yoshikawa et al. 2005). Furthermore, increased levels of inflammatory markers such as C-reactive protein and tumour necrosis factor-alpha have been reported among ST users, which could play a role in the pathogenesis of persistent hyperglycaemia, a classical manifestation of poorly controlled diabetes mellitus (DM) (Lee et al. 2012).

Metabolic syndrome (MS) is a cluster of conditions such as central obesity, hypertension, dyslipidaemia, and insulin resistance that collectively elevate the risk of CVD and DM, predominantly type-2 DM (Eckel et al. 2005; Hudish et al. 2019). A limited number of studies have investigated the association between ST use and MS or DM (Committee 1994; Kahn et al. 2005; Norberg et al. 2006). A prospective study from Northern Sweden with 10 years of follow-up used the International Diabetes Federation criteria to assess the role of ST (snuff) use in the development of MS (Norberg et al. 2006). Multivariate analysis demonstrated a higher likelihood of MS development among individuals who consumed five to six pouches of moist snuff per week (OR = 1.5, 95% CI: 1.13–2.10), with an even greater risk observed in those using seven pouches per week (OR = 2.0, 95% CI: 1.20–1.39) (Norberg et al. 2006). In contrast, individuals consuming fewer than two pouches per week or between two and four pouches per week did not exhibit a significantly increased risk (Norberg et al. 2006). Similarly, a cohort study assessed the prevalence of type-2 DM among ST-chewers and non-chewers (Eliasson et al. 2004). In "ever snus users" and "current snus users", there was not a significant increase in the OR (after adjustment of age and waist circumference) in both groups for development of type-2 DM (OR 1.21; 95% CI: 0.59 to 2.49, OR 1.06; 95% CI: 0.43–2.64). Nevertheless, a recent case-control study from India assessed the relationship between ST (*gutka*) chewing and type-2 DM (Sawane et al. 2023). The participants' ages ranged between 31 and 50 years. The results showed a statistically significant association between type-2 DM and ST-chewing (Sawane et al. 2023). The study further reported that the participants had underprivileged living standards, which may have contributed to a lack of awareness regarding the adverse impact of ST on overall health (Sawane et al. 2023). However, it is imperative to cautiously interpret these results as the data were not adjusted for potential confounders such as BMI and family history of DM, which are independent risk factors of DM (Javed et al. 2007; Karageorgi et al. 2013; Lin 2024).

In summary, the evidence linking ST with MS and DM is limited; however, a potential association between these variables mediated by nicotine-induced insulin resistance and inflammation cannot be overlooked. Given the rising prevalence of DM worldwide (Sun et al. 2022), addressing all modifiable risk factors, including ST use, is essential for effective prevention strategies. Further longitudinal studies are needed in this regard.

Key Points

- Nicotine alters glucose metabolism by activating the sympathoadrenal system, which increases blood glucose levels and impairs insulin sensitivity.
- Chronic nicotine exposure may lead to pancreatic beta-cell dysfunction, reducing insulin secretion and contributing to the development of diabetes mellitus.
- ST users often exhibit elevated inflammatory markers (e.g., CRP, TNF-alpha), which are associated with persistent hyperglycaemia and poor glycaemic control.
- Habitual snuff use (five to seven pouches per week) is significantly associated with a higher risk of developing metabolic syndrome.
- Although evidence is limited, nicotine-induced insulin resistance and inflammation suggest a possible link between ST use and metabolic syndrome/diabetes mellitus.

11.2.3 Female Reproductive System

Nicotine, a major component of combustible and non-combustible tobacco products, has been reported to affect the physiology of the female reproductive system (Kulkarni et al. 2017; Laldinsangi 2022; Totonchi et al. 2016). In addition, it has been reported that nicotine from ST products can cross the placental barrier and induce foetal tachycardia (Ashfaq et al. 2008) and cause congenital abnormalities such as cleft lip and palate. In an observational cross-sectional study, Kulkarni et al. (2017) assessed the regularity of the menstrual cycle among 1200 females from India. The study participants were approximately 34 years old. Nearly 10% of the study population comprised self-reported ST-chewers. Among the ST-chewers, nearly 86% females had dysmenorrhoea (painful menstrual cramps that occur before or during menstruation) and 42.9% had irregular menstrual periods (Oligomenorrhoea). Nearly 32% and 25% of the ST-chewers had menorrhagia (abnormally heavy or prolonged menstrual bleeding) and polymenorrhoea (frequent menstrual cycles, specifically when the cycle length is less than 21 days), respectively (Kulkarni et al. 2017). One explanation in this regard is that nicotine stimulates the release of catecholamines and disrupts the normal secretion patterns of gonadotropin-releasing hormone leading to altered levels of luteinizing and follicle-stimulating hormones. This disruption can result in irregular menstrual cycles, characterized by polymenorrhoea or oligomenorrhoea (Allen et al. 2015; Pomerleau et al. 1992). In addition, results of an *in vitro* study on human endometrial stromal primary cells showed that nicotine exposure is associated with imbalances in the expression of oestrogen and progesterone receptors thereby jeopardizing the physiology of the female reproductive system (Totonchi et al. 2016). A nationwide cohort study that encompassed data from 851,371 singleton births in Sweden (spanning from 1999 to 2010) evaluated the impact of maternal ST use during early pregnancy on the risks of stillbirth and early neonatal mortality (Baba et al. 2014). Using an *in vitro* study model, Kumar et al. (2021) assessed the effect of habitual ST chewing on placental structure, expression of hypoxia-inducible factor (HIF), and DNA damage. In this study, 51 placentae were collected from ST-chewers (n = 30) and non-chewers (n = 21) with full-term normal delivery (Kumar et al. 2021). Placental tissues were evaluated using transmission electron microscopy and immunohistochemistry. The results showed significant thickening of trophoblast basement membrane, abnormalities of the microvilli, swollen or damaged mitochondria, degenerated nuclei, and dilatation in endoplasmic reticulum cisternae in the placenta samples collected from ST-chewers than non-chewers (Kumar et al. 2021). Moreover, there was a significant reduction in the perimeter, area, and number of the stromal capillary of the tertiary villi of placenta from ST-chewers than non-chewers. Furthermore, there was an enhanced expression of HIF and oxidative DNA damage biomarker in placentae samples from ST-chewers than non-chewers (Kumar et al. 2021). The authors proposed that ST-chewing exerts harmful effects on the placenta, potentially compromising the placental barrier and limiting the transfer of nutrients and oxygen from the mother to the foetus, which could contribute to foetal growth restriction (Kumar et al. 2021). Table 11.3 provides an overview of studies that assessed the influence of ST-chewing on pregnancy and reproductive health.

Table 11.3 Impact of chronic smokeless tobacco use on pregnancy and female reproductive health

Authors et al. (Year)	Objective	Participants	Age	Main results	Conclusion
Baba et al. (2014)	To the impact of maternal ST use during early pregnancy on the risks of stillbirth and early neonatal mortality	851,371 singleton births	≤19 to ≥35 years	OR for stillbirth were higher in ST-chewers than non-chewers (1.43 [95% CI: 1.02–1.99])	ST chewing is a risk factor for stillbirth
Kulkarni et al. (2017)	To assess the association between ST use and regularity of menstrual cycles and dysmenorrhoea	1200 females	33.75 ± 9.6 years	85% of ST-chewers had dysmenorrhoea 42.9% had oligomenorrhoea 32.1% had menorrhagia 25% had polymenorrhoea	Chronic ST chewing is associated with irregularity in menstrual cycles

(continued)

Table 11.3 (continued)

Authors et al. (Year)	Objective	Participants	Age	Main results	Conclusion
Kumar et al. (2021)	To assess the effects of ST chewing on placental structure and DNA	Placentae from ST-chewers (30) and non-chewers (21)	NA	ST chewing was associated with: Endothelial cells protrusion into the capillary lumen Abnormalities of the microvilli Mitochondrial damage Reduction in the perimeter, area, and number of stromal capillary of the tertiary villi of placenta Oxidative DNA damage	ST-chewing increases villus hypoxia and oxidative DNA damage in the placenta

OR Odds ratios, *ST* Smokeless tobacco

Key Points

- Nicotine interferes with hormonal regulation by affecting gonadotropin-releasing hormone, leading to imbalances in luteinizing and follicle-stimulating hormones.
- Females chewing ST products experience high rates of menstrual imbalances.
- ST-derived nicotine can cross the placenta and has been linked to fetal tachycardia and causing cleft lip and palate.
- ST-chewing is associated with structural abnormalities in placentae including thickening of trophoblast basement membranes.
- ST-chewers show reduced perimeter, area, and number of stromal capillaries in placental villi.
- A study from Sweden has linked maternal ST use during early pregnancy to higher risks of stillbirth and early neonatal mortality.

11.2.3.1 Male Reproductive System

The ST contains mutagenic compounds including cadmium, lead, and benzo(a) pyrene diol epoxide that have been shown to be potentially toxic to normal testicular function (Aprioku and Obianime 2014; Orisakwe et al. 2014). The use of ST is associated with reduced sperm count, motility, and morphology, all of which are critical determinants of male fertility (Aprioku and Ugwu 2015; Das et al. 2016; Kimblad et al. 2022). Studies have reported that ST users exhibit significantly lower total sperm counts compared to non-users, potentially due to the disruptive effects of nicotine on the hypothalamic-pituitary-gonadal axis (Aprioku and Ugwu 2015; Das et al. 2016; Kimblad et al. 2022) (Table 11.4). Results by Aprioku and Ugwu (2015) showed that subacute exposure to ST did not significantly impact sperm morphology; however, a dose-dependent decline in sperm motility, sperm count, and testosterone levels was observed, with greater effects in prepubertal rats compared to adult rats. In this study (Aprioku and Ugwu 2015), the toxicity mechanisms may be associated with increased oxidative stress in the testes. It is important to mention that Aprioku and Ugwu (2015) did not determine whether these effects were reversible, highlighting the need for further research to assess potential recovery. Likewise, a study from India investigated the association between ST chewing and semen quality (Said et al. 2005). A total of 638 male patients undergoing infertility assessments were categorized based on the frequency of their tobacco chewing habit: mild (<3 times per day, $n = 177$), moderate (3–6 times per day, $n = 264$), and severe (>6 times per day, $n = 197$). According to the results, sperm concentration, motility percentage, morphology, and viability were significantly greater in mild than moderate ST-chewers; and in moderate compared to severe ST-chewers (Said et al. 2005). The prevalence of azoospermia increased with addiction severity (1%, 3%, and 14%), as did the prevalence of oligoasthenoteratozoospermia (2%, 8%, and 29%), though these differences were not statistically significant (Said et al. 2005). Said et al. (2005) concluded that ST chewing is significantly associated with decreased sperm quality, and infertile men should be educated about the adverse effect of ST-chewing on sperm quality. The relationship between ST use and testosterone levels is complex and appears to vary based on factors such as the specific constituents of the ST product, duration and frequency of use, and individual physiological responses. While Kimblad et al. (2022) reported elevated testosterone levels among ST users; another study on animal modes indicated a potential reduction in levels of testosterone in rats exposed to ST (Aprioku and Obianime 2014). Further research is necessary to elucidate these conflicting findings and to better understand the long-term implications of ST use on male hormonal health.

Table 11.4 Impact of chronic smokeless tobacco use on male reproductive health

Authors et al. (Year)	Objective	Participants	Age	Main results	Conclusion
Kimblad et al. (2022)	To compare the sperm counts among ST-chewers and non-chewers	613 males	18–21 years	Total sperm count was 25% lower in ST-chewers than non-chewers Testosterone levels were significantly higher in ST-chewers than non-chewers	ST chewing decreases sperm count and increases testosterone levels
Aprioku and Ugwu (2015)	To assess the effect of subacute ST exposure on rat testis	42 adult Wistar rats	5 weeks old	ST exposure reduced sperm motility by 89% Sperm count was significantly reduced in ST-exposed than unexposed rats ST exposure decreased testosterone levels There was no change in sperm morphology	Subacute exposure of ST products alters sperm characteristics, which may increase testicular oxidative stress
Said et al. (2005)	To assess the effect of ST chewing on sperm quality among Indian infertile men	638 males	18–40 years	Sperm quality and mobility were compromised in men who chewed ST 3–6 times than those who used ST <3 times daily Sperm quality and mobility were compromised in men who chewed ST >6 times than those who used ST three to six times daily	ST chewing compromises sperm quality and is possibly associated with male infertility

ST Smokeless tobacco

Key Points

- ST contains mutagenic substances such as cadmium, lead, and benzo(a) pyrene diol epoxide, which are toxic to normal testicular function.
- ST use is associated with reduced sperm count, motility, and morphology.
- The reduction in sperm quality among ST users may be due to nicotine's interference with the hypothalamic-pituitary-gonadal axis and increased oxidative stress in the testes.
- ST chewing is correlated with worse semen quality and increased prevalence of azoospermia and oligoasthenoteratozoospermia.
- The relationship between ST use and testosterone levels is unclear, with some studies showing an increase and others showing a decrease, highlighting the need for further research.

11.2.4 Respiratory System

A limited number of studies have assessed the impact of ST chewing on the respiratory system (Ahuja et al. 2018; Kumar et al. 2017). A study (conference abstract) assessed the lung function in 30 ST-chewers and 30 non-chewers (Ahuja et al. 2018). The forced expiratory volume in one second (FEV1)/forced vital capacity (FVC) was higher in non-chewers (83%) compared with ST-chewers (79.8%) (Ahuja et al. 2018). Moreover, the maximum mid-expiratory flow 75–25 was higher in non-chewers (85.4%) compared with ST-chewers (71.7%) (Ahuja et al. 2018). Similarly, results from another study showed that ST-chewers have significantly lower values for FVC, FEV1, forced expiratory flow 25–75%, and peak expiratory flow rate compared to non-chewers (Kumar et al. 2017) (Table 11.5). Moreover, a review article reported that the use of moist snuff and chewing tobacco imposes minimal risks for cancers of the upper respiratory tract, with relative risks ranging from 0.6 to 1.7. However, the use of dry snuff imposes higher risks of cancers in the upper respiratory sites (relative risk: 4–13) (Rodu and Cole 2002). Currently, no direct evidence links ST use to the development of respiratory diseases. While ST use does not involve inhaling smoke, it still exposes users to high levels of nicotine and harmful chemicals, which may potentially increase the risk of mouth and throat cancer and may have deleterious effects on the respiratory system. Moreover, the use of ST products can lead to chronic irritation and inflammation in the airways contributing to the development of respiratory conditions such as large airway inflammation or bronchitis (Schivo et al. 2014).

Table 11.5 An overview of pulmonary function parameters among smokeless tobacco chewers and non-chewers included in the study by Kumar et al. (2017)

Pulmonary function parameters	ST-chewers	Non-chewers
Forced vital capacity	88.2 ± 6.9[a]	96.2 ± 5.8
Forced expiratory volume in 1 s	100.6 ± 6.8[a]	111.2 ± 7.8
Forced expiratory flow	93.1 ± 7[a]	112.7 ± 8.9
Peak expiratory flow rate	88.2 ± 6.3[a]	105.4 ± 6.1

[a]Compared with non-chewers ($P < 0.001$)

Key Points

- ST-chewers exhibit lower lung function parameters—including FEV1/FVC ratio and mid-expiratory flow rates.
- ST use may cause chronic irritation and inflammation in the airways, contributing to bronchitis.

11.2.5 Gastrointestinal System

The International Agency for Research on Cancer (IARC) has reported that there is sufficient evidence linking ST use to oesophageal cancer (Humans et al. 2007). A recent cross-sectional observational study from India assessed the effect of ST-chewing on the upper gastrointestinal mucosa (Vaishnav et al. 2025). The study sample comprised 108 ST-chewers and 90 non-chewers. Biopsies and endoscopy were performed on tissues from the lower oesophagus, stomach, and duodenum. Macroscopic examination revealed that erosive and ulcerative lesions in the oesophagus and stomach were the most frequently observed abnormalities among ST-chewers. Barrett's oesophagus and oesophageal neoplasms were identified in 14 and 5 ST chewers, respectively, totalling 19 cases (17.59%). Histopathological analysis commonly showed chronic gastritis and duodenitis among ST-chewers. Gastric ulcers were significantly more prevalent in individuals chewing ST for over a decade compared to those who were chewing ST for less than 10 years (Vaishnav et al. 2025). Results from a systematic review reported that the risk of rectum and stomach cancer is significantly higher in Swedish snus users than non-users (Valen et al. 2023) (Table 11.6).

Table 11.6 An overview of studies that assessed the effect of smokeless tobacco chewing on gastrointestinal health

Authors et al. (Year)	Design	Type of ST product	Participants	Results
Vaishnav et al. (2025)	Cross-sectional observational	NR	108 ST chewers 90 non-chewers	Erosive and ulcerative lesions of the oesophagus and stomach were common in ST-chewers Fourteen ST-chewers had Barrett's oesophagus Five ST-chewers had oesophageal neoplasms *H. pylori* infection was identified in 62.9% of ST-chewers
Tyx et al. (2022)	Observational; shotgun metagenomic sequencing	Toombak	NA Toombak samples were subjected to microbiological assessment	Over 99% of the microbiota in toombak was bacterial Dominant bacterial taxa included: *Enteractinococcus* *Corynebacterium* *Staphylococcus* Members of the *Bacillaceae* family Such microbes can potentially jeopardize the gastrointestinal health of toombak users
Aro et al. (2010)	Population-based observational	Swedish *snus* (snuff)	1001 adults	*H. pylori* infection was not associated with snus usage Higher prevalence of macroscopic oesophagitis in snus users *Snus* use was associated with basal cell hyperplasia (OR = 1.74, 95% CI: 1.02, 3.00) *Snus* use was associated with elongation of papillae (OR = 1.79, 95% CI: 1.05–3.05) of the squamous epithelium at the oesophago-gastric junction *Snus* is not associated with gastrointestinal symptoms

CI Confidence interval, *H. pylori Helicobacter pylori*, *NA* Not applicable, *OR* Odds ratio, *ST* Smokeless tobacco

Key Points

- The IARC has classified ST as carcinogenic, with sufficient evidence linking it to oesophageal cancer.
- ST-chewing has been linked with erosive and ulcerative lesions in the oesophagus and stomach.
- Barrett's oesophagus and oesophageal neoplasms have been associated with habitual ST use.
- Chronic gastritis and duodenitis are commonly observed in ST-chewers, and long-term use (over 10 years) has been associated with a higher prevalence of gastric ulcers.
- A systematic review reported a significantly increased risk of rectal and stomach cancer among Swedish snus users compared to non-users.

11.2.5.1 Effect of Smokeless Tobacco on Gastrointestinal Microbiota

Rivera et al. (2020) performed metagenomic analysis of ST products, including moist and dry snuff used in the United States. The analysis identified bacterial, eukaryotic, and viral species across all samples, with bacteria making up 68% of the total species composition, dominated by three major phyla. Eukarya accounted for 32%, while archaea and viruses comprised 1% (Rivera et al. 2020). Moreover, 693,318 genes were identified, including those involved in nitrate and nitrite reduction, antibiotic resistance (e.g., vancomycin, β-lactamases), and multidrug transporters and efflux pumps. The analyses revealed the presence of genes encoding endo- and exotoxins, along with molecules linked to inflammatory responses. Thus, pathogenic microbes present in ST products can potentially transfer from the mouth to the gastrointestinal tract (GIT) (Rivera et al. 2020). *H. pylori* infection was detected in 68 ST-chewers (62.96%), a prevalence significantly higher than that observed in the control group ($P < 0.05$) (Vaishnav et al. 2025). The study concluded that ST chewing is associated with gross and histological changes in the upper gastrointestinal tract including neoplastic growths, chronic erosions, and peptic ulcers (Vaishnav et al. 2025). Similarly, Aro et al. (2010) assessed the effect of Swedish *snus* (snuff) on the GIT. Oesophagogastroduodenoscopy including biopsies, *H. pylori* culture, and serology were performed among *snus* users and non-users. The results showed a higher prevalence of macroscopic oesophagitis among *snus* users than non-users. In addition, *snus* use was associated with basal cell hyperplasia (OR = 1.74, 95% CI: 1.02, 3.00) and with elongation of papillae (OR = 1.79, 95% CI: 1.05–3.05) of the squamous epithelium at the oesophagogastric junction (Aro et al. 2010). However, Aro et al. (2010) found no association between *H. pylori* infection and snus usage. It is also worth mentioning that a study performed on toombak (ST product commonly used by Sudanese individuals) has suggested that this ST product possibly exerts deleterious effects on gastrointestinal health due to its high levels of TSNA (Tyx et al. 2022) (Table 11.6).

Key Points

- ST products may serve as a source of pathogenic microbes capable of transferring from the oral cavity to the gastrointestinal tract (GIT), potentially impacting gut health.
- ST products contain diverse microbial species: 68% bacterial, 32% eukaryotic, and 1% archaea and viruses.
- A significantly higher prevalence of *Helicobacter pylori* infection has been reported among ST chewers than non-users.
- One study showed a higher prevalence of macroscopic oesophagitis and epithelial changes like basal cell hyperplasia and papillae elongation in ST users; however the study showed no direct link to *H. pylori*.

11.2.6 Smokeless Tobacco and Liver and Kidney Toxicity

Use of ST has been linked to conditions such as hypertension and anaemia, which are established risk factors for chronic kidney disease (CKD) (Anand and Sk 2017). This connection can be attributed to nicotine and sodium, which are important constituents of ST products and have been implicated in hypertension (Anand and Sk 2017); which in turn increases the risk of CKD (Anand and Sk 2017). In a study from Bangladesh, Sarker et al. (2023) assessed the association between CKD and ST chewing. In this study (Sarker et al. 2023), 872 adults were recruited using a random sampling method. Individuals with an estimated glomerular filtration rate of <60 mL/min/1.73 m^2 and/or albumin to creatine ratio of ≥30 mg/g were assessed as per the CKD Epidemiology Collaboration equation (Inker et al. 2014; Sarker et al. 2023). The prevalence of ST use was 29% in this population. In the univariate analysis, several factors were found to be significantly associated with ST consumption: being aged ≥46 years (OR = 7.10; 95% CI: 4.79–10.94), female (OR = 1.64; 95% CI: 1.21–2.22), having no formal schooling (OR = 4.91; 95% CI: 3.59–6.72), family income <$100 per month (OR = 1.66; 95% CI: 1.13–2.43), sleeping <7 h per day (OR = 2.33; 95% CI: 1.70–3.19), and experiencing health issues such as undernutrition (OR = 1.63; 95% CI: 1.15–2.33), anaemia (OR = 1.94; 95% CI: 1.39–2.71), and CKD (OR = 1.62; 95% CI: 1.15–2.27). Based on these results, it seems that chewing ST products increases the risk of CKD in susceptible populations; however, it is worth mentioning that in Bangladesh, individuals with limited education exhibit lower levels of health literacy, which can limit an individual's ability to engage in self-care, make informed healthcare decisions, and adhere to medication regimes or lifestyle modifications for health promotion (Webster et al. 2017).

In an experimental study, Al-Mukhaini et al. (2017) orally administered aqueous ST extracts to male and female Wistar rats for a period of 8 weeks. The rats were divided into three groups: (a) control—distilled water instead of ST extract), (b) low-dose of ST—(3 mg nicotine/kg body weight/day and (c) high-dose of ST—6 mg nicotine/kg body weight/day. At the end of the eighth week of exposure, all animals were euthanized and their blood, liver, and kidney were collected for biochemical and histopathological investigations. Alanine aminotransferase (ALT) and aspartate aminotransferase (AST) were assayed for liver function, while blood urea nitrogen (BUN) and creatinine were assayed for kidney function. The results showed a significant increase in the ALT, AST, BUN, and creatinine levels ($P < 0.05$) in both ST-treated groups (low and high doses) compared with the control (Al-Mukhaini et al. 2017). Histopathological findings showed degenerative alterations of periportal fibrosis in the liver and oedematous and calcified changes in renal glomerulus among ST-treated groups (Al-Mukhaini et al. 2017). From a clinical perspective, these results suggest that habitual ST use jeopardizes renal and hepatic function.

Key Points

- ST use has been linked to hypertension and anemia, both of which are established risk factors for CKD.
- ST use may increase CKD risk, especially in populations with low health literacy.
- A study on rats showed that ST exposure led to elevated liver and kidney function markers (ALT, AST, BUN, creatinine) and histopathological damage in liver and kidney tissues.
- Clinical and experimental studies suggest that habitual ST use poses significant risks to kidney and liver health.

11.2.7 Smokeless Tobacco and Pancreas

The IARC has reported sufficient evidence linking ST use with various cancers including those of the pancreas (Humans et al. 2007). Table 11.7 provides a summary of four cohort studies that assessed the relationship between ST use and pancreatic cancer incidence or mortality (Boffetta et al. 2005; Luo et al. 2007; Winn et al. 1982; Zheng et al. 1993). Two studies (Winn et al. 1982; Zheng et al. 1993) were conducted in the United States and the remaining studies in Scandinavian countries (Boffetta et al. 2005; Luo et al. 2007). Studies performed in Scandinavia focused specifically on moist *snus* (snuff) use (Boffetta et al. 2005; Luo et al. 2007), and the remaining assessed the association between unspecified ST and pancreas-related mortality or cancer incidence (Winn et al. 1982; Zheng et al. 1993). Results from all cohort studies reported a significant association between ST usage and pancreatic cancer (Boffetta et al. 2005; Luo et al. 2007; Winn et al. 1982; Zheng et al. 1993). However, controversial results have also been reported (Falk et al. 1988; Farrow and Davis 1990; Ghadirian et al. 1991). Case-control studies by Falk et al. (1988), Farrow and Davis (1990), and Ghadirian et al. (1991) reported no indication of an increased risk of pancreatic cancer in

Table 11.7 An overview of cohort and case-control studies that assessed the influence of smokeless tobacco on the pancreas

Cohort studies							
Authors et al. (Year)	Location	Type of ST product	Sample-size	Follow-up	Endpoint	Adjustment factors	RR/OR (95% CI)
Winn et al. (1982)	United States	NR	~300,000 individuals[a]	15 years	Mortality	Age	1.65 (NR)
Zheng et al. (1993)	United States	NR	17,633 males	20 years	Mortality	Age, alcohol, smoking	1.70 (0.90–3.10)
Boffetta et al. (2005)	Norway	Moist snus (snuff)	10,136 males	35 years	Incidence[b]	Age, smoking	1.86 (1.13–3.05)
Luo et al. (2007)	Sweden	Moist snus (snuff)	279,897 males	26 years	Incidence	Age, BMI smoking	2.10 (1.20–3.60)
Case-control studies							
Authors et al. (year)	Location	Type of ST product	Sample-size	Study duration	Endpoint	Adjustment factors	RR/OR (95% CI)
Falk et al. (1988)	United States	Snuff	363 ST users 1234 non-users	2 years	Incidence, pancreatic cancer	NR	No excess risk[a]
Farrow et al. (1990)	United States	Snuff	168 ST users 195 non-users	4 years	Incidence, pancreatic cancer	Race, education	0.8 (NR)
Ghadirian et al. (1991)	Canada	ST-chewing (unspecified)	179 ST users 239 non-users	4 years	Diagnosis, pancreatic, bile duct or gall bladder cancer	Age, sex, smoking, education	No excess risk[a]

[a]>99.5% were male, [b]Cases diagnosed on the basis of a clinical examination or death certificate only were excluded, *BMI* Body mass index, *NR* Not reported, *RR* Relative risk, *OR* Odds ratios

relation to ST use, as shown in Table 11.7. A systematic review and meta-analysis evaluated the association between ST use and cancer of the pancreas in Europe and North America (Sponsiello-Wang et al. 2008). Random-effects estimate for ever ST use was 1.03 (95% confidence interval 0.71–1.49) based on heterogeneous estimates from included studies (Sponsiello-Wang et al. 2008). The studies included in this systematic review and meta-analysis had several limitations, such as a small number of exposed cases, reliance on baseline exposure data in cohort studies, inadequate control groups in certain case-control studies, and the absence of a clear dose–response relationship. Based on the limitations referenced above, the authors (Sponsiello-Wang et al. 2008) suggested that there might be a possible association between ST usage and pancreatic cancer; however, further well-designed studies are needed to justify this relationship.

Key Points

- The IARC has linked ST use with several cancers, including pancreatic cancers.
- Four cohort studies (two from the USA and two from Scandinavian countries) found a significant association between ST use and pancreatic cancer incidence or mortality.
- A systematic review and meta-analysis reported a non-significant pooled estimate (OR = 1.03, 95% CI: 0.71–1.49) for the association between ST use and pancreatic cancer.

11.3 Public Health Policy on Patient Education and Community-Based Health Awareness Programmes

The widespread use of ST products presents a significant public health challenge, as it contributes to oral as well as systemic health hazards, including periodontitis, oral precancer and cancer and cardiovascular diseases, metabolic disorders, reproductive complications, and an increased risk of malignancies, respectively. To address this issue, a comprehensive public health policy emphasizing patient education and community-based awareness programmes is imperative. Objectives of such a policy could include:

- *Increase Public Awareness*—Implement educational campaigns highlighting the systemic risks of ST use beyond oral health, emphasizing its role in conditions such as cardiovascular disease, diabetes, reproductive health, and cancer.
- *Target High-Risk Populations*—Design interventions tailored for high-risk groups, including adolescents, pregnant women, and individuals in lower socioeconomic strata, who have higher prevalence rates of ST use.

- *Integrate Education in Healthcare Settings*—Mandate ST-related health education in primary healthcare centres, dental clinics, and pharmacies to ensure routine counselling during medical visits.
- *Engage Community Leaders*—Collaborate with local organizations, schools, and workplaces to foster grassroots advocacy against ST use through culturally sensitive educational materials.
- *Institution-Based Prevention Programmes*—Develop educational curriculums in academic institutions such as schools, colleges, and universities that educate children, adolescents, and adults about the dangers of ST use.
- *Strengthen Regulation and Labelling*—Advocate for stricter warning labels highlighting the deleterious effects of ST products on overall health to ensure that consumers are aware of their potential health risks.
- *Accessible Cessation Support*—Establish free of charge or low-cost ST cessation programmes, including behavioural therapy, support groups, and pharmacological aids, available through public health facilities and online platforms.
- *Government ban*—The Government of India has taken multiple legislative steps to regulate the sale, production, and distribution of ST products (Adhikari et al. 2020; Mistry et al. 2015). In 2012, the Supreme Court of India upheld the ban on ST products such as gutka and pan masala reinforcing the responsibility of individual states to implement the prohibition. Following this, more than 24 Indian states and union territories imposed a ban on gutka and other ST products. While some states strictly regulate ST sales in India, others show lax enforcement due to economic and political factors (Arora and Madhu 2012; Yadav et al. 2020). Similarly, the Government of Pakistan has also imposed a ban on the sale, production, and distribution of various forms of ST products (Siddiqi et al. 2020, 2022). Despite these legal measures, the implementation of the ban remains inconsistent across South Asian countries including Bangladesh, India, and Pakistan (Abdullah et al. 2024; Siddiqi et al. 2020).

Key Points

- Effective interventions may include campaigns for high-risk groups, pregnant mothers, community involvement, and institution-based prevention programmes.
- Public health strategies could include health-care based education stronger warning labels, accessible cessation programmes, and affordable treatment options to help individuals quit ST use.
- Enforcement of strict governmental bans on ST product manufacture and sale is recommended.

11.4 Recommendations

To facilitate effective enforcement of ST control across countries, it is deemed that a multi-sectoral approach is necessary. Multimedia Awareness Campaigns (such as use of television, radio, and social media), community-based workshops and mobile clinics (including organizing local events proving free health screening and counselling), and training healthcare providers may play a role in achieving such objectives. In addition, clinicians should educate patients that ST chewing is not a safe alternate to traditional smoking and the hazards associated with the former extend beyond the oral cavity. Routine screening for hypertension, diabetes, and oral or systemic malignancies should be incorporated into clinical practice for ST users. Pregnant mothers should be informed on health risks to the fetus. Researchers should focus on longitudinal studies to better understand the causal relationships between ST use and systemic diseases while investigating potential genetic and environmental interactions.

Key Points

- Healthcare professionals and researchers should prioritize patient education on ST risks, incorporate routine health screenings for ST users, and conduct longitudinal studies to explore the systemic effects and contributing factors of ST use.
- Multimedia campaigns, community-based initiatives, and healthcare provider training are important for effective enforcement of bans on ST products across countries.

11.5 Conclusion

In conclusion, the systemic health consequences of ST use are extensive, affecting multiple organ systems, including the cardiovascular, metabolic, reproductive, respiratory, gastrointestinal, hepatic, renal, and pancreatic systems. The evidence highlights a strong association between ST use and increased risks of hypertension, myocardial infarction, metabolic syndrome, diabetes mellitus, reproductive dysfunction, and organ toxicity. Although some conflicting findings exist, particularly regarding the impact of ST on stroke, diabetes, and pancreatic cancer, the cumulative data suggest that ST use is a significant public health concern. Given the widespread use of ST products globally, there is an urgent need for stricter regulations, targeted public health campaigns, and further large-scale, well-controlled studies to elucidate the full extent of its systemic effects. Understanding these health risks is essential for developing effective interventions to reduce ST consumption and mitigate its long-term consequences.

References

Abdullah SM, Huque R, Siddiqi K, Kanaan M, Huque S, Ullah S, Garg S et al (2024) Non-compliant packaging and illicit smokeless tobacco in Bangladesh, India and Pakistan: findings of a pack analysis. Tob Control 33:333–340

Accortt NA, Waterbor JW, Beall C, Howard G (2002) Chronic disease mortality in a cohort of smokeless tobacco users. Am J Epidemiol 156:730–737

Adhikari K, Pednekar MS, Stepanov I, Singh A, Nikam S, Singhavi H, Gota V et al (2020) Observed circumvention of the Gutka smokeless tobacco ban in Mumbai, India. Tob Regul Sci 6:331–335

Ahuja AV, Uppe A, Nair G (2018) Study of lung functions in tobacco chewers. European Respiratory Society

Al-Askar M, Abduljabbar T, Vohra F, Pasumarthy S, Gholamiazizi E, Yunker M, Romanos GE et al (2017) Comparison of self-perceived oral symptoms and periodontal parameters among habitual shamma-chewers, gutka-chewers, and non-chewers. Quintessence Int 48:251–260

Allen AM, Lunos S, Heishman SJ, al'Absi M, Hatsukami D, Allen SS (2015) Subjective response to nicotine by menstrual phase. Addict Behav 43:50–53

Al-Mukhaini N, Ba-Omar T, Eltayeb E, Al-Shihi A, Al-Riyami N, Al-Belushi J, Al-Adawi K (2017) Liver and kidney toxicity induced by Afzal smokeless tobacco product in Oman. Tissue Cell 49:307–314

Anand A, Sk MIK (2017) The risk of hypertension and other chronic diseases: comparing smokeless tobacco with smoking. Front Public Health 5:255

Aprioku J, Obianime A (2014) Evaluation of the effects of Citrus aurantifolia (lime) juice in lead-induced hematological and testicular toxicity in rats. Pharmacologia 5:36

Aprioku JS, Ugwu TC (2015) Comparative evaluation of the impact of subacute exposure of smokeless tobacco and tobacco smoke on rat testis. Int J Reprod Med 2015:676245

Aro P, Ronkainen J, Storskrubb T, Vieth M, Engstrand L, Johansson SE, Bolling-Sternevald E et al (2010) Use of tobacco products and gastrointestinal morbidity: an endoscopic population-based study (the Kalixanda study). Eur J Epidemiol 25:741–750

Arora M, Madhu R (2012) Banning smokeless tobacco in India: policy analysis. Indian J Cancer 49:336–341

Ashfaq M, Channa MA, Malik MA, Khan D (2008) Morphological changes in human placenta of wet snuff users. J Ayub Med Coll Abbottabad 20:110–113

Asplund K (2003) Smokeless tobacco and cardiovascular disease. Prog Cardiovasc Dis 45:383–394

Baba S, Wikström AK, Stephansson O, Cnattingius S (2014) Influence of snuff and smoking habits in early pregnancy on risks for stillbirth and early neonatal mortality. Nicotine Tob Res 16:78–83

Bagchi M, Bagchi D, Stohs SJ (1996) In vitro effects of a smokeless tobacco extract on the production of reactive oxygen species by human oral epidermal cells and rat hepatic mitochondria and microsomes, and peritoneal macrophages. Arch Environ Contam Toxicol 30:418–422

Benowitz NL (1988) Nicotine and smokeless tobacco. CA Cancer J Clin 38:244–247

Benowitz NL (1997a) The role of nicotine in smoking-related cardiovascular disease. Prev Med 26:412–417

Benowitz NL (1997b) Systemic absorption and effects of nicotine from smokeless tobacco. Adv Dent Res 11:336–341

Benowitz NL, Gourlay SG (1997) Cardiovascular toxicity of nicotine: implications for nicotine replacement therapy. J Am Coll Cardiol 29:1422–1431

Boffetta P, Aagnes B, Weiderpass E, Andersen A (2005) Smokeless tobacco use and risk of cancer of the pancreas and other organs. Int J Cancer 114:992–995

Bolinder G, de Faire U (1998) Ambulatory 24-h blood pressure monitoring in healthy, middle-aged smokeless tobacco users, smokers, and nontobacco users. Am J Hypertens 11:1153–1163

Bolinder G, Alfredsson L, Englund A, de Faire U (1994) Smokeless tobacco use and increased cardiovascular mortality among Swedish construction workers. Am J Public Health 84:399–404
Bolinder G, Norén A, Wahren J, De Faire U (1997) Long-term use of smokeless tobacco and physical performance in middle-aged men. Eur J Clin Investig 27:427–433
Carlsson S, Andersson T, Araghi M, Galanti R, Lager A, Lundberg M, Nilsson P et al (2017) Smokeless tobacco (snus) is associated with an increased risk of type 2 diabetes: results from five pooled cohorts. J Intern Med 281:398–406
Committee NCEPC (1994) National Cholesterol Education Program. Second report of the expert panel on detection, evaluation, and treatment of high blood cholesterol in adults (Adult Treatment Panel II). Circulation 89:1333–1445
Das S, Upadhaya P, Giri S (2016) Arsenic and smokeless tobacco induce genotoxicity, sperm abnormality as well as oxidative stress in mice in vivo. Genes Environ 38:4
Eckel RH, Grundy SM, Zimmet PZ (2005) The metabolic syndrome. Lancet 365:1415–1428
Eliasson M, Asplund K, Nasic S, Rodu B (2004) Influence of smoking and snus on the prevalence and incidence of type 2 diabetes amongst men: the northern Sweden MONICA study. J Intern Med 256:101–110
Falk RT, Pickle LW, Fontham ET, Correa P, Fraumeni JF Jr (1988) Life-style risk factors for pancreatic cancer in Louisiana: a case-control study. Am J Epidemiol 128:324–336
Farrow DC, Davis S (1990) Risk of pancreatic cancer in relation to medical history and the use of tobacco, alcohol and coffee. Int J Cancer 45(5):816–820
Ghadirian P, Simard A, Baillargeon J (1991) Tobacco, alcohol, and coffee and cancer of the pancreas. A population-based, case-control study in Quebec, Canada. Cancer 67:2664–2670
Haglund B, Eliasson M, Stenbeck M, Rosén M (2007) Is moist snuff use associated with excess risk of IHD or stroke? A longitudinal follow-up of snuff users in Sweden. Scand J Public Health 35:618–622
Henley SJ, Thun MJ, Connell C, Calle EE (2005) Two large prospective studies of mortality among men who use snuff or chewing tobacco (United States). Cancer Causes Control 16:347–358
Hergens MP, Lambe M, Pershagen G, Terent A, Ye W (2008) Smokeless tobacco and the risk of stroke. Epidemiology 19:794–799
Hudish LI, Reusch JE, Sussel L (2019) Β cell dysfunction during progression of metabolic syndrome to type 2 diabetes. J Clin Invest 129:4001–4008
IARC Working Group on the Evaluation of Carcinogenic Risks to Humans, International Agency for Research on Cancer, World Health Organization (2007) Smokeless tobacco and some tobacco-specific N-nitrosamines, vol 89. World Health Organization
Inker LA, Astor BC, Fox CH, Isakova T, Lash JP, Peralta CA, Kurella Tamura M et al (2014) KDOQI US commentary on the 2012 KDIGO clinical practice guideline for the evaluation and management of CKD. Am J Kidney Dis 63:713–735
Javed F, Näsström K, Benchimol D, Altamash M, Klinge B, Engström PE (2007) Comparison of periodontal and socioeconomic status between subjects with type 2 diabetes mellitus and non-diabetic controls. J Periodontol 78:2112–2119
Javed F, Chotai M, Mehmood A, Almas K (2010) Oral mucosal disorders associated with habitual gutka usage: a review. Oral Surg Oral Med Oral Pathol Oral Radiol Endod 109:857–864
Javed F, Tenenbaum HC, Nogueira-Filho G, Nooh N, O'Bello Correa F, Warnakulasuriya S, Dasanayake AP et al (2013) Periodontal inflammatory conditions among gutka chewers and non-chewers with and without prediabetes. J Periodontol 84:1158–1164
Javed F, Al-Kheraif AA, Al Amri MD, Mikami T, Vohra F, Warnakulasuriya S, Romanos GE (2015) Periodontal parameters and whole salivary cytokine profiles among habitual gutka chewers and non-chewers. J Periodontol 86:689–695
Kahn R, Buse J, Ferrannini E, Stern M (2005) The metabolic syndrome: time for a critical appraisal. Joint statement from the American Diabetes Association and the European Association for the Study of Diabetes. Diabetologia 48:1684–1699
Karageorgi S, Alsmadi O, Behbehani K (2013) A review of adult obesity prevalence, trends, risk factors, and epidemiologic methods in Kuwait. J Obes 2013:378650

Kimblad A, Ollvik G, Lindh CH, Axelsson J (2022) Decreased sperm counts in Swedish users of oral tobacco. Andrology 10:1181–1188

Kulkarni N, Hawal N, Naik VA (2017) Tobacco use among rural women in reproductive age group and its association with the regularity of menstrual cycles and dysmenorrhoea: a community-based cross-sectional study. Int J Commun Med Public Health 5:210

Kumar D, Binawara B, Acharya MB, Maan B (2017) Effect of chewing tobacco on pulmonary functions in Bikaner city population. IRPMS

Kumar SN, Bastia B, Borgohain D, Agrawal U, Raisuddin S, Jain AK (2021) Structural changes, increased hypoxia, and oxidative DNA damage in placenta due to maternal smokeless tobacco use. Birth Defects Res 113:1198–1214

Laldinsangi C (2022) Toxic effects of smokeless tobacco on female reproductive health: a review. Curr Res Toxicol 3:100066

Lawes CM, Bennett DA, Feigin VL, Rodgers A (2004) Blood pressure and stroke: an overview of published reviews. Stroke 35:1024

Lee J, Taneja V, Vassallo R (2012) Cigarette smoking and inflammation: cellular and molecular mechanisms. J Dent Res 91:142–149

Li Y, Hecht SS (2022) Mass spectrometric quantitation of N'-Nitrosonornicotine-1N-oxide in the urine of cigarette smokers and smokeless tobacco users. Chem Res Toxicol 35:1579–1588

Lin W (2024) The association between body mass index and Glycohemoglobin (HbA1c) in the US population's diabetes status. Int J Environ Res Public Health 21:517

Luo J, Ye W, Zendehdel K, Adami J, Adami HO, Boffetta P, Nyrén O (2007) Oral use of Swedish moist snuff (snus) and risk for cancer of the mouth, lung, and pancreas in male construction workers: a retrospective cohort study. Lancet 369:2015–2020

Mistry R, Pednekar M, Pimple S, Gupta PC, McCarthy WJ, Raute LJ, Patel M et al (2015) Banning tobacco sales and advertisements near educational institutions may reduce students' tobacco use risk: evidence from Mumbai, India. Tob Control 24:e100–e107

Muthukrishnan A, Warnakulasuriya S (2018) Oral health consequences of smokeless tobacco use. Indian J Med Res 148:35–40

Nasir SM, Sultana T, Hashmi S, Ahmed M (2023) Patterns and predictors of periodontal disease and tooth loss among users of smokeless tobacco. BMC Oral Health 23:428

Norberg M, Stenlund H, Lindahl B, Boman K, Weinehall L (2006) Contribution of Swedish moist snuff to the metabolic syndrome: a wolf in sheep's clothing? Scand J Public Health 34:576–583

Orisakwe OE, Igweze ZN, Okolo KO, Ajaezi GC (2014) Heavy metal hazards of Nigerian smokeless tobacco. Tob Control 23:513–517

Peterson LA, Stanfill SB, Hecht SS (2024) An update on the formation in tobacco, toxicity and carcinogenicity of N'-nitrosonornicotine and 4-(methylnitrosamino)-1-(3-pyridyl)-1-butanone. Carcinogenesis 45:275–287

Piano MR, Benowitz NL, Fitzgerald GA, Corbridge S, Heath J, Hahn E, Pechacek TF et al (2010) Impact of smokeless tobacco products on cardiovascular disease: implications for policy, prevention, and treatment: a policy statement from the American Heart Association. Circulation 122:1520–1544

Pomerleau CS, Garcia AW, Pomerleau OF, Cameron OG (1992) The effects of menstrual phase and nicotine abstinence on nicotine intake and on biochemical and subjective measures in women smokers: a preliminary report. Psychoneuroendocrinology 17:627–638

Rivera AJ, Tyx RE, Keong LM, Stanfill SB, Watson CH (2020) Microbial communities and gene contributions in smokeless tobacco products. Appl Microbiol Biotechnol 104:10613–10629

Rodu B, Cole P (2002) Smokeless tobacco use and cancer of the upper respiratory tract. Oral Surg Oral Med Oral Pathol Oral Radiol Endod 93:511–515

Said TM, Ranga G, Agarwal A (2005) Relationship between semen quality and tobacco chewing in men undergoing infertility evaluation. Fertil Steril 84:649–653

Sarker MHR, Moriyama M, Sujon H, Rahman MM, Banu S, Chisti MJ, Ahmed T et al (2023) Smokeless tobacco consumption and its association with risk factors of chronic kidney disease in rural and peri-urban Bangladesh. Tob Induc Dis 21:138

Sawane H, Rajpurohit L, Sonawane S, Kharat P, Mathur A (2023) Smokeless tobacco use and its association with type 2 diabetes: a case control study. Asian Pac J Cancer Prev 24:4209–4217

Schivo M, Avdalovic MV, Murin S (2014) Non-cigarette tobacco and the lung. Clin Rev Allergy Immunol 46:34–53

Siddiqi K, Islam Z, Khan Z, Siddiqui F, Mishu M, Dogar O, Shah V et al (2020) Identification of policy priorities to address the burden of smokeless tobacco in Pakistan: a multimethod analysis. Nicotine Tob Res 22:2262–2265

Siddiqi K, Siddiqui F, Boeckmann M, Islam Z, Khan A, Dobbie F, Khan Z et al (2022) Attitudes of smokers towards tobacco control policies: findings from the studying tobacco users of Pakistan (STOP) survey. Tob Control 31:112–116

Simon DL, Iglauer A (1960) The acute effect of chewing tobacco and smoking in habitual users. Ann N Y Acad Sci 90:119–132

Sponsiello-Wang Z, Weitkunat R, Lee PN (2008) Systematic review of the relation between smokeless tobacco and cancer of the pancreas in Europe and North America. BMC Cancer 8:356

Stanfill SB, Hecht SS, Joerger AC, González PJ, Maia LB, Rivas MG, Moura JJG et al (2023) From cultivation to cancer: formation of N-nitrosamines and other carcinogens in smokeless tobacco and their mutagenic implications. Crit Rev Toxicol 53:658–701

Stich HF, Anders F (1989) The involvement of reactive oxygen species in oral cancers of betel quid/tobacco chewers. Mutat Res 214:47–61

Sun H, Saeedi P, Karuranga S, Pinkepank M, Ogurtsova K, Duncan BB, Stein C et al (2022) IDF diabetes atlas: global, regional and country-level diabetes prevalence estimates for 2021 and projections for 2045. Diabetes Res Clin Pract 183:109119

Teo KK, Ounpuu S, Hawken S, Pandey MR, Valentin V, Hunt D, Diaz R et al (2006) Tobacco use and risk of myocardial infarction in 52 countries in the INTERHEART study: a case-control study. Lancet 368:647–658

Totonchi H, Miladpour B, Mostafavi-Pour Z, Khademi F, Kasraeian M, Zal F (2016) Quantitative analysis of expression level of estrogen and progesterone receptors and VEGF genes in human endometrial stromal cells after treatment with nicotine. Toxicol Mech Methods 26:595–600

Tyx RE, Rivera AJ, Stanfill SB, Zaatari GS, Watson CH (2022) Shotgun metagenome sequencing of a Sudanese toombak snuff tobacco: genetic attributes of a high tobacco-specific nitrosamine containing smokeless tobacco product. Lett Appl Microbiol 74:444–451

Vaishnav B, Valiyil AS, Anand S, Ghosal A, Pailla R, Nair GR (2025) Effects of smokeless tobacco use on the upper gastrointestinal tract mucosa: gross and histopathological changes. Ann Afr Med 24:450

Valen H, Becher R, Vist GE, Holme JA, Mdala I, Elvsaas I, Alexander J et al (2023) A systematic review of cancer risk among users of smokeless tobacco (Swedish snus) exclusively, compared with no use of tobacco. Int J Cancer 153:1942–1953

Vámos O, Komora P, Gede N, Hegyi P, Kelemen K, Varga G, Mikulás K et al (2024) The effect of nicotine-containing products on Peri-implant tissues: a systematic review and network meta-analysis. Nicotine Tob Res 26:1276–1285

Vidya GS, Bhatt G, Kathiresan J, Rai S, Verma M, Goel S (2022) Predictors of hypertension among current smokeless tobacco users in India; analysis from the fourth round of National Family Health Survey (2015–2016). J Family Med Prim Care 11:5785–5791

Vu CU, Siddiqui JA, Wadensweiler P, Gayen JR, Avolio E, Bandyopadhyay GK, Biswas N et al (2014) Nicotinic acetylcholine receptors in glucose homeostasis: the acute hyperglycemic and chronic insulin-sensitive effects of nicotine suggest dual opposing roles of the receptors in male mice. Endocrinology 155:3793–3805

Warnakulasuriya S, Kerr AR (2016) Oral submucous fibrosis: a review of the current management and possible directions for novel therapies. Oral Surg Oral Med Oral Pathol Oral Radiol 122:232–241

Warnakulasuriya S, Kujan O, Aguirre-Urizar JM, Bagan JV, González-Moles M, Kerr AR, Lodi G et al (2021) Oral potentially malignant disorders: a consensus report from an international seminar on nomenclature and classification, convened by the WHO collaborating Centre for Oral Cancer. Oral Dis 27:1862–1880

Webster AC, Nagler EV, Morton RL, Masson P (2017) Chronic kidney disease. Lancet 389:1238–1252

Winn D, Walrath J, Blot W, Rogot E (1982) Chewing tobacco and snuff in relation to cause of death in a large prospective cohort. Am J Epidemiol 116. JOHNS HOPKINS UNIV SCHOOL HYGIENE PUB HEALTH 111 MARKET PLACE, STE 840 …:567–567

Yadav A, Singh PK, Yadav N, Kaushik R, Chandan K, Chandra A, Singh S et al (2020) Smokeless tobacco control in India: policy review and lessons for high-burden countries. BMJ Glob Health 5:e002367

Yoshikawa H, Hellström-Lindahl E, Grill V (2005) Evidence for functional nicotinic receptors on pancreatic beta cells. Metabolism 54:247–254

Zhao J, Qiao L, Shang P, Hua C, Xie Y, Li X, Ding M et al (2021) Effects of smokeless tobacco on cell viability, reactive oxygen species, apoptosis, and inflammatory cytokines in human umbilical vein endothelial cells. Toxicol Mech Methods 31:349–358

Zheng W, McLaughlin JK, Gridley G, Bjelke E, Schuman LM, Silverman DT, Wacholder S et al (1993) A cohort study of smoking, alcohol consumption, and dietary factors for pancreatic cancer (United States). Cancer Causes Control 4:477–482

Pharmacological Interventions for Cessation of Smokeless Tobacco Use

12

Olalekan Ayo-Yusuf and Anesu Marume

Abbreviations

CI	Confidence Interval
FCTC	Framework Convention on Tobacco Control
FTND	Fagerström Test for Nicotine Dependence
GNSBP	Glover-Nilsson Smoking Behavioural Patterns
GNSBQ	Glover-Nilsson Smoking Behavioural Questionnaire
HONC	Hooked on Nicotine Checklist
IARC	International Agency for Research on Cancer
LMICs	Low- and Middle-Income Countries
MAOI	Monoamine Oxidase Inhibitors
nAChR	Nicotinic Acetylcholine Receptor
NCD	Non-Communicable Disease
NDSS	Nicotine Dependence Syndrome Scale
NRT	Nicotine Replacement Therapy
NTCP	National Tobacco Control Programme (or Policy, depending on context)
pH	Potential of Hydrogen (a measure of acidity/alkalinity)
RCT	Randomized Controlled Trial
RR	Relative Risk
ST	Smokeless Tobacco
UHC	Universal Health Coverage

O. Ayo-Yusuf (✉) · A. Marume
Africa Centre for Tobacco Industry Monitoring and Policy Research (ATIM), School of Health Systems and Public Health, Faculty of Health Sciences, University of Pretoria, Pretoria, South Africa
e-mail: lekan.ayo-yusuf@up.ac.za; anesu.marume@up.ac.za

F. Javed, S. Warnakulasuriya (eds.), *Smokeless Tobacco and its Effects on Periodontal Health*, https://doi.org/10.1007/978-3-032-16409-4_12

WHO	World Health Organization
WHO-EML	World Health Organization's Model List of Essential Medicines
$\alpha4\beta2$	Alpha4 Beta2

Learning Goals

- Understand the global burden and cultural entrenchment of smokeless tobacco (ST) use and its implications for public health.
- Recognize the unique addiction profile of ST, including its pharmacokinetics, prolonged mucosal absorption, and sustained nicotine blood levels.
- Identify key pharmacological interventions; nicotine replacement therapy (NRT), varenicline, and bupropion and evaluate their mechanisms of action.
- Analyze the comparative effectiveness of pharmacotherapies for ST cessation through meta-analytic outcomes and relative risk estimates.
- Evaluate the safety profiles and tolerability of pharmacological agents used in ST cessation.
- Appraise the synergistic role of combining pharmacological and behavioural interventions.
- Explore health system-level factors influencing access to pharmacotherapies, including essential medicine list inclusion, regulatory challenges, and supply chain bottlenecks.
- Examine the gaps in ST cessation research, particularly among adolescents, pregnant women, rural populations, and LMICs.
- Discuss the role of oral and other primary healthcare providers in identifying ST users and initiating evidence-based cessation interventions.
- Assess the cost-effectiveness of ST cessation interventions, especially in resource-constrained settings, and the broader economic rationale for pharmacological support.
- Understand policy-level implications, including the need for national clinical guidelines, provider training, and integration of cessation services into the health system.
- Examine the role of WHO guidelines and the Model List of Essential Medicines in shaping national policies on ST cessation pharmacotherapies.
- Evaluate the contextual and cultural barriers to ST cessation.
- Identify implementation strategies for integrating cessation into existing health platforms, such as maternal and child health, oral health, and NCD programmes.
- Propose future research priorities, including RCTs tailored to ST users, novel pharmacotherapeutic agents, and innovations in personalized treatment delivery.

12.1 Introduction

Smokeless tobacco (ST) products such as snuff, chewing tobacco, and betel quid with tobacco are widely used across the globe, particularly in South Asia, parts of Africa, and among marginalized populations in high-income countries (Siddiqi et al. 2015, 2020). These products are linked to a host of adverse health outcomes, including periodontal diseases, oral and oesophageal cancers, cardiovascular disease, and nicotine addiction (Gupta and Johnson 2014; Gupta et al. 2018).

There are multiple forms and patterns of ST, which have important implications for designing and evaluating cessation interventions. While some individuals use smokeless products exclusively, such as snuff, chewing tobacco, or betel quid with tobacco, others engage in dual or poly-tobacco use, combining ST with cigarettes or other combustible products (Osibogun et al. 2020; Rath et al. 2012; Sweet et al. 2019). This dual-use pattern is particularly common in regions where cultural norms and product accessibility promote dual tobacco use. It is not uncommon for individuals to alternate between cigarette smoking and using ST based on setting or social context (Stanton and Halenar 2018). This variation in use behaviour can influence addiction severity, health outcomes, and response to behavioural and pharmacological treatment.

Evaluation of pharmacological treatment or interventions aimed at assisting those who use ST to quit also reflects this diversity in use behaviour. Some studies focus solely on individuals who use ST exclusively, tailoring interventions to the behavioural and pharmacological aspects unique to this form of tobacco (Ebbert et al. 2015; Pradhan et al. 2025). Others adopt a more integrated approach, addressing both smoking and ST cessation concurrently, especially in populations with high rates of dual use (Hecht and Hatsukami 2022). Additionally, specific trials that primarily target those who use ST still account for smoking behaviour in their design and analysis, either by adjusting for smoking status or excluding active smokers to isolate the intervention's effects (Siddiqui et al. 2024). This variability can complicate the evidence synthesis, as differences in participant profiles, intervention strategies, and outcome measures may affect study comparability. However, unlike cigarette smoking, ST use has received relatively limited attention in cessation research and policy (Ebbert et al. 2015).

In 2024, the World Health Organization (WHO) published updated guidelines on the pharmacological treatment of tobacco dependence, including recommendations for ST cessation (WHO 2024a). Several pharmacological treatments, including nicotine replacement therapy (NRT), bupropion, and varenicline, have been explored as cessation aids for those who use ST (Shang et al. 2022; Thomas et al. 2022). These interventions are grounded in evidence from smoking cessation research but have been adapted, with varying success, for those who use ST.

Additionally, contextual factors significantly improve success or failure of interventions. Low- and middle-income countries (LMICs) often face systemic barriers such as limited access to cessation services, cultural normalization of ST use, and a lack of context-specific research (Siddiqui et al. 2024). In contrast, much of the pharmacological evidence has been generated in high-income settings, raising concerns about generalizability. Similarly, young people, who represent a critical demographic for intervention due to their early initiation and potential receptivity to behaviour change, are underrepresented in current studies (Ma et al. 2021). Age-specific responses to pharmacological agents and engagement with cessation services may differ for older adults; however, data to guide youth-focused interventions remain limited.

To address persistent gaps in the response to ST use, particularly in low- and middle-income countries (LMICs) and among priority populations such as youth and those pregnant who use ST, this chapter critically examines the landscape of pharmacological interventions to help those who use ST quit. While rooted in the existing scientific evidence, the scope extends beyond traditional systematic reviews to offer a broader synthesis of clinical studies, global guidelines, and policy developments. This chapter also explores the contextual factors that shape access, adherence, and effectiveness of pharmacotherapy, with particular attention to underrepresented regions and populations.

The primary objective of this chapter is to provide an update to current evidence, and a practice-relevant overview of pharmacological interventions for ST cessation, including mechanisms of action, efficacy, safety, and implementation considerations. This chapter also identifies key challenges and directions for future research and policy. In doing so, it aims to support clinicians, researchers, and policymakers in advancing equitable and effective ST cessation strategies.

Key Points

- ST use exhibits multiple patterns, including exclusive use and dual or poly-tobacco use with combustible tobacco products. These patterns, influenced by cultural norms and accessibility, significantly impact addiction severity, health outcomes, and cessation treatment strategies.
- Pharmacological interventions for ST cessation vary in scope; some target exclusive ST users, while others address both smoking and ST cessation, introducing variability that complicates evidence synthesis and generalizability of reported results.
- Compared to cigarette smoking, ST use has historically received less attention in research and tobacco control policy, leading to insufficient evidence and support for effective cessation strategies.
- The 2024 WHO guidelines on tobacco dependence include ST-specific recommendations, endorsing pharmacotherapies such as NRT, bupropion, and varenicline.
- Systemic challenges in low- and middle-income countries, which include limited access to cessation services, cultural normalization of ST use, and a lack of localized research that hinder intervention effectiveness and adoption.
- The chapter aims to provide an evidence-based and practice-relevant synthesis of ST cessation pharmacotherapy, emphasizing the need for context-sensitive research, youth- and pregnancy-focused interventions, and equitable policy development.

12.2 Nicotine Dependence in Smokeless Tobacco Users

There is a cocktail of chemical constituents in ST, several of which are capable of contributing to dependence and addiction. These include alkaloids such as nicotine, along with additives like sugars, flavourings, and humectants, which are primarily added to enhance palatability and user satisfaction (Stepanov et al. 2008). In addition, monoamine oxidase inhibitors (MAOIs) naturally present in the tobacco leaf or formed during curing and fermentation may influence the brain's reward pathway, particularly in ST products that use whole tobacco leaf (Guillem et al. 2005). Nicotine, however, remains the most addictive component of ST. It is a potent psychoactive compound with high abuse liability, reinforcing dependence by activating nicotinic acetylcholine receptors and stimulating dopamine release in key brain regions associated with reward and reinforcement (Benowitz 2010). Compared to cigarettes, ST often provides higher nicotine bioavailability, and due to its prolonged mucosal absorption, users may experience sustained systemic nicotine levels that can exceed those achieved through cigarette smoking (Benowitz et al. 1988; Pickworth et al. 2014).

Nicotine present in smokeless tobacco products (such as oral snuff, chewing tobacco, and snus) is primarily absorbed through the oral mucosa, whereas in the case of nasal snuff, absorption occurs through the nasal mucosa (Benowitz 2010). Unlike cigarettes, which deliver nicotine via rapid pulmonary absorption, ST provides a slower, but sustained systemic exposure (Stepanov et al. 2008). The bioavailability of nicotine from ST, which is dependent on the pH of the product, is generally high, with peak plasma concentrations achieved within 30 min to an hour, depending on the product type and usage pattern (Pickworth et al. 2014).

The pharmacokinetics of ST use indicate a prolonged duration of nicotine presence in the bloodstream due to continuous absorption during oral retention of the product. The steady-state blood nicotine levels in regular ST users may be comparable to or even exceed those of smokers (Henningfield and Keenan 1993). Pharmacodynamically, nicotine from ST acts on nicotinic acetylcholine receptors in the brain, reinforcing dependence by modulating dopaminergic pathways involved in reward and reinforcement (Henningfield and Keenan 1993).

While both ST users and cigarette smokers can exhibit high levels of nicotine dependence, the behavioural patterns differ. Cigarette smoking is often linked with frequent, short bursts of nicotine intake, typically influenced by social cues and routines (Hecht and Hatsukami 2022). In contrast, ST use may involve longer sessions with fewer daily applications, but potentially higher total nicotine exposure (Hajat et al. 2021; Hecht and Hatsukami 2022). Studies show ST users often maintain higher baseline nicotine levels throughout the day, contributing to a more consistent state of dependence (Hajat et al. 2021; Hecht and Hatsukami 2022). Cravings in ST users can be less associated with situational triggers than in smokers, but more with physiological withdrawal symptoms due to sustained exposure and slower decline in plasma nicotine levels (McChargue and Collins Jr 1998).

Reliable assessment of nicotine dependence is critical in tailoring treatment approaches, whether behavioural therapy alone or combined with pharmacotherapy.

While tools like the Fagerström Test for Nicotine Dependence (FTND) are widely used for cigarette smokers, adaptations have been developed for ST users (Heatherton et al. 1991). The Fagerström Test for Nicotine Dependence Smokeless Tobacco (FTND-ST) provides a modified algorithm that includes measures like the amount of ST used per day and the time to first dip/chew upon waking (Ebbert et al. 2006). The Nicotine Dependence Syndrome Scale (NDSS) captures broader dimensions of dependence, such as drive, priority, and continuity of use (Shiffman et al. 2004). The Hooked on Nicotine Checklist (HONC), originally developed for adolescents, has versions adapted for ST, focusing on early signs of dependence (Wheeler et al. 2004). The Modified Glover-Nilsson Smoking Behavioural Questionnaire (GNSBQ) can be used to evaluate behavioural and psychological factors contributing to dependence in ST users (Glover et al. 2014).

Clinicians may consider using any of these tools when evaluating individuals who use ST, especially to determine the severity of dependence and the likelihood of benefit from pharmacological interventions such as NRT, bupropion, or varenicline.

Key Points

- ST contains addictive substances, including nicotine, sugars, flavourings, humectants, and naturally occurring MAOIs, all of which enhance its palatability and addictive potential.
- Nicotine is the most potent addictive compound in ST, exerting its effects by stimulating nicotinic acetylcholine receptors and triggering dopamine release in the brain's reward pathways.
- ST products often provide greater and more sustained nicotine levels than cigarettes due to prolonged mucosal absorption, especially through the oral and/or nasal mucosa.
- The pharmacokinetics of ST result in steady-state nicotine concentrations in users' bloodstreams, which may equal or exceed levels seen in cigarette smokers.
- Unlike the short, frequent bursts of nicotine intake during tobacco smoking, ST use tends to involve fewer but longer sessions, leading to more sustained nicotine levels and dependence patterns.
- Several validated tools have been adapted to assess nicotine dependence among ST users, including the FTND-ST, NDSS, HONC, and the Glover-Nilsson Smoking Behavioural Questionnaire.
- Accurate evaluation of nicotine dependence using these tools is essential for clinicians to tailor effective treatment strategies, including pharmacological interventions.

12.3 Challenges in Cessation of Smokeless Tobacco

Users of ST face numerous challenges when attempting to quit, many of which differ from those encountered by cigarette smokers. One key difficulty lies in the habitual and often ritualistic nature of ST use. Over time, users develop entrenched routines such as keeping a quid in the mouth for extended periods or using ST during solitary activities like working alone or relaxing indoors (Solhi et al. 2021). These behaviours can become deeply ingrained, making them harder to break than the more episodic and socially cued patterns typically associated with cigarette smoking (Ebbert et al. 2015).

Cultural and social contexts further complicate efforts to quit. In several regions, including South Asia, parts of Africa, and rural communities in the United States, ST use is embedded in traditional practices and societal norms (Mukherjea et al. 2018; Nemeth et al. 2012). It is often perceived as less harmful than smoking and is sometimes considered socially acceptable or even medicinal. For example, in India, Pakistan, and Bangladesh, ST products are commonly used after meals or during pregnancy, reinforcing their use as part of daily life (Farhadmollashahi 2014; Russo et al. 2011). Such cultural normalization diminishes users' motivation to quit and undermines the effectiveness of public health campaigns promoting cessation.

The pharmacokinetics of ST contribute to a unique dependence profile. The sustained mucosal absorption of nicotine leads to relatively stable blood nicotine levels throughout the day, fostering a steady-state dependence (Hatsukami et al. 2000). Users often report less intense but more persistent cravings compared to smokers. This continuous nicotine exposure creates a psychological environment where dependence feels "normal", reducing the urgency to quit and making cessation efforts less likely to be initiated or sustained (de Geus et al. 2019; Solhi et al. 2021).

Compared to cigarette smoking, various factors make quitting ST uniquely challenging. Unlike smoking, which is often restricted in public and carries a strong social stigma, ST can be used discreetly even indoors or in settings where smoking is prohibited (Hecht and Hatsukami 2022; Rath et al. 2012; Solhi et al. 2021). This subtle use reduces external deterrents and allows the habit to persist unnoticed, making cessation efforts harder to initiate and maintain. In an almost similar vein, most ST users underestimate its dangers, assuming that ST use is a safer alternative to smoking (Nemeth et al. 2012). They do not take into account that ST is strongly linked to oral cancers, periodontal disease, and cardiovascular conditions risk that have similar health impact as those associated with smoking (Benowitz 2010). However, health promotion efforts have traditionally emphasized the association between smoking and lung cancer, resulting in greater motivation among smokers to quit. In contrast, ST users often lack the same urgency to cease use, as they may not perceive immediate health risks associated with their behaviour.

The limited consideration of ST in health messaging is also found in regulations and public policies. ST products are often excluded from mainstream tobacco control policies, such as graphic health warnings, marketing restrictions, or taxation strategies. As a result, there is less public awareness about the risks, and fewer prompts encourage users to quit. For example, while smoking is heavily targeted in anti-tobacco campaigns, ST users often receive minimal direct messaging about cessation (Chugh et al. 2023).

Smokers often associate nicotine cravings with behavioural cues like drinking coffee or social interactions while due to the steady nicotine delivery characteristic of ST, users may experience more consistent, physiological dependence. This changes the nature of relapse whereby for smokers, it might be a social event that prompts a slip while for ST users, it may be the discomfort of withdrawal itself (Hatsukami et al. 2008). The challenges and differences in smoking and ST use highlights the need for tailored cessation strategies that account for the specific behavioural and pharmacological patterns of ST use.

Key Points

- ST users often develop deeply ingrained routines, such as prolonged quid retention or use during solitary activities, which makes cessation particularly difficult compared to the more situational habits of cigarette smokers.
- In regions such as South Asia, parts of Africa, and rural United States, ST use is embedded in traditional customs and is often viewed as socially acceptable or even medicinal.
- Due to sustained mucosal absorption, ST delivers nicotine more consistently than cigarettes, resulting in persistent but less intense cravings and a psychological normalization of dependence.
- Unlike smoking, ST can be used discreetly in indoor and public spaces without attracting social stigma, reducing external deterrents and making cessation more challenging.
- Many ST users wrongly perceive it as safer than smoking, despite strong evidence linking it to serious health risks such as oral cancers and cardiovascular diseases.
- ST is often excluded from major tobacco control initiatives such as graphic warnings, marketing bans, and taxation, leading to limited public awareness and fewer cessation cues.
- While smokers often relapse due to social triggers, ST users may relapse due to physiological withdrawal, highlighting differing mechanisms of dependence.
- Behavioural, cultural, and pharmacological uniqueness of ST use necessitates cessation strategies specifically tailored to the needs of ST users, rather than relying on approaches designed for smokers.

12.4 Research Gaps and Access to Interventions

While progress in tobacco control has been significant in many areas, there is still a major blind spot when it comes to ST. The majority of existing knowledge and available cessation support has been primarily designed with cigarette smokers as the target population. Users of ST, on the other hand, are often left navigating their quit journey with limited guidance, poorly tailored interventions, and a lack of research-backed pharmacological options.

A significant part of the problem is that ST cessation has not received the same level of research investment. Clinical trials and behavioural research have predominantly concentrated on smoking, leading to a substantially greater evidence base on effective and ineffective interventions for tobacco smoking compared to ST use. Consequently, there is a scarcity of evidence concerning the optimal efficacy, dosage, and duration of pharmacotherapies like NRT, varenicline, or bupropion when used specifically by ST users. In many instances, it remains unclear whether these treatments are effective in the same way for individuals who chew or snuff tobacco, or if they need to be delivered differently (e.g. lozenges vs. patches) to achieve effectiveness (Gupta and Johnson 2014).

Another important consideration is the need for customized or tailored interventions. Users of ST often have different patterns of use, cultural contexts, and dependence profiles than smokers; however, most cessation programmes do not reflect those differences (Hecht and Hatsukami 2022). Few behavioural interventions are designed specifically for ST users regarding content, format, or delivery method. This lack of customization diminishes the effectiveness of interventions and often leads users to perceive that mainstream programmes do not adequately address their specific needs or lived experiences.

Accessibility is another key concern, especially in LMICs and high-prevalence regions like South Asia and parts of Africa. In these areas, healthcare systems are often under-resourced, and cessation pharmacotherapies may be unavailable or unaffordable. Even when individuals are motivated to quit, they may not have access to the necessary tools or medications to succeed. Moreover, a lack of training among healthcare providers (including dentists and dental hygienists) compounds the issue. Furthermore, many clinicians receive limited training in identifying ST use or providing appropriate cessation counselling to affected patients (Mungia et al. 2025; Rasool et al. 2024). As a result, intervention opportunities are frequently missed during routine care, and ST dependence can go unaddressed despite its serious health consequences.

Lastly, at the policy level, ST is frequently overlooked in National Tobacco Control Programme (NTCP). While smoking often receives targeted campaigns, taxes, warning labels, and policy interventions, ST is left in the shadows. Few countries have comprehensive guidelines that address ST cessation specifically, and this neglect means that millions of users are left without adequate support (Chugh et al. 2023). Addressing these gaps is not merely an issue of equity; it is a critical public health imperative.

Key Points

- ST cessation remains a major blind spot, with most interventions and resources tailored for cigarette smokers rather than ST users.
- There is a significant disparity in research investment between smoking and ST, resulting in limited clinical evidence on the effectiveness, dosing, and administration methods of pharmacotherapies (e.g. NRT, varenicline, bupropion) for ST users.
- Most behavioural cessation programmes fail to consider the unique usage patterns, cultural contexts, and dependence characteristics of ST users, rendering existing interventions less effective for such population.
- There is a scarcity of behavioural interventions designed specifically for ST users in terms of content, delivery format, or cultural relevance, leading to poor user engagement and outcomes.
- In low- and middle-income countries and high-prevalence regions such as South Asia and Africa, cessation pharmacotherapies are often inaccessible or unaffordable, even for motivated users.
- Healthcare providers, including dentists and dental hygienists, are often not trained to screen for ST use or provide appropriate cessation counselling to vulnerable populations.
- National Tobacco Control Programs frequently exclude ST from targeted policy actions such as taxation, warning labels, and public health campaigns, leaving millions without adequate cessation support.
- The systemic neglect of ST cessation at clinical, research, and policy levels represents not only an equity issue but a critical public health concern.

12.5 Overview of Pharmacological Interventions

The 2024 WHO Clinical Treatment Guidelines for Tobacco Dependence provide guidance and recommendations for evidence-based interventions, including pharmacotherapy and behavioural support to all tobacco users, regardless of the form of tobacco consumed (WHO 2024a). This includes acknowledging the effectiveness of using treatment for the management and eventual cessation of ST product use.

Historically, global and national cessation efforts have disproportionately focused on combustible tobacco, leaving those who use ST with limited access to tailored cessation services. The 2021 WHO Report on the Global Tobacco Epidemic highlighted that many countries are making progress in tobacco control, but some are not addressing emerging nicotine and tobacco products and failing to regulate them (WHO 2021a).

The 2024 guidelines address this gap directly, reaffirming the need for pharmacological support for ST cessation and recommending the use of NRT, bupropion, or varenicline, depending on availability and appropriateness. The guidelines emphasize that these treatments should be accompanied by behavioural support and adapted to local health systems, cultural norms, and user needs. They also encourage national programmes to integrate ST cessation services into existing health infrastructure, including primary care and community health services (WHO 2024a).

At the national level, South Asian countries such as Bangladesh, India, Nepal, Pakistan, and Sri Lanka have taken steps to incorporate ST-specific cessation into policy frameworks (Arora and Madhu 2012; Huque et al. 2017; Nethan et al. 2018; Singh 2014). For example, India's National Tobacco Control Programme (NTCP) recommends brief advice, quitlines, and pharmacotherapy for those who use ST, although coverage and implementation vary widely across states. In contrast, many Sub-Saharan African countries, despite rising ST use, still lack formal guidelines or cessation services, a reflection of both limited resources and insufficient local evidence (Arora and Madhu 2012; Singh 2014).

This global policy lag mirrors a broader evidence gap, as few pharmacological agents have been specifically tested in ST-using populations, and regulatory approval for such indications remains limited. The 2024 WHO guidelines enable researchers and policymakers to close these gaps through context-sensitive implementation, capacity building, and integration with broader public health services, including oral health and non-communicable disease (NCD) programmes.

Key Points

- Global and national cessation initiatives have historically prioritized combustible tobacco.
- The 2024 WHO Clinical Treatment Guidelines recommend evidence-based cessation strategies and behavioural interventions for ST users.
- The new guidelines call for integrating ST cessation services into primary and community healthcare systems.
- South Asian countries like India, Pakistan, Sri Lanka, and Bangladesh have made strides in incorporating ST cessation into public health policies.
- There remains a shortage of clinical trials focused on pharmacological treatments for ST users, and few cessation medications are specifically approved for this population.

12.5.1 Mechanisms of Pharmacological Interventions

Pharmacological interventions for tobacco cessation primarily aim to counteract the neurobiological underpinnings of nicotine dependence. Among the various therapies available, the most widely used are NRT, bupropion, and varenicline. Each of these agents exerts its effects through distinct mechanisms within the central nervous system, yet they all converge on a common goal: to alleviate withdrawal symptoms, diminish the rewarding properties of nicotine, and support sustained abstinence from tobacco use. Combination therapies, such as using NRT alongside bupropion or integrating pharmacological treatment with behavioural support, have shown promise in enhancing cessation outcomes. However, such approaches remain understudied among users of ST, limiting generalizability across all forms of tobacco use.

Key Points

- Pharmacological treatments target nicotine addiction in the brain by reducing withdrawal symptoms, lessening nicotine's rewarding effects, and promoting long-term tobacco abstinence.
- Common cessation medications include NRT, bupropion, and varenicline.
- For example, NRT, with bupropion or behavioural support, improves quit rates; their effectiveness among smokeless tobacco (ST) users is not well-studied, limiting broader application.

12.5.2 Nicotine Replacement Therapy

Nicotine replacement therapy functions by delivering nicotine through non-tobacco routes, thereby avoiding the toxic constituents of tobacco while stabilizing plasma nicotine levels. This stabilization attenuates withdrawal symptoms and reduces cravings by acting on nicotinic acetylcholine receptors (nAChRs), particularly the $\alpha 4\beta 2$ subtype, which are central to the brain's reward circuitry (Molyneux 2004). By partially stimulating these receptors, NRT maintains sufficient dopaminergic activity in the mesolimbic pathway to curb withdrawal, while avoiding the rapid spikes in nicotine concentration seen with tobacco use that reinforce addiction (Molyneux 2004). For ST users, oral formulations such as nicotine gum and lozenges are particularly beneficial as they mimic the behavioural and pharmacokinetic aspects of ST consumption. Transdermal patches, though slower in onset, offer a steady delivery of nicotine, aiding in the gradual tapering of dependence (Wadgave and Nagesh 2016). The net effect of NRT is to reduce the reinforcing properties of ST and facilitate the transition to abstinence by blunting the physiological disruptions caused by nicotine discontinuation.

Key Points

- NRT works by delivering controlled doses of nicotine without the harmful by-products of tobacco, thereby reducing withdrawal symptoms and cravings through partial stimulation of $\alpha 4\beta 2$ nicotinic acetylcholine receptors.
- Oral NRT options such as gum and lozenges are especially effective for ST users as they simulate the behavioural and nicotine absorption patterns of ST use.
- NRT reduces the reinforcing effects of ST and supports a smoother transition towards nicotine abstinence.

12.5.3 Bupropion

Bupropion, originally developed as an antidepressant, exerts its tobacco cessation effects through its action as a norepinephrine and dopamine reuptake inhibitor (Dwoskin et al. 2006). By enhancing the synaptic availability of these neurotransmitters, particularly dopamine in the nucleus accumbens, bupropion helps counteract the anhedonia and dysphoria commonly experienced during nicotine withdrawal. This pharmacological profile not only mitigates craving but also stabilizes mood, which can be particularly useful for individuals with co-occurring depressive symptoms or heightened psychological dependence (Balfour 2001; Dwoskin et al. 2006). Although its efficacy in ST cessation is less robustly documented than for cigarette smoking, its dual action on mood and reward pathways suggests that it may still hold therapeutic value, especially in users with a strong affective component to their tobacco use.

Key Points

- Bupropion aids tobacco cessation by inhibiting the reuptake of norepinephrine and dopamine, which increases their levels in the brain and helps reduce nicotine withdrawal symptoms like low mood and lack of pleasure.
- Bupropion's ability to stabilize mood makes it particularly beneficial for individuals struggling with depressive symptoms or strong psychological dependence on tobacco.

12.5.4 Varenicline

Varenicline represents a more targeted approach, functioning as a partial agonist at the α4β2 nicotinic acetylcholine receptor, the same receptor subtype primarily activated by nicotine (Fagerstrom 2008). As a partial agonist, varenicline binds to the receptor and elicits a moderate release of dopamine, sufficient to alleviate withdrawal symptoms without producing the full rewarding effects of nicotine. Simultaneously, its high receptor affinity allows it to block nicotine from binding to the receptor, thereby reducing the satisfaction derived from any tobacco use during a quit attempt (Fagerstrom 2008; Hays and Ebbert 2008). This dual mechanism makes varenicline particularly effective for individuals with high levels of nicotine dependence, including ST users, by both reducing cravings and attenuating the reinforcing effects of nicotine if relapse occurs.

Key Points

- Varenicline works by partially stimulating the same brain receptors that nicotine activates, helping to ease withdrawal symptoms without producing the full pleasurable effects of nicotine.
- Varenicline not only reduces cravings but also blocks nicotine from binding to receptors, thereby making tobacco use less satisfying if a person relapses during a quit attempt.
- Varenicline is particularly beneficial for people with strong nicotine dependence.

12.5.5 Cytisine

Key Points

- Cytisine, a plant-based compound, acts as a partial agonist of the α4β2 nicotinic acetylcholine receptor providing moderate dopamine release to ease withdrawal symptoms.
- Cytisine has a shorter half-life, requiring more frequent dosing compared to varenicline.
- Cytisine's potential role in helping users quit smokeless tobacco (ST) remains untested.

Cytisine is a plant-derived alkaloid found primarily in *Cytisus laburnum* and related species, and it acts as a partial agonist of the α4β2 nicotinic acetylcholine receptor (nAChR), the same receptor targeted by varenicline (Tutka et al. 2019). Like varenicline, cytisine partially stimulates these receptors, leading to a moderate release of dopamine to alleviate withdrawal symptoms, while simultaneously blocking nicotine from binding and exerting its full rewarding effects. However, cytisine has a significantly shorter half-life and a lower receptor affinity than varenicline, necessitating more frequent dosing during the treatment regimen (Walker et al. 2014). It has been used as an over-the-counter medication in Eastern Europe and is recently starting to gain global interest mostly due to its low cost and favourable safety profile (Puljević et al. 2024b). The ASCEND trial conducted in New Zealand demonstrated that cytisine was at least as effective as NRTs in helping smokers quit, offering further evidence of its clinical utility (Rigotti et al. 2023). Given its affordability and oral formulation, cytisine is particularly promising for smoking cessation in LMICs. However, while its mechanism suggests potential utility in treating ST dependence, no trials to date have directly evaluated its efficacy for ST cessation, leaving its role in this domain speculative and in need of further research.

12.5.6 Clonidine

Clonidine, an alpha-2 adrenergic receptor agonist initially developed for the treatment of hypertension, has been investigated as a smoking cessation aid due to its ability to reduce symptoms of nicotine withdrawal, including anxiety, restlessness, and irritability (Gourlay et al. 1994). It exerts its effects by decreasing sympathetic outflow from the central nervous system, which may help stabilize the mood dysregulation associated with cessation attempts (Gourlay and Benowitz 1995). Although not considered a first-line treatment, clonidine is included in the US Clinical Practice Guideline for Treating Tobacco Use and Dependence as a second-line pharmacotherapy, typically reserved for cases where first-line agents such as NRT, bupropion, or varenicline are ineffective or contraindicated (Fiore 2009). The evidence for its effectiveness is modest, and the side effect profile particularly sedation, dry mouth, and hypotension can limit its widespread use (Wei and Young 1988). Importantly, there is a lack of studies evaluating clonidine's efficacy for ST cessation specifically, and its practical application in this context remains untested. Concerns about tolerability may further constrain its usefulness in population-level interventions, especially in resource-constrained settings.

Key Points

- Clonidine eases nicotine withdrawal symptoms such as anxiety and irritability by reducing central nervous system sympathetic activity.
- While clonidine is recognized as a second-line option in US tobacco treatment guidelines, its use is limited by side effects like sedation and hypotension, and it is generally considered when first-line therapies fail.
- There is insufficient research on clonidine's effectiveness for ST cessation and its potential role remains uncertain.

12.5.7 Novel Agents and Pathways

Scientists continue to explore approaches that are effective in maintaining tobacco use cessation. Approaches being explored include the use of nicotine vaccines, monoamine oxidase inhibitors, and psychedelic-assisted therapies (Cornuz et al. 2008; de Oca and Laucho-Contreras 2023; Nides 2008). Some of the approaches have shown preliminary promise in early-phase trials or mechanistic studies (Nides 2008). Additionally, assessment of the impact and effect of combination pharmacotherapy, such as the dual prescription of an NRT to another agent such as bupropion or that of NRT in combination with behavioural modulators, may provide a broader toolkit for addressing nicotine dependence in diverse user groups (Stitzer 1999). However, no current evidence supports the efficacy of these approaches for ST cessation specifically, and translational research is needed to assess both efficacy and contextual relevance.

Key Point

- While combining pharmacological treatments such as NRT with agents like bupropion or behavioural interventions may enhance cessation outcomes, there is currently no evidence supporting their effectiveness specifically for ST users.

12.5.8 Essential Medicines List

Most medication aimed at tobacco cessation has been included in the World Health Organization's Model List of Essential Medicines (WHO-EML) (WHO 2023) The WHO-EML provides a global reference for governments to prioritize medicines that address major public health needs (Persaud et al. 2019). Transdermal patches (NRT) and varenicline are currently included in the EML, with NRT first added in 2009 and varenicline added in the 2021 update (WHO 2021b). Their inclusion affirms these agents as clinically effective and cost-efficient tools for tobacco dependence treatment, including for those who use ST, as endorsed in the 2024 WHO Clinical Treatment Guidelines.

Importantly, inclusion in the WHO EML can expedite national-level regulatory approval, facilitate bulk procurement, and support insurance coverage or subsidy mechanisms, especially in countries that align their national EMLs with the WHO list (Persaud et al. 2019). This is particularly relevant in LMICs, where cost and supply chain constraints often hinder access to pharmacotherapies, even when national guidelines recommend their use. Access to pharmacological treatments for ST cessation is not only a clinical issue but also a regulatory and policy challenge. A critical step in improving the availability and affordability of such treatments, particularly in LMICs, lies in their inclusion in national essential medicines lists and public health formularies.

However, real-world availability remains uneven. In many countries with a high burden of ST use, regulatory frameworks often lack the provisions to import, prescribe, or subsidize cessation medications effectively (Henningfield and Slade 1998). Bupropion, although not on the WHO-EML specifically for tobacco dependence, is included as an antidepressant, and, in some settings, it is repurposed off-label for tobacco cessation. This regulatory ambiguity can hinder standardized prescribing practices (Kishore et al. 2010; Nides 2008). Another layer of complexity stems from the need for product registration and inclusion in national standard treatment guidelines (STGs). Even when a drug is on the EML, if it is not registered for use in tobacco cessation in a given country, providers may face legal or professional constraints in prescribing it.

In the context of ST cessation, regulatory and policy-level advocacy plays a critical role in bridging the gap between clinical evidence and real-world access to effective pharmacological interventions (Wadgave and Nagesh 2016). One pressing need is the alignment of national EMLs with the WHO-EML, particularly in countries where ST use remains prevalent (Kishore et al. 2010). Despite the proven efficacy of agents such as varenicline, bupropion, and cytisine in tobacco cessation, their inclusion in many national formularies remains limited, thereby constraining access especially within public health systems.

Regulatory reform is equally essential to streamline the approval and distribution of these medicines. In several low- and middle-income countries, regulatory bottlenecks hinder the availability of cessation therapies, despite international evidence supporting their use. Accelerating these pathways could expand access and encourage investment in cessation programmes tailored to both smoked and smokeless forms of tobacco. Moreover, integrating cessation pharmacotherapies into public procurement mechanisms under universal health coverage (UHC) schemes or donor-supported programmes can mitigate financial barriers and ensure equitable access. When these therapies are subsidized or provided at no cost through public health systems, uptake increases, particularly among lower-income populations, disproportionately affected by ST use.

Equally important is the inclusion of tobacco cessation pharmacotherapies in standard national treatment guidelines. Doing so helps legitimize their clinical use, foster provider confidence, and institutionalize cessation support within broader healthcare delivery. Without such formal guidance, healthcare providers may be reluctant to prescribe or recommend these agents, thereby weakening the overall infrastructure for cessation. Taken together, these advocacy priorities underscore the importance of regulatory action as a strategic lever for scaling ST cessation interventions. By complementing clinical strategies with supportive policy environments, countries can significantly enhance the reach, equity, and impact of their tobacco control efforts.

Key Points

- The WHO-EML includes NRT and varenicline, confirming their global clinical and cost-effectiveness in treating tobacco dependence, including that among ST users.
- Despite being on the WHO-EML, cessation medications are frequently inaccessible in many countries due to lack of registration, restrictive regulations, or absence from national formularies and treatment guidelines.
- Drugs like bupropion, though effective for tobacco cessation, are not universally approved for this indication in all countries, leading to inconsistent prescribing practices and limited use by healthcare providers.
- Incorporating cessation pharmacotherapies into national standard treatment guidelines legitimizes their use, builds clinician confidence, and embeds cessation support within the healthcare system.
- Improving access to cessation medications requires regulatory reforms, alignment of national essential medicines lists with WHO guidelines, and public financing strategies such as universal health coverage schemes to ensure equitable availability, especially for disadvantaged ST-using populations.

12.6 Evidence on Pharmacological Interventions for Smokeless Tobacco Cessation

To support the discussion on the effectiveness of pharmacological interventions for ST cessation, a systematic literature review and meta-analysis were conducted. The objective was to identify the most rigorous and up-to-date evidence on the use of medications such as NRT, bupropion, varenicline, and cytisine in assisting ST users to quit.

Relevant studies were identified through a comprehensive search of six major bibliographic databases: PubMed, Scopus, Embase, CINAHL, Web of Science, and the African Index Medicus. These databases were selected to ensure broad geographic representation, including studies from both high-burden and underrepresented regions. The search strategy incorporated both free-text terms and MeSH terms, combining descriptors for ST such as chewing tobacco, snuff, gutkha, betel quid, and pharmacological interventions considering either NRT, bupropion, varenicline, and cytisine pharmacotherapy. Boolean operators were used to refine the search, ensuring both sensitivity and specificity.

Studies were included if they focused on individuals using ST (either exclusively or in combination with smoked tobacco), evaluated a pharmacological cessation intervention (alone or in combination with behavioural therapy), reported outcomes related to abstinence, relapse, withdrawal symptoms, or adverse events, had a minimum follow-up duration of 3 months, and employed either randomized controlled trial (RCT) or quasi-experimental designs. Excluded were observational studies, case reports, systematic reviews, and studies focused exclusively on cigarette smoking or other combustible tobacco products.

Screening of titles, abstracts, and full texts was conducted independently by two reviewers. Discrepancies were resolved through discussion or by consulting a third reviewer. Data extraction was performed using a standardized template. The methodological quality of included studies was assessed using the Cochrane Risk of Bias tool, evaluating domains such as random sequence generation, allocation concealment, blinding, and outcome assessment reliability (Higgins et al. 2019).

For the meta-analysis, a random-effects model was used to account for variability across populations, settings, and interventions. Relative risks (RRs) and 95% confidence intervals (CIs) were either extracted directly from the studies or calculated manually when necessary. When applicable, risk estimates from studies included in the IARC Handbook 19 on Oral Cancer Prevention were used as reported, with supplemental calculations following the same definitions and procedures outlined in the handbook to ensure consistency (IARC 2023).

In total, 20 studies met the inclusion criteria. The majority (n = 16) were conducted in the United States, with others from the United Kingdom, Sweden, Norway, India, Bangladesh, and Pakistan. Most studies (n = 19) were randomized controlled trials, with one quasi-experimental design. The maximum follow-up period observed was 12 months (reported in three studies), though the majority had a 6-month follow-up; other studies reported outcomes over shorter durations, typically in weeks. One study specifically targeted adolescent ST users, while another focused on tertiary-level athletes. All remaining interventions targeted adults aged 18 years and older. Although participant recruitment was primarily through healthcare facilities, most interventions were delivered in community-based settings (Table 12.1).

Table 12.1 General description of identified studies

Reference	Year	Country	Study population	Setting	Study design	Sample size (N)	Age group	Intervention	Comparator	Follow-up (months)
Nicotine replacement therapy: Nicotine gum										
1. Hatsukami et al. (1996)	1996	USA	Intention to quit, minimum use of other forms of tobacco	Community-based	RCT	55 behaviour + gum, 50 behaviour + placebo, 51 gum, 54 placebo gum	18+	Group 1: 2 mg nicotine gum, Group 2: behaviour + placebo, Group 3 behaviour + nicotine gum	Placebo gum	12
2. Walsh et al. (1999)	1999	USA	College athletes	Rural and urban	RCT	153 intervention, 171 control	18+	2 mg nicotine gum	Brief advice	12
Nicotine replacement therapy" Nicotine patch										
3. Howard-Pitney et al. (1999)	1999	USA	Having a cell phone and willing to quit chew	Community-based	RCT	206 Experiment and 204 placebo	18+	15-mg Nicotine patches (Nicotrol)	Placebo patches	6
4. Hatsukami et al. (2000)	2000	USA	Minimum use of other forms of tobacco, intention to quit, no known medical condition or alcohol use	Community-based	RCT	100 patch and mint snuff, 101 patch and no mint snuff, 100 placebo patch and mint, 101 placebo patch no mint	18+	Transdermal and mint snuff plus counselling sessions	Counselling + placebo	12

(continued)

Table 12.1 (continued)

Reference	Year	Country	Study population	Setting	Study design	Sample size (N)	Age group	Intervention	Comparator	Follow-up (months)
5. Croucher et al. (2003)	2003	UK	Bangladesh women	Community-based	Quasi-experimental	65 NRT and behaviour, 65 behaviour	18+	15 mg Nicorette (NRT patches)	Brief advice	1
6. Ebbert et al. (2007)	2007	USA	Use of at least three cans or pouches of ST/week, intention to quit, and no known use of other forms of tobacco	Community-based	RCT	10 63 mg nicotine patch, 11 42 mg nicotine patch, 10 21 mg nicotine patch, 11 placebo	18+	63 mg Nicotine patches	Placebo	6
7. Ebbert et al. (2013a)	2013	USA	Three cans/pouches of ST daily at least	Community-based	RCT	25 nicotine patch, 27 placebo	18–55	42 mg nicotine patch daily	Placebo	6
8. Stotts et al. (2003)	2003	USA	High school adolescent males	School-based	RCT	98 active NRT patch, 100 placebo, 105 Usual care	14–19	Use-based dosage of NRT through an "intention to treat" model	Usual care and another placebo group	12

Nicotine replacement therapy: Nicotine lozenges										
9. Ebbert et al. (2009)	2009	USA	Primarily ST users with or without occasional use of other tobacco forms	Community-based	Multi-centre RCT	136 active lozenge, 134 placebo	18+	4 mg nicotine lozenges	Placebo	6
10. Ebbert et al. (2010)	2010	USA	Intention to quit	Community-based	RCT	30 nicotine lozenge, 30 placebo	18+	4 mg nicotine lozenges	Placebo	6
11. Ebbert et al. (2013b)	2013	USA	Primarily ST users with or without occasional use of other tobacco forms	Community-based	RCT	40 nicotine lozenges, 41 tobacco-free snuff	18+	4 mg nicotine lozenges	Tobacco-free snuff	6
12. Danaher et al. (2015)	2015	USA	Intention to quit	Community-based	RCT	205 lozenge + web, 202 web only	18+	4 mg lozenges	Web-based MyLastDip only	6

(continued)

Table 12.1 (continued)

Reference	Year	Country	Study population	Setting	Study design	Sample size (N)	Age group	Intervention	Comparator	Follow-up (months)
13. Severson et al. (2015)	2015	USA	Primarily ST users Intention to quit within a month	Community-based	RCT	356 lozenge, 354 coaching, 357 lozenge + coaching	18+	4 mg lozenges tapered use over time with coaching	Coaching	6
14. Siddiqui et al. (2024)	2024	Bangladesh, India, Pakistan	Planned quit attempt within 30 days, not dual users, i.e. ST and cigarettes	Health facility-based	RCT	NRT 66, behavioural intervention 66, NRT + Behavioural intention 66, brief advice 66	18+	4 mg NRT (option for choosing flavour) with option for behavioural therapy	Very brief advice (3As)	6
15. Schiller et al. (2012)	2011	USA	Set a quit date within 90 days	Community-based	Quasi-experimental	163 immediate cessation +169 reduction	18+	4 mg Nicotine lozenges 14 mg nicotine patch	Lozenge for reduction	6
Non-nicotine replacement therapy: Bupropion										
16. Glover et al. (2002)	2002	USA	Dipped or rubbed moist snuff, motivated to quit, not using other forms of tobacco smoking and chewing	Community-based	RCT	35 Bupropion tablets, 35 placebo	18+	150 mg AM and 150 mg PM	Placebo	3

17. Dale et al. (2002)	2002	USA	ST user	Community-based	RCT	34 Bupropion, 34 placebo	18+	150 mg twice day bupropion	Placebo	6
18. Dale et al. (2007)	2007	USA	Intention to quit, no history of substance misuse	Community-based	RCT	Bupropion 113, placebo 112	18+	150 mg bupropion SR titrated from one tablet to two tablets a day	Placebo	12
Non-nicotine replacement therapy: Varenicline										
19. Fagerström et al. (2010)	2010	Sweden and Norway	Intention to quit no other forms of tobacco	Multi-centre community-based	RCT	213 varenicline, 218 placebo	18+	0.5 mg once daily for 3 days, then twice daily for 4 days followed by 1 mg twice daily through week 12	Placebo	6
20. Ebbert et al. (2011)	2011	USA	Primarily ST users	Community-based	RCT	38 varenicline, 38 placebo	18+	0.5 mg varenicline daily for 3 days increased to 0.5 mg twice daily for days 4–7 with a target of 1 mg twice daily for 12 weeks + behaviour change	placebo	6
21. Jain et al. (2014)	2014	India	ST clients to the dental care centre in India	Health facility-based	RCT	118 placebo, 119 varenicline	18+	0.5 mg varenicline daily for 11 weeks with counselling	Placebo	3

* *USA* United States of America, *RCT* Randomized control trial, *NR* Not reported, *NRT* Nicotine replacement therapy, *ANC* Ante-natal care, *PNC* Post-natal care, *NICU* Neonatal intensive care unit, *IQR* Inter-quartile range

12.7 Methodological Characteristics of Identified Studies

Key Points

- A systematic review and meta-analysis evaluated studies, which aimed to evaluate the effectiveness of pharmacological interventions (NRT, bupropion, varenicline, and cytisine) for ST cessation.
- Solely RCTs or quasi-experimental studies focusing on ST users and assessing pharmacological interventions with or without behavioural support were included.
- Methodological quality was assessed using the Cochrane Risk of Bias tool.
- Twenty studies were assessed, of which 80% were conducted in the United States.
- Nineteen studies were RCTs and one had a quasi-experimental design.
- The majority of studies targeted adult ST users, with interventions delivered mainly in community settings and follow-up periods ranging from a few weeks to 12 months.

12.7.1 Inclusion and Exclusion Criteria

Across the included studies, participant selection was generally guided by clearly defined inclusion and exclusion criteria aimed at minimizing confounding variables and ensuring homogeneity in baseline tobacco use. A common exclusion criterion was the concurrent use of other tobacco products such as cigarettes, cigars, e-cigarettes, or marijuana, with one study specifying that they also excluded individuals who used another form of ST.

Most studies included only adults aged 18 years and older, although a few focused on specific subgroups such as rural or disadvantaged populations and South Asian women. Another key inclusion criterion was a stated willingness or intent to quit ST use. In many cases, participants had to set a quit date before or shortly after study enrolment. Additional issues considered for exclusion were a history of psychiatric illness, current use of pharmacotherapy for any other addiction, pregnancy, or known contraindications to the pharmacological intervention regimen such as NRT, bupropion, or varenicline.

12.7.2 Outcome Measurement

Across the studies included in this review, the primary outcome of interest was abstinence from ST. In most cases, participants self-reported abstinence, but the majority of studies enhanced the credibility of these reports through biological verification methods. Cotinine, a nicotine metabolite, was the most commonly used biomarker and was primarily measured through saliva. Cotinine levels served a dual purpose: they were used not only to verify self-reported abstinence but also to monitor adherence to nicotine replacement therapies such as patches, gum, or lozenges. In some cases, cotinine results were also employed to identify continued or undisclosed use of other nicotine-containing substances.

In addition to abstinence, several studies reported on withdrawal symptoms as a key secondary outcome. Withdrawal was assessed using standardized tools such as the Minnesota Nicotine Withdrawal Scale or symptom-specific checklists. Common symptoms documented included irritability, strong cravings, restlessness, difficulty concentrating, and sleep disturbances. Interventions that combined pharmacotherapy with behavioural components appeared more effective in mitigating the intensity of these symptoms, although this was not always statistically tested across studies.

The safety and tolerability of pharmacological interventions were evaluated through the documentation of adverse events. For nicotine replacement therapies, reported side effects were generally mild and included localized skin reactions from patches, gastrointestinal discomfort, and throat irritation from gum or lozenges. Varenicline was more frequently associated with nausea and vivid dreams, while bupropion use was linked to insomnia and dry mouth. Serious adverse events were rare, and most studies concluded that the interventions were well tolerated within the study populations. However, adherence to pharmacotherapy could be influenced by these side effects, with some studies noting dropouts attributable to tolerability issues.

A smaller subset of studies explored additional outcomes such as reduction in tobacco use among participants who did not achieve full abstinence. These reductions were typically self-reported and included decreases in the frequency or amount of ST consumed per day. Some studies also measured participants' motivation to quit, their readiness to change behaviour, and satisfaction with the intervention, though these were often secondary or exploratory in nature and not uniformly reported.

Overall, while abstinence remained the central focus across trials, the inclusion of withdrawal severity, adverse events, treatment adherence, and behavioural readiness provided a more comprehensive picture of intervention effectiveness and feasibility. However, the diversity in outcome measures introduced challenges for cross-study comparison and meta-analysis, particularly where tools or time points differed significantly. There is a pressing need for increased research focused on ST, not only to develop effective pharmacological interventions but also to create culturally sensitive behavioural strategies. National tobacco control policies should integrate ST into their guidelines and funding priorities. Bridging these gaps is essential to ensure that ST users receive evidence-based, accessible, and contextually appropriate care.

Key Points

- Most studies assessed ST cessation primarily through self-reported abstinence, which was often validated biologically using salivary cotinine levels.
- Combined pharmacological and behavioural interventions were more effective in alleviating these symptoms.
- Pharmacological treatments were generally well tolerated. Nicotine replacement therapies caused minor side effects such as skin irritation and throat discomfort, while varenicline and bupropion were linked to nausea and insomnia, respectively.
- Some studies documented partial successes, such as reduced ST use in those not achieving full abstinence.
- Other secondary measures, such as motivation to quit, behavioural readiness, and participant satisfaction, were inconsistently reported.
- National tobacco control strategies should formally include ST in their priorities and guidelines to improve care access and intervention effectiveness.

12.8 Effectiveness of Pharmacological Interventions in ST Cessation

There were multiple interventions conducted, with some integrating pharmacological components into broader behavioural strategies, while others were either standalone pharmacological or behavioural interventions. The behavioural elements varied widely, some were grounded in theoretical frameworks such as Cognitive Behavioural Therapy, while others employed practical approaches such as one-on-one coaching, brief educational sessions, or digital health messages delivered via mobile phones or web platforms. Overall pharmacological interventions in all their different components significantly contribute to ST cessation (RR 1.15; 95% CI: 1.05, 1.27) (Fig. 12.1).

Study	logRR	SE(logRR)	Risk Ratio	RR	95%-CI	Weight (common)	Weight (random)
Walsh 1999	0.7764	0.1978		2.17	[1.47; 3.20]	3.4%	4.5%
Siddiqui 2024	0.2513	0.4729		1.29	[0.51; 3.25]	0.6%	0.9%
Siddiqui 2024	1.0986	0.6435		3.00	[0.85; 10.59]	0.3%	0.5%
Siddiqui 2024	-0.5596	0.6021		0.57	[0.18; 1.86]	0.4%	0.6%
Siddiqui 2024	0.2877	0.7437		1.33	[0.31; 5.73]	0.2%	0.4%
Ebbert 2013	0.0247	0.5921		1.03	[0.32; 3.27]	0.4%	0.6%
Ebbert 2013a	0.5470	0.4980		1.73	[0.65; 4.59]	0.5%	0.8%
Stotts 2003	-0.3529	0.2570		0.70	[0.42; 1.16]	2.0%	2.9%
Stotts 2003	0.0606	0.3214		1.06	[0.57; 1.99]	1.3%	1.9%
Fagerstorm 2010	0.1823	0.1096		1.20	[0.97; 1.49]	10.9%	10.3%
Dale 2002	0.5108	0.3449		1.67	[0.85; 3.28]	1.1%	1.7%
Dale 2007	-0.1424	0.2674		0.87	[0.51; 1.46]	1.8%	2.7%
Danaher 2015	0.0862	0.0990		1.09	[0.90; 1.32]	13.4%	11.5%
Ebbert 2002	0.4418	0.3541		1.56	[0.78; 3.11]	1.0%	1.6%
Ebbert 2009	0.3335	0.2372		1.40	[0.88; 2.22]	2.3%	3.3%
Ebbert 2009a	-0.3185	0.3863		0.73	[0.34; 1.55]	0.9%	1.4%
Ebbert 2011	0.3483	0.2992		1.42	[0.79; 2.55]	1.5%	2.2%
Hatsukami 1996	0.2180	0.2874		1.24	[0.71; 2.18]	1.6%	2.3%
Hatsukami 1996	0.2842	0.3023		1.33	[0.73; 2.40]	1.4%	2.1%
Hatsukami 1996	-0.4537	0.3737		0.64	[0.31; 1.32]	0.9%	1.4%
Hatsukami 2000	0.0351	0.2245		1.04	[0.67; 1.61]	2.6%	3.6%
Howard-Pitney 1999	0.1128	0.1325		1.12	[0.86; 1.45]	7.5%	8.1%
Ebbert 2007	0.4680	0.6985		1.60	[0.41; 6.28]	0.3%	0.4%
Jain 2013	0.2573	0.2448		1.29	[0.80; 2.09]	2.2%	3.1%
Severson 2015	0.1536	0.0793		1.17	[1.00; 1.36]	20.9%	14.2%
Severson 2015	-0.0297	0.0858		0.97	[0.82; 1.15]	17.9%	13.2%
Boyle 1992	0.2231	0.2236		1.25	[0.81; 1.94]	2.6%	3.7%
Common effect model				**1.14**	**[1.06; 1.22]**	**100.0%**	**.**
Random effects model (HK)				**1.15**	**[1.05; 1.27]**	**.**	**100.0%**

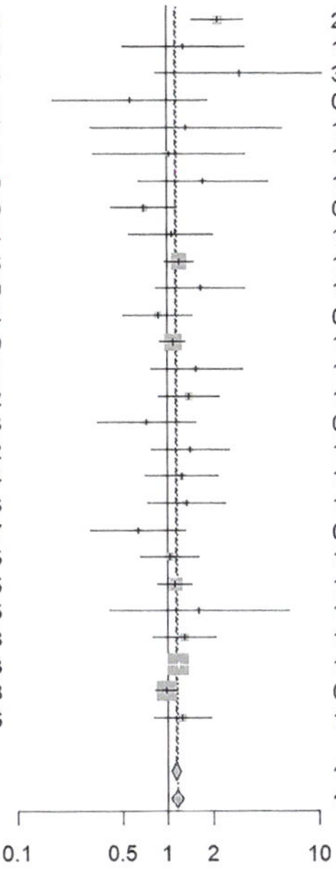

Heterogeneity: $I^2 = 18.6\%$, $\tau^2 = 0.0089$, $p = 0.1944$

Fig. 12.1 Effectiveness of pharmacological interventions in ST cessation

12.8.1 Nicotine Replacement Therapy (NRT)

Key Points
- Pharmacological interventions significantly improve ST cessation outcomes.
- Combining pharmacotherapy with behavioural strategies enhances the impact of cessation interventions.

The most frequently studied pharmacological interventions were NRT ($n = 22$). There were various NRTs considered with a majority being nicotine lozenges ($n = 5$), followed by nicotine patches ($n = 4$), and lastly nicotine gum ($n = 2$). While there were different dosages considered, the most common regimen per NRT were 4 mg of nicotine Lozenges, 15 mg of nicotine patches, and 2 mg of nicotine gum. A meta-analysis of studies conducted suggests a statistically significant benefit of NRT for ST cessation. NRT use had a statistically significant effect on ST cessation (RR 1.13; 95% CI: 1.00–1.28) (Fig. 12.2).

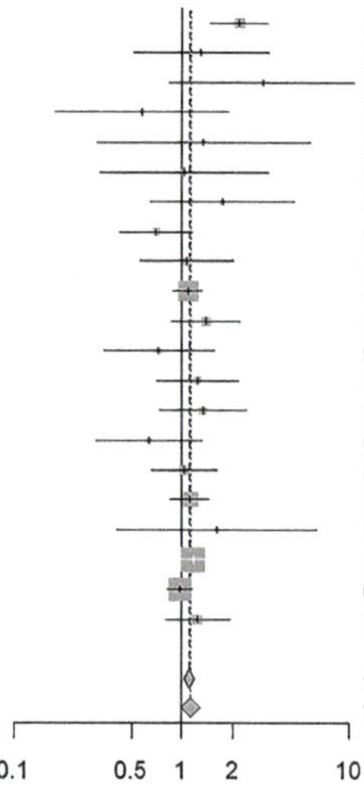

Study	logRR	SE(logRR)	RR	95%-CI	Weight (common)	Weight (random)
Walsh 1999	0.7764	0.1978	2.17	[1.47; 3.20]	4.1%	6.2%
Siddiqui 2024	0.2513	0.4729	1.29	[0.51; 3.25]	0.7%	1.4%
Siddiqui 2024	1.0986	0.6435	3.00	[0.85; 10.59]	0.4%	0.8%
Siddiqui 2024	-0.5596	0.6021	0.57	[0.18; 1.86]	0.4%	0.9%
Siddiqui 2024	0.2877	0.7437	1.33	[0.31; 5.73]	0.3%	0.6%
Ebbert 2013	0.0247	0.5921	1.03	[0.32; 3.27]	0.5%	0.9%
Ebbert 2013a	0.5470	0.4980	1.73	[0.65; 4.59]	0.7%	1.3%
Stotts 2003	-0.3529	0.2570	0.70	[0.42; 1.16]	2.4%	4.1%
Stotts 2003	0.0606	0.3214	1.06	[0.57; 1.99]	1.6%	2.8%
Danaher 2015	0.0862	0.0990	1.09	[0.90; 1.32]	16.5%	13.6%
Ebbert 2009	0.3335	0.2372	1.40	[0.88; 2.22]	2.9%	4.7%
Ebbert 2009a	-0.3185	0.3863	0.73	[0.34; 1.55]	1.1%	2.0%
Hatsukami 1996	0.2180	0.2874	1.24	[0.71; 2.18]	2.0%	3.4%
Hatsukami 1996	0.2842	0.3023	1.33	[0.73; 2.40]	1.8%	3.1%
Hatsukami 1996	-0.4537	0.3737	0.64	[0.31; 1.32]	1.2%	2.2%
Hatsukami 2000	0.0351	0.2245	1.04	[0.67; 1.61]	3.2%	5.1%
Howard-Pitney 1999	0.1128	0.1325	1.12	[0.86; 1.45]	9.2%	10.3%
Ebbert 2007	0.4680	0.6985	1.60	[0.41; 6.28]	0.3%	0.7%
Severson 2015	0.1536	0.0793	1.17	[1.00; 1.36]	25.7%	15.8%
Severson 2015	-0.0297	0.0858	0.97	[0.82; 1.15]	21.9%	15.1%
Boyle 1992	0.2231	0.2236	1.25	[0.81; 1.94]	3.2%	5.1%
Common effect model			**1.12**	**[1.03; 1.21]**	**100.0%**	.
Random effects model (HK)			**1.13**	**[1.00; 1.28]**	.	**100.0%**

Heterogeneity: $I^2 = 27.7\%$, $\tau^2 = 0.0147$, $p = 0.1178$

Fig. 12.2 Effectiveness of NRTs in ST cessation

12.8.2 Non-nicotine Pharmacotherapies: Varenicline

Key Points

- NRT is the most frequently studied pharmacological intervention for ST cessation, with nicotine lozenges being the most commonly evaluated form, followed by patches and gum.
- Meta-analysis findings indicate that NRT significantly improves cessation outcomes among ST users, with a relative risk of 1.13 (95% CI: 1.00–1.28), confirming its efficacy.

Three studies evaluated the efficacy of 0.5 mg Varenicline, a partial agonist at the α4β2 nicotinic acetylcholine receptor. Varenicline reduces withdrawal symptoms and block the reinforcing effects of nicotine. Participants were typically titrated up to 0.5 mg twice daily after an initial introductory period to monitor tolerance and reduce side effects such as nausea or vivid dreams. Outcomes measured included both biochemical and self-reported abstinence at follow-ups ranging from 4 weeks to 6 months. The pooled estimate indicates a statistically significant increase in cessation success among those using varenicline compared to control (RR 1.23; 95% CI: 1.05–1.45) (Fig. 12.3).

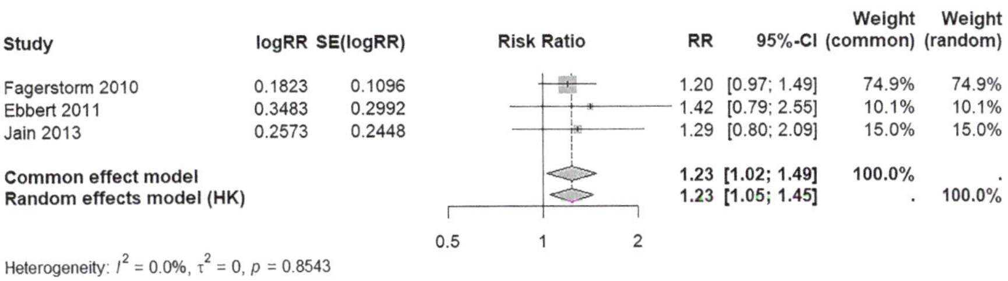

Fig. 12.3 Effectiveness of varenicline in ST cessation

12.8.3 Non-nicotine Pharmacotherapies: Bupropion

Key Point

- Varenicline improves ST cessation outcomes by reducing withdrawal symptoms and blocking nicotine's reinforcing effects, with a pooled relative risk of 1.23 (95% CI: 1.05–1.45).

Three studies assessed 150 mg sustained-release Bupropion, an atypical antidepressant that acts as a norepinephrine and dopamine reuptake inhibitor. Bupropion is thought to reduce cravings and withdrawal symptoms by modulating reward pathways involved in nicotine addiction. Studies typically initiated treatment 1–2 weeks before the target quit date, continuing for up to 12 weeks. Some studies reported modest increases in quit rates compared to placebo, though dropout due to adverse events such as insomnia or dry mouth was a noted limitation. The pooled estimate indicates a non-significant effect of varenicline on ST cessation (RR 1.24; 95% CI: 0.49–3.16). There was no observed heterogeneity among the included studies (Fig. 12.4).

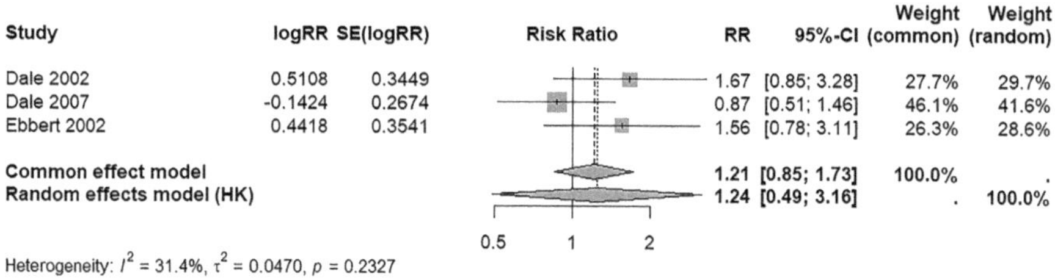

Fig. 12.4 Effectiveness of Bupropion for ST cessation

12.9 Integrating Pharmacological and Behavioural Interventions

While pharmacological strategies such as, bupropion and varenicline form the cornerstone of medical approaches to ST cessation, evidence strongly supports the integration of behavioural interventions to enhance treatment efficacy (Ebbert et al. 2015; Hatsukami et al. 1996). Tobacco dependence is both physiological and behavioural, and addressing one without the other often leads to suboptimal outcomes (Benowitz 2010; Hatsukami et al. 2008).

Combining pharmacotherapy with behavioural support has consistently been shown to improve quit rates compared to either approach alone. In studies involving those who use ST, those receiving medications alongside structured counselling or quit-line support demonstrated higher abstinence rates and lower relapse risk than those using pharmacological treatment alone (Rasool et al. 2024; Siddiqui et al. 2024; Stitzer 1999). The synergy arises from a dual-action mechanism. Pharmacological agents target the neurochemical basis of nicotine dependence. Behavioural support addresses habits, cues, and psychological reinforcements sustaining ST use.

This integrated model is endorsed by cessation guidelines from the WHO and national bodies in countries like India and Bangladesh, where ST prevalence is high (Huque et al. 2017; Siddiqi et al. 2020; Singh 2014). For instance, combining nicotine gum with brief motivational counselling in rural Indian settings has shown promising quit rates among daily gutkha users (Kumbhalwar et al. 2022).

Behavioural therapies complementing pharmacological cessation include brief advice from oral healthcare providers (dentists and dental hygienists), often delivered during routine clinical visits. Motivational interviewing enhances internal motivation to quit through patient-centred dialogue, making it particularly useful for ambivalent or low-readiness users. Cognitive-behavioural therapy aids users in identifying triggers, developing coping skills, and restructuring their thinking patterns concerning ST use (Perkins et al. 2013). Digital technologies have further expanded the reach of behavioural support, with mobile cessation apps tailored for those who use ST, such as mCessation, providing reminders, tips, and motivational messaging (Su et al. 2023).

Additionally, interactive voice response and text messaging services have shown effectiveness in rural or low-literacy populations, particularly when combined with pharmacotherapy (Scott-Sheldon et al. 2016). Importantly, these tools are not only cost-effective but also scalable, making them valuable in resource-constrained settings. Community and healthcare provider perspectives emphasize that sustained cessation often requires multi-level support, highlighting the necessity of insights from both community members and healthcare providers for designing culturally appropriate interventions.

Community engagement can significantly reduce stigma, shift social norms, and enhance the acceptability of cessation efforts, especially in regions where ST use is culturally entrenched or influenced by gender. Frontline health workers, particularly in low-resource settings, play a crucial role in delivering both behavioural support and pharmacotherapy; their training and confidence in counselling those who use ST are vital for the effectiveness of programmes.

There were selected studies that were conducted that had a behavioural component together with NRT. None of the studies that used varenicline or bupropion as a pharmacological intervention reported whether they had a behavioural component within their intervention. The behavioural package ranged from a simple brief message to a theoretical intervention which may be the cause for high heterogeneity. There was no statistically significant effect of the interventions on ST cessation (RR = 1.28; 95% CI: 0.98–1.67). However, the prediction interval includes the possibility of no effect, suggesting that future studies may yield varied results (Fig. 12.5). The intervention appears moderately effective overall, but the evidence base is limited in size and precision.

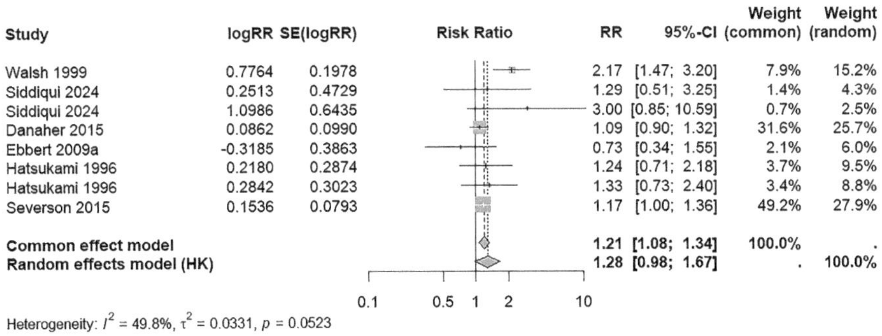

Fig. 12.5 Combination of pharmacological approach and behaviour for ST-cessation

Key Points

- Combining pharmacological treatments (e.g., bupropion, varenicline) with behavioural interventions improves cessation outcomes more effectively than either approach alone.
- WHO and national health agencies, especially in high-burden countries like India and Bangladesh, support integrated cessation strategies, including the combined use of nicotine gum and motivational counselling.
- Effective behavioural supports include brief advice by dental professionals, motivational interviewing, cognitive-behavioural therapy, and digital tools like mobile apps (e.g., mCessation).
- Interactive voice response systems and text messaging services have demonstrated success in rural and low-literacy populations, offering cost-effective and scalable support.
- Community involvement and frontline health worker training are essential for reducing stigma, increasing intervention acceptability, and delivering culturally appropriate care.
- Meta-analysis showed moderate but statistically non-significant effects, highlighting a need for further research with better design and precision.

12.10 Health Service Provision of Pharmacological Interventions for ST Cessation

Oral hygienists, dental therapists and dentists, and other primary care physicians contribute significantly by identifying dependent users, initiating cessation discussions, and recommending suitable pharmacological aids (Rasool et al. 2024). However, despite these opportunities, many users report inadequate access to cessation services, and healthcare providers often feel ill-equipped to support ST cessation due to limited training, unclear guidelines, or a lack of medication availability.

Selected studies specifically stated that they were conducted in health-facility settings, these were either done through coordination by health-facility staff, when a client went for dental care or managed by the pharmacist. There could be more studies conducted within health facility settings but they did not mention the setting or the service provider. The pooled effect for the health facility-based study shows a non-significant overall effect (RR 1.30; 95% CI: 0.88 to 1.91). Heterogeneity among the included studies was substantial, with an I^2 of 64.1%, $\tau^2 = 0.048$ suggesting that a considerable proportion of the variability in effect sizes is due to between-study differences rather than chance (Fig. 12.6).

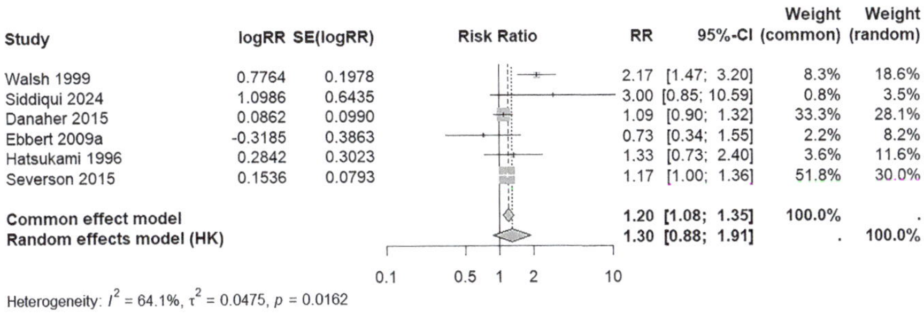

Fig. 12.6 Health-facility-based pharmacological interventions

12.11 Adverse Events and Safety of Pharmacological Interventions

Pharmacological interventions for ST cessation were generally well tolerated across studies, with a low incidence of serious or treatment-limiting adverse events. NRT formulations such as nicotine gum, lozenges, and patches were associated with mostly mild to moderate adverse events. The most reported symptoms included local irritation, such as mouth or throat discomfort, nausea, dizziness, hiccups, and sleep disturbances. These effects were typically transient and resolved without medical intervention. No serious or life-threatening events directly linked to NRT use were reported in the included studies. Importantly, the safety profile of NRT in ST users appeared consistent with that observed in cigarette smokers, although the literature remains limited regarding long-term safety in this specific population.

Varenicline was also well tolerated in most studies, with no reports of serious adverse events attributable to the medication. The most frequent side effects included nausea, vivid dreams, insomnia, and headache. While these symptoms were occasionally cited as reasons for discontinuation, they were generally manageable and did not require cessation of treatment. No evidence emerged linking varenicline to psychiatric or cardiovascular events within the scope of the reviewed trials.

Bupropion use was associated with a favourable safety profile. Common adverse effects included insomnia, dry mouth, headache, and nausea. These symptoms were typically mild and self-limiting. None of the reviewed studies reported seizures or other severe outcomes, and there were no documented instances of major psychiatric or cardiovascular complications during treatment.

Across all interventions, serious adverse events were rare and, when reported, were not deemed causally related to the pharmacotherapy. The consistency of safety profiles across studies reinforces the acceptability of these agents for ST cessation. Nonetheless, a notable limitation is the lack of long-term safety data specific to ST users, who may differ in nicotine metabolism and exposure patterns compared to cigarette smokers.

Key Points

- Pharmacological interventions for ST cessation are generally well-tolerated.
- NRTs (gum, lozenges, patches) are associated mainly with mild to moderate side effects such as mouth/throat irritation, nausea, dizziness, hiccups, and sleep disturbances.
- Varenicline is well-tolerated, with manageable side effects like nausea, vivid dreams, insomnia, and headaches.
- Bupropion presents a favourable safety profile, with mild and self-limiting side effects (e.g., insomnia, dry mouth, headache, nausea), and no reports of seizures or major complications.

12.12 Pharmacological Interventions for Vulnerable Populations in ST Cessation

While ST use affects the broader population, certain groups are disproportionately burdened due to increased vulnerability, restricted access to cessation support, or higher associated health risks (Ganz and Delnevo 2020; Puljević et al. 2024a). These populations more often require targeted intervention strategies that address their specific contexts. Understanding what makes these groups "priority populations" allows for a more equitable and effective allocation of cessation resources, especially where pharmacological treatments are underutilized or inaccessible. Addressing the needs of priority populations is essential for advancing equity in ST cessation efforts. Pharmacological interventions offer significant promise but must be adapted to the specific risks, barriers, and cultural contexts each population faces. Without such tailoring, interventions risk leaving behind those most in need. Future policies, guidelines, and research must explicitly consider these groups to ensure comprehensive and inclusive tobacco control strategies.

12.12.1 Adolescents

Adolescence marks a critical window for tobacco prevention and cessation, as ST use often begins during this developmental stage (Orlandi and Boyd 1989). In several high-burden regions, ST is culturally accepted and viewed as a safer alternative to smoking, contributing to early initiation. Nicotine exposure during adolescence, however, can interfere with brain development, increase susceptibility to long-term dependence, and impair executive function (Orlandi and Boyd 1989; Sinha et al. 2017).

Despite these risks, few pharmacotherapies are approved for use in adolescents. Most clinical guidelines recommend behavioural interventions such as motivational interviewing or cognitive behavioural therapy as first-line approaches (Moolchan et al. 2000). Off-label use of NRT may be cautiously considered in cases of significant dependence, particularly with supervision and in combination with behavioural support (Stotts et al. 2003). Youth-centred engagement strategies including school-based cessation programmes, social media outreach, and mobile health platforms can improve accessibility and acceptability.

Key Points

- Nicotine exposure during adolescence can interfere with brain development, increase susceptibility to long-term dependence, and impair executive function.
- Youth-centred engagement strategies, including school-based cessation programmes, social media outreach, and mobile health platforms, can improve accessibility and acceptability.

12.12.2 Pregnancy

The use of ST products during pregnancy has been linked to multiple adverse outcomes, including preterm birth, low birth weight, and stillbirth (Baraona et al. 2017). Nevertheless, the safety and efficacy of pharmacological cessation therapies during pregnancy remain poorly understood, especially in the context of ST, where data are particularly scarce (Claire et al. 2020). Behavioural counselling remains the standard of care for pregnant individuals seeking to quit ST. For those with strong nicotine dependence where behavioural strategies are insufficient, short-acting forms of NRT such as lozenges or gum may be used after a risk-benefit assessment, especially when the risk of continued ST use is high (Baraona et al. 2017; Claire et al. 2020; Haddad and Davis 2016). However, the lack of clear clinical guidelines and limited research in this area hampers consistent care. There is a pressing need for rigorous RCTs and safety evaluations of pharmacotherapies for ST cessation during pregnancy.

Key Points

- ST use during pregnancy is linked with adverse outcomes, including preterm birth, low birth weight, and stillbirth.
- There is a dire need for rigorous RCTs and safety evaluations of pharmacotherapies for ST cessation during pregnancy.

12.12.3 Rural Populations

Rural areas bear a disproportionate burden of ST use due to affordability, accessibility, and cultural normalization. Unfortunately, access to cessation services in rural settings is often limited by healthcare workforce shortages, geographic isolation, and under-resourced health facilities (Noonan et al. 2025). To overcome these barriers, innovative approaches are required. Task-shifting to trained community health workers, integration of cessation interventions into existing primary care or maternal health services, and delivery of support via telehealth or mobile health platforms can enhance reach. Making pharmacological interventions available at the community level, supported by culturally sensitive educational campaigns may increase both uptake and adherence in rural populations (Nemeth et al. 2012; Noonan et al. 2025; Trigg et al. 2023).

Key Points

- Access to cessation services in rural settings is often limited by healthcare workforce shortages, geographic isolation, and under-resourced health facilities.
- Availability of ST session pharmacologic interventions supported by culturally sensitive educational campaigns may increase uptake and adherence in rural populations.

12.12.4 Populations in LMICs

The use of ST products is often deeply rooted in cultural practices and bolstered by weak regulatory environments within LMICs, resulting in them having the highest burden of ST use (Nadkarni et al. 2025). Products are frequently inexpensive, widely available, and perceived as less harmful than smoked tobacco. Moreover, regulatory policies that restrict advertising, increase taxation, or mandate warning labels are often poorly enforced or absent (Ayo-Yusuf and Burns 2012; Mehrotra et al. 2019). In these settings, cost and supply chain barriers limit access to pharmacological cessation tools. Providing free or subsidized medications such as NRT, bupropion, or varenicline through public health systems or donor-supported initiatives has shown promise in increasing uptake (Nadkarni et al. 2025; Thakur and Choudhari 2024). Interventions embedded in existing health services, such as tuberculosis or diabetes care, have also proven effective, especially when combined with health worker training and community outreach (Aryanpur et al. 2016; Wang and Shen 2009).

Key Points

- Cultural norms and weak regulatory enforcement in LMICs contribute to the widespread use of ST products.
- Integrating subsidized pharmacological cessation tools like NRT, bupropion, and varenicline into existing health services has shown promise in improving ST cessation outcomes.

12.12.5 Other Priority Populations

Indigenous populations in several countries experience high rates of ST use, often linked to historical marginalization and trauma (Bonevski et al. 2017; Carson et al. 2014). Culturally safe interventions co-designed with these communities are critical for long-term success. Similarly, individuals with mental health conditions are more likely to use tobacco, including ST, and may benefit from integrated treatment models that address both dependence and mental health needs. Occupational groups such as agricultural or construction workers also exhibit elevated ST use, often driven by workplace stress or misconceptions about performance benefits. Workplace-based cessation programmes could be an effective avenue for engagement in these populations.

Key Points

- Cultural norms and weak regulatory enforcement in LMICs contribute to the widespread use of ST products.
- Integrating subsidized pharmacological cessation tools like NRT, bupropion, and varenicline into existing health services has shown promise in improving ST cessation outcomes.

12.13 Cost-Effectiveness of Pharmacological Interventions and Health System Integration

The cost-effectiveness of pharmacological interventions for ST cessation, while less extensively studied than for combustible tobacco, is gaining recognition (Brett et al. 2019; Ebbert and Fagerstrom 2012; Nethan et al. 2018). Such growing body of evidence suggests that investment in ST cessation not only delivers health benefits but also represents a financially sound public health strategy, especially in high-prevalence, resource-constrained settings.

The implementation of NRT, when delivered in conjunction with behavioural counselling, has emerged as a cost-effective intervention in several contexts (Siddiqui et al. 2024; Stitzer 1999). Studies in ST-endemic countries have demonstrated that such combined interventions yield favourable outcomes relative to their costs, particularly when delivered through community platforms (Nethan et al. 2018; Siddiqui et al. 2024). These models leverage existing health infrastructure and reach populations that may otherwise lack access to cessation services. In some trials, brief advice administered by frontline health workers, followed by pharmacotherapy support, has shown a compelling cost-benefit profile in LMICs, suggesting that relatively modest investments can produce significant gains in terms of quit rates and future disease prevention.

A key dimension of sustainability lies in how these interventions are integrated into health systems. Stand-alone cessation programmes are often donor-driven and limited in scope and duration, which raises concerns about long-term viability. In contrast, embedding ST cessation within routine primary care through maternal and child health services, non-communicable disease clinics, or community outreach programmes has been shown to enhance both equity and continuity of care (Arora and Madhu 2012; Huque et al. 2017; Singh 2014). Such integration ensures that cessation support becomes a routine part of patient engagement, rather than a niche service, and reduces costs through economies of scale.

Beyond immediate cost metrics, the broader economic case for ST cessation is compelling. ST use is associated with a range of chronic conditions, including oral and oropharyngeal cancers, cardiovascular disease, poor birth outcomes, and periodontal diseases. These illnesses place a significant and growing burden on already stretched health systems in LMICs. Effective cessation can avert many of these downstream costs, offering not just personal health benefits, but systemic financial savings. Investing in pharmacological cessation support today can therefore be viewed as a cost-containment measure for tomorrow's healthcare challenges.

While additional high-quality economic evaluations specific to ST cessation are urgently needed especially in diverse cultural and regulatory contexts, the emerging evidence provides a strong rationale for integrating pharmacotherapy into national tobacco control strategies. In doing so, governments and global health actors can enhance the value-for-money of public health investments while addressing an often-overlooked aspect of the tobacco epidemic.

Key Points

- Pharmacological interventions for ST cessation are increasingly being recognized as cost-effective, especially in high-burden and resource-limited settings.
- NRT, when coupled with behavioural counselling, yields favourable outcomes and demonstrates strong cost-effectiveness, particularly when delivered through existing community health platforms.
- Embedding ST cessation into routine primary care and public health services (e.g., maternal–child health, NCD clinics) improves both cost-efficiency and continuity of care, unlike donor-dependent, stand-alone initiatives.
- ST use contributes to significant healthcare costs through its association with chronic diseases.
- Effective cessation efforts can mitigate these expenses, positioning pharmacological support as a long-term cost-containment strategy.
- While preliminary evidence supports the economic rationale for ST cessation pharmacotherapy, more context-specific economic evaluations are necessary to inform national tobacco control strategies and maximize public health investment returns.

12.14 Implementation Considerations for Smokeless Tobacco Cessation Interventions

Translating evidence-based ST cessation interventions into practice requires more than establishing clinical efficacy. It demands attention to real-world implementation. Despite strong evidence supporting the effectiveness of pharmacological and behavioural therapies, their uptake and sustained delivery remain constrained by systemic, logistical, and contextual challenges. These challenges are particularly pronounced in LMICs, where ST use is most prevalent and health systems often operate under significant resource limitations.

One of the most persistent barriers is the accessibility and affordability of pharmacotherapies. NRT and varenicline while effective are often unavailable or underutilized in many LMICs. National essential medicines lists frequently omit tobacco cessation medications, and out-of-pocket costs can be prohibitive, especially for rural or socio-economically disadvantaged populations who form the majority of ST users (IARC 2023). Even when these products are available, their use is hampered by low public awareness and scepticism about their effectiveness, often fuelled by cultural beliefs that ST is either harmless or beneficial to health (Sinha et al. 2014).

The integration of cessation support into primary healthcare systems offers a pathway to scalable, equitable intervention delivery. Primary care settings, including dental clinics, maternal and child health services and non-communicable disease clinics, serve as the first point of contact for many ST users, making them ideal platforms for routine screening and brief intervention. Effective integration involves training oral healthcare and other healthcare providers to identify ST users using validated tools, deliver brief cessation advice, and initiate or refer for pharmacological support as appropriate. In practice, however, many countries lack structured ST-specific protocols at the primary care level, and existing tobacco cessation guidelines often focus exclusively on smoked forms of tobacco, leaving those who use ST underserved (Aung et al. 2016; Gupta et al. 2005).

Building provider capacity is the key cornerstone of successful implementation. Clinicians, nurses, and community health workers must receive targeted training on the unique patterns of ST use, associated health risks, and cessation strategies. Without adequate training, healthcare providers may underestimate the harm caused by ST or believe that it requires less intensive intervention than cigarette smoking (Siddiqui et al. 2024). Addressing these misconceptions through in-service training, supervision, and mentorship is essential to ensure the consistent and competent delivery of cessation services.

A robust monitoring and evaluation framework is also critical for effective implementation. Without standardized tools to capture ST-specific indicators, health systems struggle to assess coverage, effectiveness, and quality of interventions. Key metrics should include the number of individuals screened for ST use, the proportion offered cessation support, uptake of pharmacotherapy, and follow-up outcomes such as quit rates at 3, 6, and 12 months. However, many LMICs currently lack the infrastructure to routinely collect and analyse such data, making it difficult to evaluate programme impact or identify areas for improvement (Arora and Gupta 2019; WHO 2024b).

Overall, bridging the gap between evidence and practice for ST cessation requires a comprehensive approach that strengthens health system readiness, improves access to affordable pharmacotherapy, equips providers with the necessary skills, and embeds cessation support into existing service delivery platforms. These steps are essential not only to scale up ST cessation efforts but also to ensure that interventions reach the populations most affected by the burden of ST use.

Key Points

- Despite strong clinical evidence supporting pharmacological and behavioural therapies for ST cessation, real-world application remains limited due to systemic, logistical, and contextual barriers, especially in LMICs.
- A major obstacle is the inaccessibility and high cost of effective pharmacotherapies such as NRT and varenicline, which are often excluded from essential medicine lists and are unaffordable for rural and disadvantaged populations.
- Even where treatments are available, low public awareness and cultural beliefs that ST is harmless or beneficial hinder their use and reduce treatment uptake.
- Integrating cessation support into primary healthcare systems, including dental, maternal, and NCD clinics, offers an opportunity for routine screening, brief advice, and initiation of pharmacotherapy.
- Many national healthcare systems lack structured protocols for ST cessation at the primary care level, focusing instead on smoked tobacco, thus neglecting a large segment of affected users.
- Effective implementation requires targeted training of clinicians and community health workers to recognize the specific risks and patterns of ST use and to deliver appropriate cessation interventions.
- A robust monitoring system is essential to track intervention coverage, pharmacotherapy uptake, and quit outcomes.
- Bridging the gap between evidence and practice demands a multifaceted strategy that includes health system readiness, affordable pharmacotherapies, trained providers, and integrated service platforms to ensure equitable reach and impact.

12.15 Policy Implications and Recommendations

Strengthening ST cessation requires targeted policy action that goes beyond individual-level interventions to address systemic and structural enablers. Despite the rising global awareness of ST's health harms, policy responses have often lagged behind those aimed at combustible tobacco (Mehrotra et al. 2019). A strategic, multi-sectoral policy framework is needed to integrate pharmacological cessation support into national tobacco control agendas and health system planning particularly in countries where ST use is endemic.

By advancing these policy priorities, countries can move towards a comprehensive approach to ST cessation that is equitable, effective, and sustainable. These actions will not only reduce the burden of ST-related disease but also contribute to broader goals of universal health coverage and health system strengthening.

In many countries, tobacco control legislation primarily focuses on smoking, leaving ST regulation fragmented or absent. National tobacco control strategies should explicitly include ST cessation and allocate dedicated resources to support implementation (Huque et al. 2017; Nethan et al. 2018; Singh 2014). This includes updating treatment guidelines to reflect ST-specific approaches, integrating pharmacotherapy into national essential medicines lists, and establishing clear clinical protocols for cessation across all levels of care (WHO 2008).

Access to affordable pharmacological treatment remains a cornerstone of effective cessation yet cost and availability remain major barriers in LMICs. Policymakers should prioritize the inclusion of NRT and other cessation aids in public health supply chains and consider subsidization or price regulation to enhance affordability. Innovative financing mechanisms such as using tobacco tax revenues to fund cessation programmes can ensure sustainability while aligning with broader tobacco control objectives (WHO 2021c).

Building the capacity of healthcare providers is critical to operationalizing cessation at scale. National curricula for dental, medical, nursing, and public health professionals should incorporate ST-specific content, including pharmacological and behavioural strategies. Continuing professional development programmes should emphasize skill-building in screening, counselling, and medication initiation, particularly for providers in primary and community settings (Gupta and Johnson 2014). Task-shifting models, where trained community health workers support cessation delivery, offer a scalable solution in resource-limited environments.

Public health messaging around ST cessation must be grounded in cultural relevance and informed by community contexts. Policies should support large-scale communication campaigns, such as social marketing, that challenge myths surrounding ST safety, highlight the benefits of cessation, and promote available treatment options. Engaging local influencers, including educators, faith leaders, and traditional healers can help shift social norms and enhance trust in evidence-based interventions (Sinha et al. 2014). Reliable data must guide policy development. Governments should institutionalize the collection of ST-specific indicators through health information systems, household surveys, and routine monitoring frameworks. Investments in implementation research are also needed to test scalable models of pharmacological cessation in diverse settings, particularly among underrepresented populations such as adolescents, pregnant women, and rural residents (WHO 2021c).

International tools such as the WHO Framework Convention on Tobacco Control (FCTC) provide a roadmap for coordinated action on ST (McInerney 2019; Zaatari and Bazzi 2019). Countries should fully implement Article 14, which emphasizes tobacco dependence treatment, and adapt their guidance to reflect ST realities (WHO FCTC 2005). Global health partners can support through technical assistance, funding, and capacity-building initiatives aimed at integrating cessation support into broader health agendas, including non-communicable disease (NCD) and maternal–child health programmes.

Key Points

- Despite growing awareness of ST-related harms, policy responses remain inadequate necessitating more comprehensive and specific strategies for ST control.
- A strategic, multi-sectoral policy framework is essential to incorporate pharmacological cessation support into national tobacco control agendas, especially in countries with high ST prevalence.
- Integrating ST cessation into broader health systems is expected to reduce disease burden and promote equity, sustainability, and progress towards universal health coverage.
- National tobacco control policies must explicitly address ST, updating treatment guidelines, integrating cessation pharmacotherapy into essential medicines lists, and ensuring clinical protocols across care levels.
- Policymakers should address affordability barriers by including cessation medications like NRT in public supply chains and considering subsidies or tobacco-tax-funded programmes.
- Strengthening provider capacity through education and task-shifting to trained community health workers is critical for scaling ST cessation services.
- Effective public health messaging should be context-specific, challenge misconceptions, and engage local influencers to shift social norms and increase uptake of cessation interventions.
- Full implementation of the WHO FCTC—particularly Article 14—along with international funding, technical assistance, and integration into NCD and maternal–child health programmes is key to advancing ST cessation globally.

12.16 Future Directions and Research Gaps

Despite increasing recognition of the health risks posed by ST use, the evidence base for effective pharmacological cessation interventions remains limited and uneven. Findings from our meta-analysis, alongside recent systematic reviews such as the Cochrane assessment, reveal critical gaps that constrain clinical practice, policy development, and health system implementation (IARC 2023; Livingstone-Banks et al. 2025; Pradhan et al. 2025). Addressing these gaps is essential to strengthening the impact and reach of ST cessation programmes globally.

A foremost priority is the development of high-quality, ST-specific RCTs. Much of the current evidence is extrapolated from studies focused on combustible tobacco, with limited consideration of the unique patterns of ST use, such as frequency, mode of administration, and cultural context. Existing trials often suffer from small sample sizes, short follow-up periods, and inconsistent use of outcome measures, particularly the lack of biochemical verification of abstinence (Ebbert et al. 2015; Gupta and Johnson 2014; Nethan et al. 2018). Future research should prioritize sufficiently powered RCTs that are culturally and contextually tailored to those who use ST, with a rigorous methodology that includes long-term follow-up, standardized outcome reporting, and the inclusion of diverse population groups especially adolescents, women, and rural populations, who are frequently underrepresented in clinical trials.

Moreover, comparative effectiveness research is needed to determine the optimal pharmacological regimen for ST cessation. Head-to-head trials of available therapies including NRT, bupropion, and varenicline either as monotherapy or in combination with behavioural interventions, would provide more definitive guidance for clinical and public health practice. The heterogeneity of ST products globally necessitates localized investigations to ensure interventions are relevant and scalable within specific epidemiological contexts (Livingstone-Banks et al. 2025; Siddiqui et al. 2024).

Advancements in pharmacotherapy delivery methods, such as buccal films, sublingual tablets, and long-acting implants, present promising avenues for enhancing adherence to ST cessation treatments. These novel delivery systems can improve bioavailability and align more closely with users' preferences and consumption behaviours, potentially increasing treatment efficacy (Macedo et al. 2020). In parallel, the field of precision medicine offers opportunities to tailor cessation therapies based on individual genetic and metabolic profiles. Genetic variations, particularly in enzymes like CYP2A6 that influence nicotine metabolism, have been associated with differential responses to cessation medications, suggesting that pharmacogenetic profiling could inform personalized treatment strategies (Chen et al. 2018). While the implementation of such personalized approaches remains aspirational in many LMICs, ongoing research and investment in this area could lay the groundwork for more effective, individualized cessation options in the future.

Use of ST products is a risk factor for various oral health conditions which include periodontal disease, oral cancers, and oral potentially malignant disorders such as oral submucous fibrosis and leukoplakia. This makes the consideration of health services such as oral health services key in ST cessation (Chan et al. 2023). The WHO sees the integration of tobacco cessation programmes in routine oral care as a key intervention (IARC 2023). However, oral health services are often siloed from broader tobacco control programmes, particularly in LMICs. Embedding ST screening, brief advice, and pharmacotherapy referral pathways into routine dental and oral health visits could provide a dual benefit enabling early detection of

ST-related pathology while facilitating cessation support. This approach is especially relevant in settings where access to dental specialists is limited, but where individuals may still engage with primary care or community-based health services.

While NRTs, varenicline, and bupropion remain the most widely studied and approved pharmacological agents for tobacco cessation, there is growing interest in exploring the utility of other agents either already approved for smoking cessation or under investigation for their potential application in ST cessation. Notably, no RCTs or high-quality studies have yet evaluated the efficacy of these agents including cytisine, specifically among those who use ST, but their mechanisms and success in smoking populations warrant future investigation.

In summary, the future of ST cessation depends on both strengthening the evidence base and fostering systemic innovation in increasing affordability and wide access to effective cessation interventions. This includes investing in robust clinical trials, embracing novel technologies and personalized care models, and integrating cessation efforts with existing healthcare platforms, such as oral health services. These research and policy priorities will be essential to advancing equitable and effective ST cessation in diverse global settings.

Key Points

- The current evidence base for pharmacological cessation interventions remains limited, uneven, and largely extrapolated from smoking cessation research.
- There is an urgent need for well-powered, culturally tailored RCTs that focus specifically on ST users, including underrepresented groups such as adolescents, women, and rural populations.
- RCTs comparing NRT, bupropion, and varenicline (individually and in combination with behavioural interventions) are essential for optimizing treatment strategies across diverse contexts.
- Emerging pharmacotherapy delivery systems (e.g., buccal films, sublingual tablets, long-acting implants) may improve treatment adherence and efficacy by aligning with user preferences and behaviours.
- Advances in pharmacogenetics, such as CYP2A6-based profiling, hold promise for developing individualized ST cessation treatments.
- Embedding cessation services into routine oral healthcare systems present a critical opportunity for dual benefit—early disease detection and cessation support.
- NRT, varenicline, and bupropion are widely studied; however, agents like cytisine remain underexplored in ST cessation, despite promising mechanisms seen in smoking populations.
- The future of ST cessation hinges on building a stronger research foundation and integrating affordable, accessible pharmacological interventions into broader healthcare systems, especially in resource-limited settings.

12.17 Conclusion

Pharmacological interventions remain a critical yet underutilized component in the global response to ST use. While behavioural strategies have formed the backbone of cessation efforts particularly in settings where access to medications is limited, evidence consistently points to the enhanced efficacy of combined pharmacological and behavioural approaches. As the burden of ST-related morbidity continues to rise, particularly in LMICs, the case for integrating pharmacotherapy into broader cessation programmes and primary care services becomes increasingly compelling.

This chapter has highlighted the distinct pharmacological and behavioural dimensions of ST dependence, which differ significantly from cigarette smoking and therefore demand tailored treatment strategies. Current evidence supports the use of NRT and varenicline as promising pharmacological options, though the field remains hampered by a paucity of high-quality, ST-specific trials. Robust RCTs, culturally grounded in the contexts where ST use is most entrenched, are urgently needed to close these knowledge gaps and strengthen clinical guidance.

Beyond clinical efficacy, the success of pharmacological interventions depends heavily on implementation readiness. Barriers such as cost, availability, health system integration, and provider training must be addressed to ensure that interventions reach those most in need. Innovative delivery models including integration into primary and oral health care, digital platforms, and task-shifting to community health workers offer scalable and sustainable pathways for expanding access, particularly in resource-constrained environments.

For clinicians, this calls for a more proactive, culturally competent approach to identifying and treating ST dependence. This includes routine screening, understanding local ST products and patterns of use, and being equipped to offer or refer for appropriate pharmacotherapy. For researchers, the challenge lies in designing trials that not only meet methodological rigour but also reflect the lived realities of diverse ST-using populations. And for policymakers, investing in pharmacological cessation especially when delivered alongside behavioural support offers a cost-effective opportunity to reduce the long-term burden of ST-related diseases.

Finally, from both a public health and clinical dentistry perspective, pharmacological interventions offer unique value in mitigating the substantial oral health harms associated with ST use. When implemented effectively, these tools serve a dual function: preventing the onset of ST-related oral diseases and supporting recovery among those already affected. In doing so, they align with the broader goals of universal health coverage and the integration of non-communicable disease prevention into primary care systems.

Closing the gap between what we know and what we do in ST cessation will require bold, coordinated action. With the right investments in research, policy, and system capacity, pharmacological interventions can move from the margins to the mainstream of global tobacco control strategies delivering both health gains and equity in the fight against ST.

Key Points

- Combining pharmacological and behavioural interventions offers superior outcomes for ST cessation compared to either approach alone, especially in low-resource settings.
- Although NRT and varenicline show promise, there is a critical shortage of high-quality, culturally relevant RCTs specific to ST users.
- Widespread use of pharmacological interventions is hindered by challenges such as cost, availability, lack of provider training, and weak health system integration, particularly in LMICs.
- When embedded into primary and oral healthcare services, pharmacological interventions may reduce ST-related morbidity, aligning with broader goals of universal health coverage and non-communicable disease prevention.

References

Arora S, Gupta S (2019) Monitoring tobacco use and prevention policies: perspective of WHO report on the global tobacco epidemic, 2017. J Nurs Sci Pract 9:39–45

Arora M, Madhu R (2012) Banning smokeless tobacco in India: policy analysis. Indian J Cancer 49:336–341

Aryanpur M, Hosseini M, Masjedi MR, Mortaz E, Tabarsi P, Soori H, Emami H, Heidari G, Dizagie MK, Baikpour M (2016) A randomized controlled trial of smoking cessation methods in patients newly-diagnosed with pulmonary tuberculosis. BMC Infect Dis 16:369. https://doi.org/10.1186/s12879-016-1727-4

Aung MN, Yuasa M, Moolphate S, Kitajima T, Fukuda H, Lorga T, Marui E (2016) Challenges for smoking cessation intervention as part of primary health care services in developing countries. J Smok Cessat 11:211–218

Ayo-Yusuf OA, Burns DM (2012) The complexity of 'harm reduction'with smokeless tobacco as an approach to tobacco control in low-income and middle-income countries. Tob Control 21:245–251

Balfour D (2001) The pharmacology underlying pharmacotherapy for tobacco dependence: a focus on bupropion. Int J Clin Pract 55:53–57. https://doi.org/10.1111/j.1742-1241.2001.tb10974.x

Baraona LK, Lovelace D, Daniels JL, McDaniel L (2017) Tobacco harms, nicotine pharmacology, and pharmacologic tobacco cessation interventions for women. J Midwifery Womens Health 62:253–269. https://doi.org/10.1111/jmwh.12616

Benowitz NL (2010) Nicotine addiction. N Engl J Med 362:2295–2303. https://doi.org/10.1056/NEJMra0809890

Benowitz NL, Porchet H, Sheiner L, Jacob P (1988) Nicotine absorption and cardiovascular effects with smokeless tobacco use: comparison with cigarettes and nicotine gum. Clin Pharmacol Ther 44:23–28. https://doi.org/10.1038/clpt.1988.107

Bonevski B, Borland R, Paul CL, Richmond RL, Farrell M, Baker A, Gartner CE, Lawn S, Thomas DP, Walker N (2017) No smoker left behind: it's time to tackle tobacco in Australian priority populations. Med J Aust 207:141–142

Brett K, Yeung SS, Ford C (2019) Pharmacist-led interventions for tobacco smoking cessation: a review of clinical effectiveness and cost-effectiveness. Canadian Agency for Drugs and Technologies in Health, Ottawa

Carson K, Jayasinghe H, Smith B, Newchurch J, Brinn M, Veale A, Peters M, Esterman A, Singh K (2014) Smoking cessation and tobacco prevention in indigenous populations. Evid Base J Evid Rev Key Policy Areas 2014:1–55

Chan HL, Chan AKY, Chu CH, Tsang YC (2023) Smoking cessation in dental setting: a narrative review on dental professionals' attitude, preparedness, practices and barriers. Front Oral Health 4. https://doi.org/10.3389/froh.2023.1266467

Chen L-S, Zawertailo L, Piasecki TM, Kaprio J, Foreman M, Elliott HR, David SP, Bergen AW, Baurley JW, Tyndale RF (2018) Leveraging genomic data in smoking cessation trials in the era of precision medicine: why and how. Nicotine Tob Res 20:414–424

Chugh A, Arora M, Jain N, Vidyasagaran A, Readshaw A, Sheikh A, Eckhardt J, Siddiqi K, Chopra M, Mishu MP (2023) The global impact of tobacco control policies on smokeless tobacco use: a systematic review. Lancet Glob Health 11:e953–e968

Claire R, Chamberlain C, Davey M-A, Cooper SE, Berlin I, Leonardi-Bee J, Coleman T (2020) Pharmacological interventions for promoting smoking cessation during pregnancy. Cochrane Database Syst Rev 3:CD010078

Cornuz J, Zwahlen S, Jungi WF, Osterwalder J, Klingler K, van Melle G, Bangala Y, Guessous I, Müller P, Willers J (2008) A vaccine against nicotine for smoking cessation: a randomized controlled trial. PLoS One 3:e2547

Croucher R, Islam S, Jarvis MJ, Garrett M, Rahman R, Shajahan S, Howells G (2003) Oral tobacco cessation with UK resident Bangladeshi women: a community pilot investigation. Health Educ Res 18:216–223

Dale LC, Ebbert JO, Schroeder DR, Croghan IT, Rasmussen DF, Trautman JA, Cox LS, Hurt RD (2002) Bupropion for the treatment of nicotine dependence in spit tobacco users: a pilot study. Nicotine Tob Res 4:267–274

Dale LC, Ebbert JO, Glover ED, Croghan IT, Schroeder DR, Severson HH, Hurt RD (2007) Bupropion SR for the treatment of smokeless tobacco use. Drug Alcohol Depend 90:56–63

Danaher BG, Severson HH, Crowley R, van Meter N, Tyler MS, Widdop C, Lichtenstein E, Ebbert JO (2015) Randomized controlled trial examining the adjunctive use of nicotine lozenges with MyLastDip: an eHealth smokeless tobacco cessation intervention. Internet Interv 2:69–76

de Geus J-L, Wambier L-M, Loguercio A-D, Reis A (2019) The smokeless tobacco habit and DNA damage: a systematic review and meta-analysis. Med Oral Patol Oral Cir Bucal 24:e145

de Oca MM, Laucho-Contreras ME (2023) Smoking cessation and vaccination. Eur Respir Rev 32:220187

Dwoskin LP, Rauhut AS, King-Pospisil KA, Bardo MT (2006) Review of the pharmacology and clinical profile of bupropion, an antidepressant and tobacco use cessation agent. CNS Drug Rev 12:178–207. https://doi.org/10.1111/j.1527-3458.2006.00178.x

Ebbert JO, Fagerstrom K (2012) Pharmacological interventions for the treatment of smokeless tobacco use. CNS Drugs 26:1–10. https://doi.org/10.2165/11598450-000000000-00000

Ebbert JO, Patten CA, Schroeder DR (2006) The Fagerström test for nicotine dependence-smokeless tobacco (FTND-ST). Addict Behav 31:1716–1721

Ebbert JO, Dale LC, Patten CA, Croghan IT, Schroeder DR, Moyer TP, Hurt RD (2007) Effect of high-dose nicotine patch therapy on tobacco withdrawal symptoms among smokeless tobacco users. Nicotine Tob Res 9:43–52

Ebbert JO, Severson HH, Croghan IT, Danaher BG, Schroeder DR (2009) A randomized clinical trial of nicotine lozenge for smokeless tobacco use. Nicotine Tob Res 11:1415–1423

Ebbert JO, Severson HH, Croghan IT, Danaher BG, Schroeder DR (2010) A pilot study of mailed nicotine lozenges with assisted self-help for the treatment of smokeless tobacco users. Addict Behav 35:522–525

Ebbert JO, Croghan IT, Severson HH, Schroeder DR, Hays JT (2011) A pilot study of the efficacy of varenicline for the treatment of smokeless tobacco users in Midwestern United States. Nicotine Tob Res 13:820–826

Ebbert JO, Croghan IT, Schroeder DR, Hurt RD (2013a) A randomized phase II clinical trial of high-dose nicotine patch therapy for smokeless tobacco users. Nicotine Tob Res 15:2037–2044

Ebbert JO, Severson HH, Croghan IT, Danaher BG, Schroeder DR (2013b) Comparative effectiveness of the nicotine lozenge and tobacco-free snuff for smokeless tobacco reduction. Addict Behav 38:2140–2145

Ebbert JO, Elrashidi MY, Stead LF (2015) Interventions for smokeless tobacco use cessation. Cochrane Database Syst Rev 2015:CD004306

Fagerstrom K (2008) Varenicline in the treatment of tobacco dependence. Neuropsychiatr Dis Treat 4(2):353–363. https://doi.org/10.2147/NDT.S927

Fagerström K, Gilljam H, Metcalfe M, Tonstad S, Messig M (2010) Stopping smokeless tobacco with varenicline: randomised double blind placebo controlled trial. BMJ 341:c6549

Farhadmollashahi L (2014) Sociocultural reasons for smokeless tobacco use behavior. Int J High Risk Behav Addict 3:e20002

Fiore, M., 2009. Treating tobacco use and dependence: 2008 update: clinical practice guideline. Diane Publishing

Ganz O, Delnevo CD (2020) Young adults as a tobacco control priority population in the US. JAMA Netw Open 3:e2019365–e2019365

Glover ED, Glover PN, Sullivan CR, Cerullo CL, Hobbs G (2002) A comparison of sustained-release bupropion and placebo for smokeless tobacco cessation. Am J Health Behav 26:386–393

Glover ED, Nilsson F, Westin Å, Glover PN, Laflin MT, Persson B (2014) Glover-Nilsson smoking behavioral questionnaire. Am J Health Behav 29:443–455

Gourlay SG, Benowitz NL (1995) Is clonidine an effective smoking cessation therapy? Drugs 50:197–207. https://doi.org/10.2165/00003495-199550020-00001

Gourlay S, Forbes A, Marriner T, Kutin J, McNeil J (1994) A placebo-controlled study of three clonidine doses for smoking cessation. Clin Pharmacol Ther 55:64–69. https://doi.org/10.1038/clpt.1994.11

Guillem K, Vouillac C, Azar MR, Parsons LH, Koob GF, Cador M, Stinus L (2005) Monoamine oxidase inhibition dramatically increases the motivation to self-administer nicotine in rats. J Neurosci 25:8593–8600

Gupta B, Johnson NW (2014) Systematic review and meta-analysis of association of smokeless tobacco and of betel quid without tobacco with incidence of oral cancer in South Asia and the Pacific. PLoS One 9:e113385

Gupta PC, Pednekar MS, Parkin DM, Sankaranarayanan R (2005) Tobacco associated mortality in Mumbai (Bombay) India. Results of the Bombay cohort study. Int J Epidemiol 34:1395–1402

Gupta S, Gupta R, Sinha DN, Mehrotra R (2018) Relationship between type of smokeless tobacco & risk of cancer: a systematic review. Indian J Med Res 148:56–76

Haddad A, Davis AM (2016) Tobacco smoking cessation in adults and pregnant women: behavioral and pharmacotherapy interventions. JAMA 315:2011–2012

Hajat C, Stein E, Ramstrom L, Shantikumar S, Polosa R (2021) The health impact of smokeless tobacco products: a systematic review. Harm Reduct J 18:123. https://doi.org/10.1186/s12954-021-00557-6

Hatsukami D, Jensen J, Allen S, Grillo M, Bliss R (1996) Effects of behavioral and pharmacological treatment on smokeless tobacco users. J Consult Clin Psychol 64:153

Hatsukami DK, Grillo M, Boyle R, Allen S, Jensen J, Bliss R, Brown S (2000) Treatment of spit tobacco users with transdermal nicotine system and mint snuff. J Consult Clin Psychol 68:241

Hatsukami DK, Stead LF, Gupta PC (2008) Tobacco addiction. Lancet 371:2027–2038

Hays JT, Ebbert JO (2008) Varenicline for tobacco dependence. N Engl J Med 359:2018–2024. https://doi.org/10.1056/NEJMct0800146

Heatherton TF, Kozlowski LT, Frecker RC, Fagerstrom K (1991) The Fagerström test for nicotine dependence: a revision of the fagerstrom tolerance questionnaire. Br J Addict 86:1119–1127. https://doi.org/10.1111/j.1360-0443.1991.tb01879.x

Hecht SS, Hatsukami DK (2022) Smokeless tobacco and cigarette smoking: chemical mechanisms and cancer prevention. Nat Rev Cancer 22:143–155

Henningfield JE, Keenan RM (1993) Nicotine delivery kinetics and abuse liability. J Consult Clin Psychol 61:743

Henningfield JE, Slade J (1998) Tobacco-dependence medications: public health and regulatory issues. Food Drug LJ 53:75

Higgins JP, Savović J, Page MJ, Elbers RG, Sterne JA (2019) Assessing risk of bias in a randomized trial. In: Higgins JPT, Thomas J, Chandler J, Cumpston M, Li T, Page MJ, Welch VA (eds) Cochrane handbook for systematic reviews of interventions. Wiley, pp 205–228. https://doi.org/10.1002/9781119536604.ch8

Howard-Pitney B, Killen JD, Fortmann SP (1999) Quitting chew: results from a randomized trial using nicotine patches. Exp Clin Psychopharmacol 7:362

Huque R, Zaman MM, Huq SM, Sinha DN (2017) Smokeless tobacco and public health in Bangladesh. Indian J Public Health 61:18–24

IARC (2023) IARC handbooks on cancer prevention. IARC Handb Cancer Prev 19:1–358

Jain R, Jhanjee S, Jain V, Gupta T, Mittal S, Goelz P, Wileyto EP, Schnoll RA (2014) A double-blind placebo-controlled randomized trial of varenicline for smokeless tobacco dependence in India. Nicotine Tob Res 16:50–57

Kishore SP, Bitton A, Cravioto A, Yach D (2010) Enabling access to new WHO essential medicines: the case for nicotine replacement therapies. Glob Health 6:22. https://doi.org/10.1186/1744-8603-6-22

Kumbhalwar A, Hegde S, Kakodkar P, Mehta V, Gupte H, Jadhav S (2022) Effectiveness of behavioral counseling in smokeless tobacco cessation among adult users reporting to a dental hospital in Pune: a randomized controlled trial. Cureus 14(4):e24041

Livingstone-Banks J, Vidyasagaran AL, Croucher R, Siddiqui F, Zhu S, Kidwai Z, Parkhouse T, Mehrotra R, Siddiqi K (2025) Interventions for smokeless tobacco use cessation. Cochrane Database Syst Rev 4(4):CD015314

Ma C, Xi B, Li Z, Wu H, Zhao M, Liang Y, Bovet P (2021) Prevalence and trends in tobacco use among adolescents aged 13–15 years in 143 countries, 1999–2018: findings from the Global Youth Tobacco Surveys. Lancet Child Adolesc Health 5:245–255

Macedo AS, Castro PM, Roque L, Thomé NG, Reis CP, Pintado ME, Fonte P (2020) Novel and revisited approaches in nanoparticle systems for buccal drug delivery. J Control Release 320:125–141. https://doi.org/10.1016/j.jconrel.2020.01.006

McChargue DE, Collins FL Jr (1998) Differentiating withdrawal patterns between smokers and smokeless tobacco users. Exp Clin Psychopharmacol 6:205

McInerney TF (2019) The WHO FCTC and global governance: effects and implications for future global public health instruments. Tob Control 28:s89–s93

Mehrotra R, Yadav A, Sinha DN, Parascandola M, John RM, Ayo-Yusuf O, Nargis N, Hatsukami DK, Warnakulasuriya S, Straif K, Siddiqi K, Gupta PC (2019) Smokeless tobacco control in 180 countries across the globe: call to action for full implementation of WHO FCTC measures. Lancet Oncol 20:e208–e217. https://doi.org/10.1016/S1470-2045(19)30084-1

Molyneux A (2004) Nicotine replacement therapy. BMJ 328:454–456

Moolchan ET, Ernst M, Henningfield JE (2000) A review of tobacco smoking in adolescents: treatment implications. J Am Acad Child Adolesc Psychiatry 39:682–693

Mukherjea A, Modayil MV, Tong EK (2018) Moving toward a true depiction of tobacco behavior among Asian Indians in California: prevalence and factors associated with cultural smokeless tobacco product use. Cancer 124:1607–1613. https://doi.org/10.1002/cncr.31102

Mungia R, Gelfond JA, Valenzuela EJ, Sangdahl CE, Taverna M, Farokhi MR (2025) Understanding dental practitioners' knowledge and practices of smokeless tobacco: South Texas Oral Health Network study. Patient Educ Couns 130:108448

Nadkarni A, Gaikwad L, Sequeira M, Javeri P, Benoy D, Pacheco MG, Velleman R, Murthy P, Naughton F (2025) Behavioral interventions for tobacco cessation in low-and middle-income countries: a systematic review and meta-analysis. Nicotine Tob Res 27:575–585

Nemeth JM, Liu ST, Klein EG, Ferketich AK, Kwan M-P, Wewers ME (2012) Factors influencing smokeless tobacco use in rural Ohio Appalachia. J Community Health 37:1208–1217. https://doi.org/10.1007/s10900-012-9556-x

Nethan ST, Sinha DN, Chandan K, Mehrotra R (2018) Smokeless tobacco cessation interventions: a systematic review. Indian J Med Res 148:396–410

Nides M (2008) Update on pharmacologic options for smoking cessation treatment. Am J Med 121:S20–S31

Noonan D, Silva SG, Fish LJ, Simmons LA, Nwankwo N, Scherr K, Da Costa M, Sang E, Sanders C, Swinkels C (2025) Randomized controlled trial of a text-based smokeless tobacco cessation intervention for rural and medically underserved communities. Nicotine Tob Res 27:132–142

Orlandi MA, Boyd G (1989) Smokeless tobacco use among adolescents: a theoretical overview. NCI Monogr 8:5–12

Osibogun O, Bursac Z, Mckee M, Li T, Maziak W (2020) Cessation outcomes in adult dual users of e-cigarettes and cigarettes: the population assessment of tobacco and health cohort study, USA, 2013–2016. Int J Public Health 65:923–936. https://doi.org/10.1007/s00038-020-01436-w

Perkins KA, Conklin CA, Levine MD (2013) Cognitive-behavioral therapy for smoking cessation: a practical guidebook to the most effective treatments. Routledge

Persaud N, Jiang M, Shaikh R, Bali A, Oronsaye E, Woods H, Drozdzal G, Rajakulasingam Y, Maraj D, Wadhawan S (2019) Comparison of essential medicines lists in 137 countries. Bull World Health Organ 97:394

Pickworth WB, Rosenberry ZR, Gold W, Koszowski B (2014) Nicotine absorption from smokeless tobacco modified to adjust pH. J Addict Res Ther 5:1000184

Pradhan S, Priyadarshini SR, Panda S, Misra SR, Panigrahi R, Choudhury BK (2025) Efficacy of pharmacological intervention for smokeless tobacco cessation in adults: a systematic review and meta-analysis. Arch Public Health 83:105

Puljević C, Feulner L, Hobbs M, Erku D, Bonevski B, Segan C, Baker A, Hefler M, Cho A, Gartner C (2024a) Tobacco endgame and priority populations: a scoping review. Tob Control 33:e231–e239

Puljević C, Stjepanović D, Meciar I, Kang H, Chan G, Morphett K, Bendotti H, Kunwar G, Gartner C (2024b) Systematic review and meta-analyses of cytisine to support tobacco cessation. Addiction 119:1713–1725. https://doi.org/10.1111/add.16592

Rasool S, Holliday R, Khan Z, Dobbie F, Bauld L (2024) Behavior change intervention for smokeless tobacco cessation delivered through dentists in dental settings: a pragmatic pilot trial. Nicotine Tob Res 26:878–887

Rath JM, Villanti AC, Abrams DB, Vallone DM (2012) Patterns of tobacco use and dual use in us young adults: the missing link between youth prevention and adult cessation. J Environ Public Health 2012:1–9. https://doi.org/10.1155/2012/679134

Rigotti NA, Benowitz NL, Prochaska J, Leischow S, Nides M, Blumenstein B, Clarke A, Cain D, Jacobs C (2023) Cytisinicline for smoking cessation: a randomized clinical trial. JAMA 330:152–160

Russo P, Nastrucci C, Alzetta G, Szalai C (2011) Tobacco habit: historical, cultural, neurobiological, and genetic features of people's relationship with an addictive drug. Perspect Biol Med 54:557–577

Schiller KR, Luo X, Anderson AJ, Jensen JA, Allen SS, Hatsukami DK (2012) Comparing an immediate cessation versus reduction approach to smokeless tobacco cessation. Nicotine Tob Res 14:902–909

Scott-Sheldon LA, Lantini RC, Jennings EG, Thind H, Rosen RK, Salmoirago-Blotcher E, Bock BC (2016) Text messaging-based interventions for smoking cessation: a systematic review and meta-analysis. JMIR Mhealth Uhealth 4:e5436

Severson HH, Danaher BG, Ebbert JO, Van Meter N, Lichtenstein E, Widdop C, Crowley R, Akers L, Seeley JR (2015) Randomized trial of nicotine lozenges and phone counseling for smokeless tobacco cessation. Nicotine Tob Res 17:309–315

Shang X, Guo K, E F, Deng X, Wang Y, Wang Z, Wu Y, Xu M, Yang C, Li X (2022) Pharmacological interventions on smoking cessation: a systematic review and network meta-analysis. Front Pharmacol 13:1012433

Shiffman S, Waters AJ, Hickcox M (2004) The nicotine dependence syndrome scale: a multidimensional measure of nicotine dependence. Nicotine Tob Res 6:327–348

Siddiqi K, Shah S, Abbas SM, Vidyasagaran A, Jawad M, Dogar O, Sheikh A (2015) Global burden of disease due to smokeless tobacco consumption in adults: analysis of data from 113 countries. BMC Med 13:194. https://doi.org/10.1186/s12916-015-0424-2

Siddiqi K, Husain S, Vidyasagaran A, Readshaw A, Mishu MP, Sheikh A (2020) Global burden of disease due to smokeless tobacco consumption in adults: an updated analysis of data from 127 countries. BMC Med 18:222. https://doi.org/10.1186/s12916-020-01677-9

Siddiqui F, Kanaan M, Croucher R, Bauld L, Fieroze F, Kumar P, Mazhar L, Pandey V, Jackson C, Huque R, Iqbal R, Siddiqi K, ASTRA Global Health Research Group (2024) Behavioural support and nicotine replacement therapy for smokeless tobacco cessation in Bangladesh, India and Pakistan: a pilot randomized controlled trial. Addiction 119:1366–1377. https://doi.org/10.1111/add.16515

Singh PK (2014) Smokeless tobacco use and public health in countries of South-East Asia Region. Indian J Cancer 51:1

Sinha DN, Palipudi KM, Gupta PC, Singhal S, Ramasundarahettige C, Jha P, Indrayan A, Asma S, Vendhan G (2014) Smokeless tobacco use: a meta-analysis of risk and attributable mortality estimates for India. Indian J Cancer 51:S73–S77

Sinha DN, Kumar A, Bhartiya D, Sharma S, Gupta PC, Singh H, Mehrotra R (2017) Smokeless tobacco use among adolescents in global perspective. Nicotine Tob Res 19:1395–1396

Solhi M, Fattahi E, Manzari ZS, Gupta PC, Kargar M, Kasmei P, Barati H (2021) The reasons for using smokeless tobacco: a review. Iran J Public Health 50:492–501. https://doi.org/10.18502/ijph.v50i3.5589

Stanton CA, Halenar MJ (2018) Patterns and correlates of multiple tobacco product use in the United States. Nicotine Tob Res 20:S1–S4

Stepanov I, Jensen J, Hatsukami D, Hecht SS (2008) New and traditional smokeless tobacco: comparison of toxicant and carcinogen levels. Nicotine Tob Res 10:1773–1782. https://doi.org/10.1080/14622200802443544

Stitzer ML (1999) Combined behavioral and pharmacological treatments for smoking cessation. Nicotine Tob Res 1:S181–S187

Stotts RC, Roberson PK, Hanna EY, Jones SK, Smith CK (2003) A randomised clinical trial of nicotine patches for treatment of spit tobacco addiction among adolescents. Tob Control 12:iv11–iv15. https://doi.org/10.1136/tc.12.suppl_4.iv11

Su Z, Wei X, Cheng A, Zhou X, Li J, Qin R, Liu Y, Xia X, Song Q, Liu Z (2023) Utilization and effectiveness of a message-based tobacco cessation program (mCessation) in the Chinese general population: longitudinal, real-world study. J Med Internet Res 25:e44840

Sweet L, Brasky TM, Cooper S, Doogan N, Hinton A, Klein EG, Nagaraja H, Quisenberry A, Xi W, Wewers ME (2019) Quitting behaviors among dual cigarette and e-cigarette users and cigarette smokers enrolled in the tobacco user adult cohort. Nicotine Tob Res 21:278–284

Thakur J, Choudhari SG (2024) Effectiveness of healthcare interventions on smoking cessation in adolescents in low-and middle-income countries: a narrative review. Cureus 16(2):e54051

Thomas KH, Dalili MN, López-López JA, Keeney E, Phillippo DM, Munafò MR, Stevenson M, Caldwell DM, Welton NJ (2022) Comparative clinical effectiveness and safety of tobacco cessation pharmacotherapies and electronic cigarettes: a systematic review and network meta-analysis of randomized controlled trials. Addiction 117:861–876. https://doi.org/10.1111/add.15675

Trigg J, Skelton E, Lum A, Guillaumier A, McCarter K, Handley T, Judd L, Lye A, Bonevski B (2023) Smoking cessation interventions and abstinence outcomes for people living in rural, regional, and remote areas of three high-income countries: a systematic review. Nicotine Tob Res 25:1709–1718

Tutka P, Vinnikov D, Courtney RJ, Benowitz NL (2019) Cytisine for nicotine addiction treatment: a review of pharmacology, therapeutics and an update of clinical trial evidence for smoking cessation. Addiction 114:1951–1969. https://doi.org/10.1111/add.14721

Wadgave U, Nagesh L (2016) Nicotine replacement therapy: an overview. Int J Health Sci 10:425

Walker N, Howe C, Glover M, McRobbie H, Barnes J, Nosa V, Parag V, Bassett B, Bullen C (2014) Cytisine versus nicotine for smoking cessation. N Engl J Med 371:2353–2362. https://doi.org/10.1056/NEJMoa1407764

Walsh MM, Hilton JF, Masouredis CM, Gee L, Chesney MA, Ernster VL (1999) Smokeless tobacco cessation intervention for college athletes: results after 1 year. Am J Public Health 89:228–234. https://doi.org/10.2105/AJPH.89.2.228

Wang J, Shen H (2009) Review of cigarette smoking and tuberculosis in China: intervention is needed for smoking cessation among tuberculosis patients. BMC Public Health 9:292. https://doi.org/10.1186/1471-2458-9-292

Wei H, Young D (1988) Effect of clonidine on cigarette cessation and in the alleviation of withdrawal symptoms. Br J Addict 83:1221–1226. https://doi.org/10.1111/j.1360-0443.1988.tb03029.x

Wheeler KC, Fletcher KE, Wellman RJ, Difranza JR (2004) Screening adolescents for nicotine dependence: the hooked on nicotine checklist. J Adolesc Health 35:225–230

WHO (2008) MPOWER: a policy package to reverse the tobacco epidemic

WHO (2021a) WHO report on the global tobacco epidemic, 2021: addressing new and emerging products: executive summary. In: WHO report on the global tobacco epidemic, 2021: addressing new and emerging products: executive summary

WHO (2021b) WHO model list of essential medicines—22nd List

WHO (2021c) WHO report on the global tobacco epidemic 2021

WHO (2023) WHO model list of essential medicines–23rd list, 2023

WHO (2024a) WHO clinical treatment guideline for tobacco cessation in adults. World Health Organization

WHO (2024b) WHO global report on trends in prevalence of tobacco use 2000–2030. World Health Organization

WHO FCTC (2005) Framework Convention on Tobacco Control (FCTC). WHO, Geneva

Zaatari GS, Bazzi A (2019) Impact of the WHO FCTC on non-cigarette tobacco products. Tob Control 28:s104–s112

Behavioural Interventions for Smokeless Tobacco Cessation

13

Shaista Rasool and Richard Holliday

Abbreviations

BCT	Behavior Change Technique
BCT Taxonomy v1	Behavior Change Technique Taxonomy version 1
CONSORT	Consolidated Standards of Reporting Trials
COPD	Chronic Obstructive Pulmonary Disease
FCTC	Framework Convention on Tobacco Control
LMICs	Low- and Middle-Income Countries
MI	Motivational Interviewing
NCSCT	NHS Centre for Smoking Cessation and Training
RCT	Randomized Controlled Trial
TPB	Theory of Planned Behavior
TTM	Transtheoretical Model
U.S.	United States
VBA	Very Brief Advice
WHO	World Health Organization

Behavioural Interventions for ST Cessation

S. Rasool
Institute of Public Health and Social Sciences, Khyber Medical University, Peshawar, Pakistan
e-mail: drshaista.iph@kmu.edu.pk

R. Holliday (✉)
School of Dental Sciences, Faculty of Medical Sciences, Newcastle University, Newcastle upon Tyne, UK
e-mail: richard.holliday@newcastle.ac.uk

F. Javed, S. Warnakulasuriya (eds.), *Smokeless Tobacco and its Effects on Periodontal Health*, https://doi.org/10.1007/978-3-032-16409-4_13

Learning Goals

- *Understand the public health burden of smokeless tobacco (ST) use*: Gain insight into the prevalence and health consequences of smokeless tobacco use, especially in South Asia, and its association with oral and systemic diseases.
- *Recognize the role of dental professionals in ST cessation*: Appreciate the unique position of dental professionals in identifying tobacco-related oral lesions and delivering cessation interventions.
- *Differentiate between behavioural intervention strategies*: Learn the distinctions among various behavioural approaches such as brief advice, motivational interviewing, individual and group counselling, and self-help strategies.
- *Comprehend the theoretical frameworks underpinning behavioural interventions*: Explore behaviour change theories like the Transtheoretical Model and Social Cognitive Theory that inform the design of tobacco cessation interventions.
- *Identify and apply behaviour change techniques:* Understand the significance of BCTs in intervention design and delivery, and how identifying specific techniques enhances reproducibility and effectiveness.
- *Assess the evidence base and effectiveness of ST cessation interventions:* Review the current evidence from Cochrane reviews and clinical trials on the efficacy of behavioural interventions in both high-income and low-resource settings.
- *Analyse barriers to implementation in dental and low- and middle-income countries:* Identify practical constraints such as lack of time, space, and cultural stigmas that affect intervention delivery in low- and middle-income countries.
- *Evaluate the feasibility and impact of telephone and self-help interventions:* Understand how telephone-based counselling and self-help materials serve as scalable, cost-effective cessation tools.
- *Explore emerging and alternative behavioural strategies;* Examine the potential role of culturally integrated approaches like yogic breathing and physical activity in supporting cessation.
- *Develop context-specific, scalable cessation strategies:* Learn how to adapt and implement behavioural interventions tailored to local sociocultural and infrastructural realities, particularly in high-burden countries.

13.1 Background

Cessation of smokeless tobacco (ST) use poses unique challenges due to the wide variation in product types, patterns of use, and health risks across regions. Interventions for ST cessation typically involve behavioural support, pharmacotherapy, or a combination of both (Livingstone-Banks et al. 2025). However, the diversity of ST products, such as gutkha/gutka/ghutka, naswar, paan (betel-quid), zarda, and khaini in South Asia; and Swedish snus in Northern Europe, complicates both the design of cessation strategies and the generalizability of global research. For instance, ST products used in South Asia and some parts of Africa often contain high levels of bioavailable nicotine, making them particularly addictive, and are significantly associated with oral cancers and periodontal disease (Coyle et al. 2024; Javed et al. 2008, 2010, 2013, 2015; Palipudi et al. 2014; Siddiqi et al. 2015). These regional differences in both product composition and health burden highlight the need for context-specific intervention strategies.

While evidence is beginning to emerge from South Asia, including trials evaluating dentist-delivered behavioural interventions (Kumbhalwar et al. 2022; Rasool et al. 2024c), the majority of research to date still comes from high-income countries, especially the United States. The latest Cochrane review of smokeless tobacco cessation interventions (Livingstone-Banks et al. 2025) included only two studies conducted in dental settings from South Asia (Kumbhalwar et al. 2022; Rasool et al. 2024c). Whereas the latest Cochrane review on tobacco cessation interventions delivered by dental professionals (Holliday et al. 2021) included six trials on smokeless tobacco, all conducted in the United States. Not a single study from South Asia was represented highlighting a persistent gap in regionally relevant evidence within the global literature. This lack of regional representation limits the applicability of findings in the very settings where the need is most urgent.

Within clinical settings, dental professionals are uniquely positioned to contribute to tobacco cessation. Dental practitioners are often the first to observe any oral changes associated with tobacco use, including staining, leukoplakia, gingival recession, and mucosal lesions. More than 60% of tobacco users visit a dentist or dental hygienist annually, offering opportunities for brief interventions or referrals to cessation services. In alignment with the World Health Organization (WHO) Framework Convention on Tobacco Control (FCTC) Article 14, all dental professionals are encouraged to incorporate cessation support into routine care. Evidence, including findings from a Cochrane review (Holliday et al. 2021), suggests that tobacco cessation interventions delivered by dental professionals can significantly increase quit rates, though results vary based on intervention intensity and delivery context.

Key Points

- The wide variation in smokeless tobacco (ST) products, such as gutkha, naswar, paan, and khaini in South Asia, and snus in Northern Europe complicates cessation strategies due to differences in composition, nicotine content, and health risks.
- ST products in South Asia are highly addictive due to high levels of bioavailable nicotine and are strongly associated with oral cancers and periodontal disease.
- Most ST cessation research has been conducted in high-income countries, particularly the United States, while South Asia remains underrepresented in global literature, limiting the applicability of existing evidence to high-burden regions.
- Dentists and dental hygienists are often the first to detect tobacco-related oral health issues.
- The Cochrane reviews on ST cessation and dental professional-delivered interventions highlight a dearth of studies from South Asia, reinforcing the urgent need for region-specific research.
- Due to cultural, logistical, and infrastructural constraints in South Asia, there is a pressing need for contextually relevant, feasible, and effective behavioural interventions that can be integrated into routine dental practice.

In this chapter, we explore the role of dental settings in supporting ST cessation, with a focus on behavioural interventions. We examine existing evidence, and also touch upon the practical implementation barriers and opportunities for integrating cessation support into routine dental care.

13.1.1 How Do Behavioural Interventions Work?

Tobacco dependency is classified by the Diagnostic and Statistical Manual of Mental Disorder's (DSM-5) as "tobacco use disorder", which is placed in the same category as other substance use disorders. The diagnosis of the disorder is made on the basis of symptoms such as craving, withdrawal, impaired control over use of the substance, and continued use despite knowledge of health risks (American Psychiatric Association 2013). Understanding these diagnostic criteria is important because the initiation and continued use of tobacco is governed by a complex interplay of biological, psychological, and sociocultural factors. Theories underpinning tobacco use and its cessation are based upon understanding the complex interplay between these proximal determinants of the user's decisions and attempts to quit. Evidence suggests that interventions that are guided by theoretical frameworks are more effective in promoting healthy behaviours as compared to those that are not (Godin et al. 1992). Today, the most popular theories underlying tobacco cessation interventions are behaviour change theories which have their origin in social psychology including "Behaviourism", "Social Cognitive Theory", the "Theory of Planned Behaviour" (TPB), the "Transtheoretical Model" (TTM), and the "Social–Ecological Model". These behaviour change approaches to health promotion focus on the modification of the individual's health-related behaviours and the primary feature of these approaches is a consideration of the role of self-efficacy and motivation and the importance of barriers and facilitators to change, the norms, attitudes, and cues to action (Roberts et al. 2013).

Behavioural interventions for ST cessation are complex and highly context-sensitive, often determined by the type of product, the user's social environment, cultural norms, and level of addiction. A growing body of evidence suggests that the effectiveness of available interventions depends not just on whether support is provided, but how it is delivered, in other words, on the specific components that make up the intervention. These components, known as Behaviour Change Techniques (BCTs), are the active ingredients designed to drive behaviour change. They are observable, replicable, and irreducible techniques, such as goal setting, providing feedback, or increasing self-efficacy—that underpin effective interventions (Davidson et al. 2003; Michie et al. 2013). Recognizing and describing these BCTs clearly is critical for both understanding *what works* and for enabling researchers and clinicians to replicate and adapt successful interventions in new settings.

However, a major challenge in synthesizing and applying evidence across studies is that intervention descriptions are often vague or incomplete. While guidelines like the CONSORT recommend that interventions be described in detail (Boutron et al. 2008), the guidelines do not specify what the description should be (Michie et al. 2013).

To address this, researchers have developed BCT taxonomies, structured systems for classifying the techniques used in behavioural interventions. The most comprehensive of these, BCT Taxonomy v1, includes 93 distinct techniques across 16 categories (Michie et al. 2013). While a simple intervention may include just one or two BCTs, most effective tobacco cessation programmes use a combination of 10–20 or more, often blending motivational, cognitive, and environmental strategies (Black et al. 2020; de Bruin et al. 2021).

Key Points

- Tobacco use is classified as a substance use disorder in the DSM-5, characterized by symptoms such as craving, withdrawal, and continued use despite health risks.
- Behavioural interventions are more effective when grounded in behaviour change theories such as Behaviourism, Social Cognitive Theory, Theory of Planned Behaviour, Transtheoretical Model, and Social–Ecological Model.
- Interventions must account for contextual factors, including the type of smokeless tobacco product used, cultural norms, and levels of addiction.
- Effective interventions use specific, observable, and replicable techniques known as BCTs, such as goal setting or feedback.

- Many studies fail to adequately describe the components of their interventions, which hinders replication and limits understanding of what works and why.
- Tools like the BCT Taxonomy v1 help classify intervention techniques system.
- Most effective interventions combine multiple BCTs, blending motivational, cognitive, and environmental strategies to address the multifaceted nature of tobacco addiction.

In the context of ST cessation, especially in dental or low-resource settings, clearly identifying which BCTs are used allows us to better assess which techniques are most feasible and effective, and how they might be tailored to the sociocultural and clinical realities of different populations. For example, knowing whether an intervention focused on "problem solving" versus "social support" can help practitioners replicate or adapt that approach in culturally appropriate ways. In summary, understanding and reporting BCTs is essential for translating evidence into practice. Especially in regions like South Asia, where most ST users reside and resources are limited, knowing what works and how to reproduce it is crucial for scaling effective cessation support. In the following section, we will explore different types of behavioural interventions for ST cessation.

13.1.2 Brief Avice

Brief advice from health professionals has been shown to increase quit attempts and is recommended for all patients using any form of tobacco (Aveyard et al. 2012; Fiore and Baker 2008). Early efforts by the US National Cancer Institute led to the development of the 4A's model—Ask, Advise, Assist, Arrange—which helped integrate tobacco cessation into routine clinical care (Manley et al. 1992; Solberg et al. 1990). A fifth step, Assess, was later added, forming the widely adopted 5A's model (Fiore and Baker 2008). This structured intervention takes 3–5 min and is considered feasible and effective in primary care settings. The WHO recommends that all health professionals use the 5A's: Ask about tobacco use, Advise users to quit, Assess readiness to quit, Assist with a quit plan or referral, and Arrange follow-up. For patients not ready to quit, the 5R's model—Relevance, Risks, Rewards, Roadblocks, and Repetition—is recommended to enhance motivation, with emphasis tailored to individual barriers or doubts (WHO 2017). Despite its effectiveness, time constraints often limit the delivery of brief advice in clinical practice (McEwen et al. 2012). To address this, a "Very Brief Advice" (VBA) model was developed, emphasizing the 3 A's—Ask, Advise, Act—and taking under 60 s to deliver (Aveyard and West 2007). This approach shifts the focus from assessing motivation to offering help to all tobacco users, highlighting positive support rather than judgment (NHS Centre for Smoking Cessation and Training (NCSCT)).

According to a study conducted in 2025, brief advice is moderately effective in promoting ST cessation compared to no support (Livingstone-Banks et al. 2025). This highlights its value as a simple yet impactful intervention in routine healthcare (Holliday et al. 2021).

The latest Cochrane review on tobacco cessation interventions delivered via dental professionals provides encouraging evidence in favour of brief behavioural interventions. Single-session counselling was associated with a significant increase in quit rates (seven studies; RR 1.86, 95% CI: 1.01–3.34), and multi-session interventions yielded a comparable effect (four studies; RR 1.90, 95% CI: 1.17–3.11), suggesting that extended duration may not always be necessary for effectiveness (Holliday et al. 2021).

Among the six trials on ST via dental professionals, all were conducted in the United States (Andrews et al. 1999; Gansky et al. 2005; Severson et al. 2009; Stevens et al. 1995; Walsh et al. 1999, 2003). These studies were conducted in dental clinics or dental-affiliated settings (including school-based settings). Each study integrated brief advice but were supplemented by additional elements, such as video-based programmes, printed self-help resources, telephone follow-up, or peer-led support, to reinforce quit efforts. Delivery personnel ranged from dentists and dental hygienists to athletic trainers, showing that even in non-specialist dental settings, ST cessation interventions can be effectively incorporated into patient care.

It is important to note that this evidence comes from high-income settings, where referral pathways to dedicated cessation services are well established and often free at the point of care. In contrast, in low- and middle-income countries (LMICs), where the burden of ST use is greatest, such infrastructure is often lacking. Cessation clinics are limited, and where available, the services may not be covered by public health insurance, requiring users to pay out-of-pocket (Rasool et al. 2024a, b). This presents a major barrier to the "Assist" and "Arrange" components of the 5A's model, making referrals difficult or ineffective. In these settings, dental professionals may be the only point of contact for tobacco users, further emphasizing the need for feasible, stand-alone interventions that can be totally delivered within dental clinics.

These issues highlight a critical gap in the global implementation of tobacco cessation guidelines and point to the importance of context-adapted strategies that reflect the healthcare delivery constraints in LMICs. While the US-based evidence illustrates what can work under almost-ideal conditions, it may not be directly applicable in resource-limited environments where cessation systems are underdeveloped or financially inaccessible to patients.

Key Points

- Brief advice is an evidence-based approach that aims to encourage tobacco users to quit by providing them with simple, structured, and effective guidance.
- It typically follows the 3A model—Ask, Advise, and Act—where health-care professionals identify tobacco use, provide clear advice to quit, and assist or refer users for further support.
- Dental professionals are in a unique position to deliver brief advice, particularly because tobacco use has direct and visible effects on oral health.
- Even a short conversation—as little as 30 s to 3 min—can significantly increase the chances of a quit attempt and long-term cessation.
- The use of visual aids, such as clinical photographs of oral lesions and the oral effects of tobacco, can strengthen the message and motivate users to quit.
- The tone of the advice should be non-judgmental, empathetic, and supportive, focusing on the benefits of quitting rather than guilt or blame.
- Brief advice is cost-effective and time-efficient, making it highly feasible for routine incorporation into dental and medical consultations.
- Training in delivering brief advice is essential to build confidence and consistency among dental professionals, ensuring that the intervention is both patient-centred and impactful.

13.1.3 Individual and Group-Based Behavioural Counselling

Evidence supports the effectiveness of individual behavioural counselling in helping people quit ST, with outcomes consistently showing higher quit rates compared to minimal support or usual care (Holliday et al. 2021; Livingstone-Banks et al. 2025). This type of intervention typically involves face-to-face sessions delivered by trained tobacco cessation specialists (Lancaster and Stead 2017; Roberts et al. 2013). This approach is patient-centred and tailored to the user's history of tobacco use, motivational level, and considering risk factors for relapse. Common elements include assessing tobacco use, offering motivation and guidance, identifying high-risk situations, and developing strategies to manage them (Lifrak et al. 1997; Nohlert et al. 2013). Support materials such as written, audio, or video resources are often included, and some follow-up sessions may be conducted via telephone to maintain engagement over time (Tønnesen et al. 2006). In contrast to brief advice, which is often generic and limited in duration, individual counselling allows for a more in-depth exploration of each user's behavioural patterns and motivations. A key strength of this approach lies in its adaptability across stages of change (described by Prochaska), with interventions often designed to support users from pre-contemplation through to maintenance.

Key Points

- Individual behavioural counselling, especially when delivered face-to-face significantly improves quit rates for ST users compared to minimal or usual care.
- This approach is personalized, addressing the user's tobacco history, motivation, and relapse risks, and includes motivation building, identifying high-risk situations, and developing coping strategies.
- Although longer sessions (over 3 h) show consistent results, shorter or single-session interventions, particularly in dental settings, are also effective when contextually tailored and well-integrated into routine care.
- Brief yet structured counselling may be both feasible and effective.

While most evidence for behavioural counselling comes from smoking cessation studies, findings from ST-specific trials reinforce its applicability. For example, counselling interventions delivered in healthcare settings in South Asia, where the majority of the world's ST users reside, have demonstrated positive outcomes in terms of quit rates and reductions in frequency of use (Rasool et al. 2024c; Siddiqui et al. 2024). While subgroup analysis from a recent Cochrane review of behavioural interventions for ST (Livingstone-Banks et al. 2025) suggested that interventions exceeding 3 h in duration yielded more consistent outcomes across trials, this does not imply that shorter interventions are ineffective. On the contrary, findings from another review of interventions delivered via dental professionals (Holliday et al. 2021) showed that both single-session and multi-session behavioural interventions in dental settings produced similar increases in quit rates. This suggests that, in busy clinical environments like dental practices, brief but structured counselling may be both feasible and effective, provided it is contextually relevant and embedded within routine care. The key determinant may not be duration alone, but the quality, skills and enthusiasm of the operator, delivery context, and alignment with patient needs.

It is also worthwhile to mention that the delivery of extended behavioural counselling may face practical limitations in busy dental settings, especially in LMICs, where dental settings face infrastructure limitations, such as a lack of private consultation space, heavy patient loads, and insufficient time to conduct counselling sessions. Social and cultural dynamics also influence feasibility. In South Asia, for example younger patients and women may feel uncomfortable disclosing their use of ST during dental visits, due to stigma, fear of judgement, or concern about repercussions within their families.

This raises important considerations about the feasibility of high-intensity interventions within routine dental care. Rather than arguing against such interventions altogether, these constraints highlight the need to select intervention approaches that align with available resources. For example, brief but structured interventions can still be effective, particularly when delivered consistently and paired with referral pathways or self-help materials.

Importantly, as mentioned earlier, much of the existing evidence on behavioural interventions for ST cessation via dental professionals, originates from high-income countries, particularly the United States, where patterns of use, availability of products, and healthcare infrastructure differ significantly from those in South Asia. Thereby limiting the generalizability of findings to settings where ST use is often more culturally entrenched, socially concealed, and normalized. A recent process evaluation of a pragmatic feasibility trial in Pakistan (Rasool et al. 2024b) highlighted these contextual barriers. The study, conducted in dental hospitals, found that while dentist-delivered behavioural support was well received, dentists struggled with logistical challenges such as time constraints and lack of private space, and patients expressed concerns about confidentiality. Some younger participants even avoided taking printed materials home, fearing family discovery of their tobacco use. Despite these challenges, the intervention led to positive changes in behaviour among those who engaged with it, suggesting that dental professionals in South Asia can play a meaningful role in ST cessation if interventions are tailored to the cultural and clinical realities of their settings. There remains, however, a pressing need for more regionally relevant research to guide the development and implementation of effective cessation strategies in high-burden countries.

Ultimately, the choice between single sessions and more intensive counselling should be guided by clinical context, patient readiness, and system capacity, recognizing that even low-intensity single session interventions can play a meaningful role in prompting quit attempts, particularly in under-resourced or high-burden environments.

Key Points

- Practical and cultural barriers hinder intensive counselling in dental settings, especially in LMICs like South Asia, due to limited infrastructure, time constraints, and sociocultural stigma, particularly among youth and women.
- Tailored brief interventions, when delivered consistently and supported with referral systems or self-help materials, can be effective and more feasible than extended counselling in resource-limited settings.
- Evidence from high-income countries may not generalize to regions like South Asia, where ST use is deeply rooted and socially concealed, underscoring the need for context-specific research.
- Even low-intensity interventions can be impactful, especially when aligned with clinical capacity and patient readiness, offering a viable approach in high-burden, under-resourced environments.

Group-based behavioural counselling has been used less frequently than individual counselling in ST cessation, and evidence from dental settings remains limited. Most documented group counselling interventions have been delivered in general healthcare or community environments, often led by psychologists, health educators, or addiction specialists (Roberts et al. 2013; Stead et al. 2017). This approach offers opportunities for social learning, mutual support, and the sharing of coping strategies. The group dynamics can enhance motivation and accountability, particularly when participants engage with others facing similar challenges (Hajek 1996; Stead et al. 2017). Although group counselling generally requires fewer resources per participant compared to individual sessions, its content still covers core behavioural strategies such as cognitive-behavioural skills training, relapse prevention, and motivational enhancement.

Evidence on group counselling for smoking cessation shows clear benefits over no intervention, self-help materials, and brief advice (Stead et al. 2017). Among young people in particular, group support has shown moderate effectiveness (Fanshawe et al. 2017). While similar trials on ST cessation are fewer, available evidence suggests that group interventions may be as effective as individual counselling, although one trial found no significant difference between the two (Savant et al. 2013). Within dental settings, there is a notable lack of research evaluating the stand-alone effectiveness of group counselling for ST cessation. However, one well-designed, cluster-randomized controlled trial (RCT) from the United States (Gansky et al. 2005) demonstrated how dental professionals can play a key role in a multi-component intervention that includes both individual and group elements. The study targeted male collegiate baseball athletes and incorporated dental oral cancer screenings, brief counselling by dental hygienists, and peer-led education sessions. While the individual counselling component was delivered in dental contexts during preseason health checks, follow-up was conducted by athletic trainers through group booster sessions, where athletes discussed quit attempts, shared coping strategies, and addressed challenges in a supportive environment.

Although the dental professionals delivered care outside traditional dental clinics, the intervention still relied on oral health messaging and brief counselling techniques rooted in dental practice. While the intervention did not significantly increase cessation rates compared to control colleges, it significantly reduced new initiation of ST use, highlighting the preventive value of such efforts.

While group counselling offers potential benefits such as peer reinforcement and cost-effectiveness, it has seen limited implementation in dental care environments, and evidence for its effectiveness in these settings remains scarce. Overall, both individual and group-based behavioural counselling can play important roles in ST cessation strategies; however, in dental settings, individual counselling remains the predominant and more established mode of intervention. The decision to incorporate individual or group-based approaches should be guided by factors such as clinical workflow, practitioner capacity, patient preference, and setting-specific feasibility.

Key Points

- Group-based counselling is used less frequently than individual counselling in ST cessation, and its application in dental settings remains under-researched.
- This approach fosters social learning, peer support, and accountability, and is more resource-efficient per participant compared to individual counselling.
- While group counselling has proven effective for smoking cessation and moderately effective among young people, evidence for ST cessation is limited.
- Despite potential benefits, group counselling is rarely implemented in dental care; and individual counselling remains the preferred method due to factors like clinical feasibility, patient preference, and practitioner capacity.

13.1.4 Motivational Interviewing

Motivational interviewing (MI) is a patient-centred counselling approach that can be delivered in both individual and group formats. As such, it represents a flexible strategy within the broader category of behavioural counselling, offering tailored support whether in one-on-one dental consultations or in peer-group sessions. MI is potentially useful in changing oral health behaviours and has been increasingly applied in dental settings (Gao et al. 2014; Kay et al. 2016). Unlike brief advice, which typically involves delivering generic information and normative guidance, MI adopts a counselling-based strategy aimed at fostering sustained behaviour change. It follows these key steps: engaging (building rapport), focusing (identifying the target behaviour), evoking (helping the patient uncover intrinsic motivation), planning (supporting patients to find their own solutions and set realistic goals with appropriate guidance).

While MI may offer some benefit for smoking cessation (Lindson et al. 2019), its role in ST (ST) cessation, particularly in dental practice, is an emerging area of interest. Some studies suggest that group-based motivational strategies may be more effective than individual counselling, particularly when focused on tobacco-related harms (Patel et al. 2020). Notably, a RCT by Kumbhalwar et al. (2022), conducted in a dental hospital setting in India, demonstrated that participants who received MI-based behavioural counselling were more likely to quit ST compared to those who received only brief advice (Kumbhalwar et al. 2022). The intervention combined personalized counselling with self-help materials and follow-up contact, highlighting the feasibility of incorporating such approaches into routine dental care. These findings suggest that MI, when delivered in dental settings and supported by ongoing behavioural reinforcement, may enhance cessation outcomes for ST users. However, further research is needed to establish the best practices for its implementation and long-term effectiveness.

Key Points

- Motivational interviewing (MI) is a patient-centred counselling method that can be effectively delivered in both individual and group settings.
- While MI shows promise for smoking cessation, its effectiveness in ST cessation within dental settings is a growing area of research.
- A randomized trial from India found that MI-based behavioural counselling, supported by follow-up and self-help tools, led to higher quit rates in ST users, indicating its potential integration into routine dental care.

13.1.5 Quitline and Telephone Counselling

Telephone-based counselling is a flexible behavioural intervention that can support users in quitting tobacco, including smokeless forms. In dental settings, it has been used both as a stand-alone follow-up tool and as a complement to face-to-face counselling provided during dental visits. Telephone support can be offered as a stand-alone intervention or used in conjunction with face-to-face counselling, self-help materials, or pharmacotherapy. It plays an instrumental role in planning quit attempts and providing relapse prevention support during early abstinence (Matkin et al. 2019). It is typically delivered in either a reactive format, where individuals initiate contact via quitlines or helplines, or a proactive format, where trained counsellors call users as per a pre-arranged plan. Among these, proactive counselling has shown greater effectiveness in increasing smoking quit rates compared to reactive approaches (Ebbert et al. 2007; Zhu et al. 2002). While most evidence for telephone-based counselling originates from smoking cessation research, its potential application to ST users is supported by findings from several trials. Evidence from trials in the United States show that adding proactive phone counselling to mailed resources encourages greater use of recommended behavioural strategies, resulting in higher quit rates for smokeless use (Severson et al. 2000). These findings highlight the public health potential of low-cost, scalable interventions that combine printed materials with personalized telephone support.

In terms of dental settings, several studies have demonstrated the feasibility and utility of telephone counselling in dental contexts for ST users. For instance, in one such study (Stevens et al. 1995), dental hygienists and dentists delivered brief in-clinic advice supplemented with follow-up telephone calls, which reinforced the behavioural messages initially given during dental appointments. Similarly, Walsh et al. (1999, 2003) implemented school and college-based interventions, where dental professionals provided brief counselling in person, followed by proactive telephone support often focusing on quit planning and relapse prevention (Walsh et al. 1999, 2003). These studies show that dental professionals, particularly dental hygienists, can play an effective role in maintaining engagement and motivation through telephone counselling after initial in-person contact. Such findings highlight the potential for dental settings to serve as entry points for such cessation interventions. The integration of brief behavioural advice during routine oral health appointments followed by structured telephone counselling, offers a scalable, low-cost model particularly suited for populations with limited access to continuous in-person support. As part of a comprehensive tobacco control strategy, this approach enables dental teams to extend their preventive role beyond the clinic, helping users sustain quit attempts over time.

Key Points

- Telephone-based counselling, offered in proactive (counsellor-initiated) or reactive (user-initiated) formats, effectively supports tobacco cessation by planning quit attempts and preventing relapse.
- In dental contexts, it can be used as a stand-alone tool or as follow-up to in-person counselling.
- Dental professionals, especially hygienists, play a key role in reinforcing cessation messages through follow-up calls.
- US-based trials found that proactive calls combined with mailed materials improve quit rates by encouraging evidence-based cessation strategies.
- Integrating brief in-clinic counselling with structured follow-up telephone support in dental settings offers a low-cost, scalable intervention—particularly beneficial for underserved populations.

13.1.6 Self-Help Materials

Self-help materials were initially developed in printed form and continue to be widely used. In dental settings, where brief interventions are often necessary, these materials can offer a practical and low-cost method to support ST users in quitting. Over time, however, alternative formats have emerged, including video and audio recordings, as well as web-based and digital content. These materials typically consist of structured manuals or guides designed for independent use, without the direct involvement of trained professionals. Dental practitioners can integrate these resources into routine preventive care, either by directly distributing them to patients or referring users to appropriate platforms.

Self-help resources can be disseminated through mass media campaigns targeting the general population of tobacco users or tailored to address the needs of specific subgroups. Evidence suggests that self-help interventions can be effective in supporting ST users to quit. Studies have shown that even minimal interventions, such as printed materials, can lead to meaningful quit rates. Adding components like videos or brief telephone support can further enhance outcomes (Hartmann-Boyce et al. 2014; Lancaster and Stead 2005; Livingstone-Banks et al. 2019; Severson et al. 2000). A notable large-scale trial demonstrated that low-cost self-help interventions, delivered by mail and phone, can significantly increase quit rates among ST users. The study showed that adding brief telephone counselling and video content to a printed self-help manual led to higher cessation rates for both ST and all tobacco use. These enhanced outcomes appeared to be driven by increased engagement with behavioural cessation strategies, encouraged by the support elements (Severson et al. 2000). Similarly, in a study by (Rasool et al. 2024c) conducted in Pakistan, participants in both the intervention and control groups received printed self-help materials. However, the intervention group also received additional structured behavioural support. Quit rates were higher in the intervention group compared to the control group; however the quit rates observed in the control arm, who received only self-help materials highlight the potential utility of these resources as a stand-alone strategy for ST cessation in dental settings. However, the study also highlighted important implementation barriers: younger patients expressed reluctance to take the materials home, fearing their tobacco use would be discovered by family members, and low literacy levels further limited the usefulness of printed materials for some participants, reducing their ability to engage with the content effectively.

Key Points

- Self-help materials are practical and low-cost tools that can be integrated into dental settings to support ST users in quitting, especially when time for direct counselling is limited.
- Formats have evolved from printed manuals to include video, audio, and web-based resources, allowing for independent use without the need for professional supervision.
- Evidence supports their effectiveness, with studies showing that even basic printed materials can lead to meaningful quit rates, and that supplementing them with video content or brief telephone support can significantly enhance outcomes.
- Barriers such as stigma and low literacy can limit the utility of printed materials among certain populations, particularly younger users and individuals with limited reading skills, underscoring the need for tailored and accessible approaches.

13.1.7 Other Behavioural Interventions

Beyond conventional counselling and support strategies, researchers have explored a range of other behavioural interventions to promote ST cessation. These approaches aim to address the physical, psychological, and emotional aspects of addiction through alternative techniques, often complementing standard cessation support. One such approach is the use of exercise and related practices as a means of reducing withdrawal symptoms and enhancing motivation to quit. The evidence on adding exercise to ST cessation support is mixed. A review of multiple studies found no clear benefit of general physical activity in increasing tobacco quit rates

(Ussher et al. 2019). However, other research suggests that incorporating specific practices such as yogic breathing may improve outcomes when combined with brief advice (Sarkar et al. 2017). There is no published evidence on the use of these alternative behavioural strategies, such as physical activity or yogic breathing, within dental settings, where time and structural constraints may further limit their feasibility. This highlights a potential area for future exploration, particularly in regions where culturally rooted practices like yoga are widely accepted and could be integrated into oral health promotion.

Key Points

- Alternative behavioural interventions, such as exercise and yogic breathing support ST cessation by addressing the psychological and physical components of addiction.
- Evidence on the effectiveness of physical activity in promoting tobacco cessation is mixed, with some studies showing limited benefits, while others suggest potential advantages when specific practices like yogic breathing are included.
- Culturally accepted practices like yoga may offer promising avenues for integration into oral health promotion, especially in settings where such interventions align with local beliefs and behaviours.
- There is currently no published evidence supporting the use of these alternative strategies in dental settings.

13.2 Conclusion

This chapter has examined a range of behavioural interventions designed to support ST cessation in dental/dental affiliated settings, including brief advice, motivational interviewing, individual and group-based counselling, telephone support, self-help materials, and alternative behavioural strategies. The evidence suggests that these approaches can improve quit rates and help sustain long-term abstinence. However, most of this research has been conducted in high-income countries, particularly the United States, and may not fully reflect the cultural, social, and healthcare contexts of South Asia—home to the majority of ST users.

Dental professionals are uniquely positioned to contribute to ST cessation efforts, as they often encounter early signs of tobacco-related harm and maintain regular contact with patients. Incorporating tailored behavioural interventions into routine dental care, whether through brief interventions, structured counselling, or referral pathways, can play a meaningful role in addressing tobacco use. Yet, the successful implementation of such strategies requires attention to practical constraints in dental settings, such as limited time, privacy, and cultural sensitivities around tobacco disclosure.

Going forward, there is a critical need to adapt and evaluate these interventions within dental care frameworks, particularly in low-resource and high-burden contexts. By integrating evidence-based behavioural support into dental practice in a way that aligns with local realities, oral health professionals can help reduce the burden of ST use and its associated oral and systemic harms.

References

American Psychiatric Association (2013) Diagnostic and statistical manual of mental disorders (DSM-5®). American Psychiatric Publications

Andrews JA, Severson HH, Lichtenstein E, Gordon JS, Barckley MF (1999) Evaluation of a dental office tobacco cessation program: effects on smokeless tobacco use. Ann Behav Med 21:48–53

Aveyard P, West R (2007) Managing smoking cessation. BMJ 335:37–41

Aveyard P, Begh R, Parsons A, West R (2012) Brief opportunistic smoking cessation interventions: a systematic review and meta-analysis to compare advice to quit and offer of assistance. Addiction 107:1066–1073

Black N, Johnston M, Michie S, Hartmann-Boyce J, West R, Viechtbauer W, Eisma MC et al (2020) Behaviour change techniques associated with smoking cessation in intervention and comparator groups of randomized controlled trials: a systematic review and meta-regression. Addiction 115:2008–2020

Boutron I, Moher D, Altman DG, Schulz KF, Ravaud P (2008) Extending the CONSORT statement to randomized trials of nonpharmacologic treatment: explanation and elaboration. Ann Intern Med 148:295–309

Coyle K, Singh PK, Kaushik R, Huque R, Khan Z, Mehrotra R, Siddiqi K et al (2024) The lifetime health and economic burden of smokeless tobacco use in Bangladesh, India, and Pakistan: results from ASTRAMOD. Nicotine Tob Res 27:684–692

Davidson KW, Goldstein M, Kaplan RM, Kaufmann PG, Knatterud GL, Orleans CT, Spring B et al (2003) Evidence-based behavioral medicine: what is it and how do we achieve it? Ann Behav Med 26:161–171

de Bruin M, Black N, Javornik N, Viechtbauer W, Eisma MC, Hartman-Boyce J, Williams AJ et al (2021) Underreporting of the active content of behavioural interventions: a systematic review and meta-analysis of randomised trials of smoking cessation interventions. Health Psychol Rev 15:195–213

Ebbert JO, Carr AB, Patten CA, Morris RA, Schroeder DR (2007) Tobacco use quitline enrollment through dental practices: a pilot study. J Am Dent Assoc 138:595–601

Fanshawe TR, Halliwell W, Lindson N, Aveyard P, Livingstone-Banks J, Hartmann-Boyce J (2017) Tobacco cessation interventions for young people. Cochrane Database Syst Rev 11(11):CD003289

Fiore MCJC, Baker TB (2008) Treating tobacco use and dependence: 2008 update U.S. Public Health Service clinical practice guideline executive summary. Respir Care 53:1217–1222

Gansky SA, Ellison JA, Rudy D, Bergert N, Letendre MA, Nelson L, Kavanagh C et al (2005) Cluster-randomized controlled trial of an athletic trainer-directed spit (smokeless) tobacco intervention for collegiate baseball athletes: results after 1 year. J Athl Train 40:76–87

Gao X, Lo ECM, Kot SCC, Chan KCW (2014) Motivational interviewing in improving oral health: a systematic review of randomized controlled trials. J Periodontol 85:426–437

Godin G, Valois P, Lepage L, Desharnais R (1992) Predictors of smoking behaviour: an application of Ajzen's theory of planned behaviour. Br J Addict 87:1335–1343

Hajek P (1996) Current issues in behavioral and pharmacological approaches to smoking cessation. Addict Behav 21:699–707

Hartmann-Boyce J, Lancaster T, Stead LF (2014) Print-based self-help interventions for smoking cessation. Cochrane Database Syst Rev 3(6):CD001118

Holliday R, Hong B, McColl E, Livingstone-Banks J, Preshaw PM (2021) Interventions for tobacco cessation delivered by dental professionals. Cochrane Database Syst Rev 2:Cd005084
Javed F, Altamash M, Klinge B, Engström PE (2008) Periodontal conditions and oral symptoms in gutka-chewers with and without type 2 diabetes. Acta Odontol Scand 66:268–273
Javed F, Chotai M, Mehmood A, Almas K (2010) Oral mucosal disorders associated with habitual gutka usage: a review. Oral Surg Oral Med Oral Pathol Oral Radiol Endod 109:857–864
Javed F, Tenenbaum HC, Nogueira-Filho G, Nooh N, O'Bello Correa F, Warnakulasuriya S, Dasanayake AP et al (2013) Periodontal inflammatory conditions among gutka chewers and non-chewers with and without prediabetes. J Periodontol 84:1158–1164
Javed F, Al-Kheraif AA, Al Amri MD, Mikami T, Vohra F, Warnakulasuriya S, Romanos GE (2015) Periodontal parameters and whole salivary cytokine profiles among habitual gutka chewers and non-chewers. J Periodontol 86:689–695
Kay E, Vascott D, Hocking A, Nield H (2016) Motivational interviewing in general dental practice: a review of the evidence. Br Dent J 221:785–791
Kumbhalwar A, Hegde S, Kakodkar P, Mehta V, Gupte H, Jadhav S (2022) Effectiveness of behavioral counseling in smokeless tobacco cessation among adult users reporting to a dental hospital in Pune: a randomized controlled trial. Cureus 14(4):e24041
Lancaster T, Stead LF (2005) Self-help interventions for smoking cessation. Cochrane Database Syst Rev 2000(2):CD001118
Lancaster T, Stead LF (2017) Individual behavioural counselling for smoking cessation. Cochrane Database Syst Rev 3(3):CD001292
Lifrak P, Gariti P, Alterman AI, McKay J, Volpicelli J, Sparkman T, O'Brien C (1997) Results of two levels of adjunctive treatment used with the nicotine patch. Am J Addict 6:93–98
Lindson N, Thompson TP, Ferrey A, Lambert JD, Aveyard P (2019) Motivational interviewing for smoking cessation. Cochrane Database Syst Rev 7:CD006936
Livingstone-Banks J, Ordóñez-Mena JM, Hartmann-Boyce J (2019) Print-based self-help interventions for smoking cessation. Cochrane Database Syst Rev 1:CD001118
Livingstone-Banks J, Vidyasagaran AL, Croucher R, Siddiqui F, Zhu S, Kidwai Z, Parkhouse T et al (2025) Interventions for smokeless tobacco use cessation. Cochrane Database Syst Rev 2015(10):CD004306
Manley MW, Epps RP, Glynn TJ (1992) The clinician's role in promoting smoking cessation among clinic patients. Med Clin North Am 76:477–494
Matkin W, Ordóñez-Mena JM, Hartmann-Boyce J (2019) Telephone counselling for smoking cessation. Cochrane Database Syst Rev 5:CD002850
McEwen A, Mclivar M, Locker J (2012) Very brief advice on smoking. Nurs Times 108(9):23
Michie S, Richardson M, Johnston M, Abraham C, Francis J, Hardeman W, Eccles MP et al (2013) The behavior change technique taxonomy (v1) of 93 hierarchically clustered techniques: building an international consensus for the reporting of behavior change interventions. Ann Behav Med 46:81–95
NHS Centre for Smoking Cessation and Training (NCSCT) Very brief advice on smoking: training module
Nohlert E, Helgason ÁR, Tillgren P, Tegelberg Å, Johansson P (2013) Comparison of the cost-effectiveness of a high-and a low-intensity smoking cessation intervention in Sweden: a randomized trial. Nicotine Tob Res 15:1519–1527
Palipudi K, Rizwan S, Sinha D, Andes L, Amarchand R, Krishnan A, Asma S (2014) Prevalence and sociodemographic determinants of tobacco use in four countries of the World Health Organization: South-East Asia region: findings from the Global Adult Tobacco Survey. Indian J Cancer 51:S24–S32
Patel K, Deshpande A, Jain A, Shah Y, Kalyan P (2020) Tobacco cessation effects on oral health by group and individualized motivational therapy in 12 to 18 years old boys–a randomized controlled study. J Indian Soc Pedod Prev Dent 38:280–288
Rasool S, Dobbie F, Ahmad F, Khan Z, Holliday R, Bauld L (2024a) Smokeless tobacco cessation support in dental hospitals in Pakistan: dentists and dental patients' perspectives on current practices, support needed, and opportunities available. Nicotine Tob Res 26:63–71

Rasool S, Dobbie F, Khan Z, Holliday R, Khalid F, Khan T, Bauld L (2024b) Process evaluation of a pragmatic feasibility trial on smokeless tobacco cessation intervention delivered in dental hospitals. BMC Public Health 24:1327

Rasool S, Holliday R, Khan Z, Dobbie F, Bauld L (2024c) Behavior change intervention for smokeless tobacco cessation delivered through dentists in dental settings: a pragmatic pilot trial. Nicotine Tob Res 26:878–887

Roberts NJ, Kerr SM, Smith SM (2013) Behavioral interventions associated with smoking cessation in the treatment of tobacco use. Health Serv Insights 6:HSI. S11092

Sarkar BK, West R, Arora M, Ahluwalia JS, Reddy KS, Shahab L (2017) Effectiveness of a brief community outreach tobacco cessation intervention in India: a cluster-randomised controlled trial (The BABEX Trial). Thorax 72:167–173

Savant SC, Hegde-Shetiya S, Agarwal D, Shirhatti R, Shetty D (2013) Effectiveness of individual and group counseling for cessation of tobacco habit amongst industrial workers in pimpri, Pune-an interventional study. Asian Pac J Cancer Prev 14:1133–1139

Severson HH, Andrews JA, Lichtenstein E, Gordon JS, Barckley M, Akers L (2000) A self-help cessation program for smokeless tobacco users: comparison of two interventions. Nicotine Tob Res 2:363–370

Severson HH, Peterson AL, Andrews JA, Gordon JS, Cigrang JA, Danaher BG, Hunter CM et al (2009) Smokeless tobacco cessation in military personnel: a randomized controlled trial. Nicotine Tob Res 11:730–738

Siddiqi K, Shah S, Abbas SM, Vidyasagaran A, Jawad M, Dogar O, Sheikh A (2015) Global burden of disease due to smokeless tobacco consumption in adults: analysis of data from 113 countries. BMC Med 13:194

Siddiqui F, Kanaan M, Croucher R, Bauld L, Fieroze F, Kumar P, Mazhar L et al (2024) Behavioural support and nicotine replacement therapy for smokeless tobacco cessation in Bangladesh, India and Pakistan: a pilot randomized controlled trial. Addiction 119:1366–1377

Solberg LI, Maxwell PL, Kottke TE, Gepner GJ, Brekke ML (1990) A systematic primary care office-based smoking cessation program. J Fam Pract 30:647–654

Stead LF, Carroll AJ, Lancaster T (2017) Group behaviour therapy programmes for smoking cessation. Cochrane Database Syst Rev 3(3):CD001007

Stevens VJ, Severson H, Lichtenstein E, Little SJ, Leben J (1995) Making the most of a teachable moment: a smokeless-tobacco cessation intervention in the dental office. Am J Public Health 85:231–235

Tønnesen P, Mikkelsen K, Bremann L (2006) Nurse-conducted smoking cessation in patients with COPD using nicotine sublingual tablets and behavioral support. Chest 130:334–342

Ussher MH, Faulkner GEJ, Angus K, Hartmann-Boyce J, Taylor AH (2019) Exercise interventions for smoking cessation. Cochrane Database Syst Rev 2019(10):CD002295

Walsh MM, Hilton JF, Masouredis CM, Gee L, Chesney MA, Ernster VL (1999) Smokeless tobacco cessation intervention for college athletes: results after 1 year. Am J Public Health 89:228–234

Walsh MM, Hilton JF, Ellison JA, Gee L, Chesney MA, Tomar SL, Ernster VL (2003) Spit (smokeless) tobacco intervention for high school athletes: results after 1 year. Addict Behav 28:1095–1113

WHO (2017) Toolkit for oral health professionals to deliver brief tobacco interventions in primary care. WHO

Zhu SH, Anderson CM, Tedeschi GJ, Rosbrook B, Johnson CE, Byrd M, Gutiérrez-Terrell E (2002) Evidence of real-world effectiveness of a telephone quitline for smokers. N Engl J Med 347:1087–1093

GPSR Compliance

The European Union's (EU) General Product Safety Regulation (GPSR) is a set of rules that requires consumer products to be safe and our obligations to ensure this.

If you have any concerns about our products, you can contact us on ProductSafety@springernature.com

In case Publisher is established outside the EU, the EU authorized representative is:

Springer Nature Customer Service Center GmbH
Europaplatz 3
69115 Heidelberg, Germany

Batch number: 10732044

Printed by Printforce, the Netherlands